SEX: A MAN'S GUIDE
includes important, up-to-date information on...

Afterplay: Why you should stay awake a little longer after sex.

Positions: Dozens of couplings that can turn lovemaking into a dance.

Harassment: Where to draw the line, professionally and socially.

Aphrodisiacs: How to use chocolate to entice your partner.

One-Night Stands: Why men are so open to casual sex.

Stress: How to keep the daily grind from hurting your love life.

Bondage: Why it's not as kinky and weird as you might think.

Lingerie: A visual glossary of what lies in a woman's underwear drawer.

Sex Drive: Why it's natural for men to be sexually hungry.

And much more!

SEX

A MAN'S GUIDE

*Stefan Bechtel, Laurence Roy Stains, and
the editors of* Men's Health *books*

Reviewed by E. Douglas Whitehead, M.D., associate clinical professor of urology
at Mount Sanai School of Medicine of the City University of New York,
and Bernie Zilbergeld, Ph.D., an Oakland, California, sex
therapist and author of The New Male Sexuality

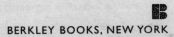
BERKLEY BOOKS, NEW YORK

NOTICE: This book is intended as a reference volume only, not as a medical manual. The information given here is designed to help you make informed decisions about your health and sex life. It is not intended as a substitute for any treatment that may have been prescribed by your doctor. If you suspect that you have a medical problem, we urge you to seek competent help.

SEX: A MAN'S GUIDE
A Berkley Book / published by arrangement with
Rodale Press, Inc.

PRINTING HISTORY
Rodale Press, Inc., edition published 1996
Berkley edition / October 1998

The Penguin Putnam Inc. World Wide Web site address is
http://www.penguinputnam.com

ISBN: 0-425-16580-9

BERKLEY®
Berkley Books are published by The Berkley Publishing Group,
a division of Penguin Putnam Inc.,
375 Hudson Street, New York, New York 10014.
BERKLEY and the "B" design
are trademarks belonging to Penguin Putnam Inc.

PRINTED IN THE UNITED STATES OF AMERICA

10 9 8 7

SEX AND VALUES AT RODALE PRESS

We believe that an active and healthy sex life, based on mutual consent and respect between partners, is an important component of physical and mental well-being. We also respect that sex is a private matter, and that each person has a different opinion of what sexual practices or levels of discourse are appropriate. Rodale Press is committed to offering responsible, practical advice about sexual matters, supported by accredited professionals and legitimate scientific research. Our goal—for sex and all other topics—is to publish information that empowers people's lives.

We dedicate this book to the 2,514 brave, foolish souls who responded to our surveys, and whose wisdom, creativity and devotion to the art of love are reflected throughout.

For an interactive experience, visit our web site at
http://www.sexamansguide.com

CONTENTS

INTRODUCTION
Why We Did What We Did, and How

You could be in complete control of your life, awash in success and happiness, a master of the universe. In fact, we hope you are.

But be honest now: Is there a single person you could comfortably ask, face-to-face, without paying any money, these vital questions: "Know any ways I could improve my oral sex technique?" or "Have you ever figured out any way to help your partner consistently reach orgasm?"

It's sad, really. Your father or doctor probably are out of the question. Your friends and colleagues would respond, at best, with a sneer or a wisecrack; sex talk among guys is mostly winks and nods, bravado and innuendo. Then there are the women of our lives, but we all know our track record of communicating openly with them. That leaves radio and TV talk show hosts.

For some reason, despite that we live in a culture absolutely saturated with sex (or at least the kind of faux sex used in advertising), Americans—and especially men—don't really talk to each other honestly about it. "Men do not have anyone to talk to about their sex lives . . . everyone wants to know and to share, but not with anyone they know," one 72-year-old farmer told us.

The proof is that a billion-dollar industry has emerged to answer all those questions we refrain from asking each other. Mountains of sex books are for sale, the *Penthouse* letters section is the stuff of legends and thousands of sex videos are heaped on the shelves. And any time a new medium gets invented, it's instantly eroticized—you can get on the Internet this afternoon, identify yourself as a dog who loves bondage and hold intimate conversations with some like-minded collie logged on in Finland.

Some of this is legitimately informative and helpful. But much of the sex-oriented stuff for sale out there is just a kind of cotton candy for the libido: A blast of pure sugar that's gone in a flash. All show, no substance.

Which means that when it comes to legitimate sexual information for men, it's either candy or horse manure (like the stuff you hear in locker rooms). What's lacking is the sort of honest, useful, practical talk about male sexuality that our farmer—along with millions of other men—is longing for.

So that's what we decided we'd give you. A bunch of

ARE WE GETTING IT?

A fair amount. More than half of respondents say their sex lives are good or excellent. The question: "How would you characterize your sex life?"

	All	Married	Not Married
Excellent	18.0%	20.0%	15.2%
Good	39.7%	43.4%	36.4%
Fair	22.0%	20.8%	23.1%
Poor	12.9%	12.5%	13.6%
Nonexistent	5.7%	2.1%	9.5%
No answer	1.7%	1.2%	2.2%

DOES HEALTH MATTER?

Absolutely. The better the respondents rated their health, the better they also rated the status of their sex lives.

Excellent	65.9%
Good	54.1%
Fair	22.2%

HOW IMPORTANT IS SEX TO A RELATIONSHIP?

Considerably. And that's true for all ages and income levels. We asked: "In general, how important is good sex to a happy long-term marriage or relationship?"

Absolutely critical	19.3%
Very important	55.4%
Moderately important	22.9%
Not very important	1.0%
No answer	1.4%

Men's Health editors, writers, cronies and hangers-on got together in a conference room, kicked off our shoes and brainstormed every sexual topic a guy could possibly want to know about. Then we set out to find the answers.

Of course, being clever boys, we also brainstormed ways to guarantee our success. Our solution? Have you write a whole lot of the book.

DO YOU USE EROTIC TOOLS?

You sure do, particularly videos and lingerie. We asked: "Have you ever used any of the following erotic items?" Below are those who answered yes.

Videos	55.4%
Lingerie	46.1%
Fantasy	27.4%
Toys	27.2%
Never used any	22.3%
Games	11.0%

ARE YOU TOO TIRED FOR SEX?

More often than you'd like, apparently. Fatigue is the number one impediment to better sex. The question: "In your own life what do you feel are the biggest barriers to great sex?"

Fatigue	54.0%
Lack of time	42.3%
Partner not interested	37.0%
Presence of children	23.8%
Lack of personal interest	16.8%

We Asked, You Answered

Sure, we talked to dozens of doctors, therapists and sexologists, read tons of books, ran database searches to dig up hundreds of studies. We made certain we had a handle on the best current thinking among the "sexperts."

But to make this truly rich, truly yours, we went to the readers of *Men's Health* magazine for tales from the frontlines. And boy, did they respond.

We conducted two studies, actually. One was a written survey mailed to 3,000 randomly selected *Men's Health*

WHAT DO WE FEAR?

Number one among men is impotence. The question: "What are your greatest sexual fears?"

Impotence	31.4%
Contracting AIDS	26.8%
Losing interest with age	22.3%
Losing your partner	14.8%
Getting a sexually transmitted disease	8.8%

ARE YOU HURT?

Sometimes we get upset about this stuff. The question: "Do you ever get angry about sex?"

Yes	27.1%
No	45.4%
No answer	27.5%

subscribers, representing a statistically valid sampling of the magazine's readership. Now, you may think the world does not need another survey about sex, but we respectfully beg to differ. We think our survey is particularly relevant because of who we surveyed: healthy, smart, physical men like you. If any survey is going to reflect the collective wisdom of your peer group, this is the one.

We received 776 useable responses, which were carefully tabulated and analyzed. Results of this written survey are sprinkled throughout the book. We've also put many of the findings in boxes throughout this introduction.

Actually, though, we were really more interested in another, shorter version of the survey that ran in the magazine itself, consisting of 12 open-ended essay questions (the kind you used to hate in high school). We got more than 1,800 responses to this survey—some faxed to us, some e-mailed, some sent by ordinary mail, often with additional

DOES SHE MEAN IT?

This one surprised us. The question: "When a woman says no to a sexual advance, do you think she always means it?"

Yes	47.7%
No	47.4%
No answer	4.9%

HAVE YOU EVER SAID NO?

This surprised us, too. The question: "Have you ever said no to a woman who wanted to have sex with you?"

Yes	73.1%
No	23.6%
No answer	3.3%

ARE YOU EMBARRASSED?

For a fourth of us guys, sex comes with some bad mental luggage. The question: "Do you ever feel guilty or ashamed about sex?"

Yes	23.2%
No	73.5%
No answer	3.3%

pages attached. One guy sent us a play. Others scribbled their deepest secrets on yellow legal pads or the backs of envelopes. A few people lectured or preached at us, but most just told us their stories with a candor that was amazing. Taken together, all these responses filled two big boxes and weighed in at more than 30 pounds. (Okay, sure: Some of these guys were probably embellishing things a bit, but we decided to take everybody at their word.)

Many took the job very seriously, confirming what we said at the top: that men have nowhere to turn to talk truly about sex. One 47-year-old civil servant told us, "I have answered very truthfully and honestly and may not be able to share this with but one true friend. So don't take it casually."

We've tried to honor that request.

Unlike the written survey, which conformed to the science of statistical sampling, this "fax poll" in the magazine had no science to it at all. It's what statisticians call a self-selected sample—these guys responded just because they felt like it or had something they wanted to say. Well, so what? We don't care. All we wanted were men's voices. Men's stories. Men's techniques. Men's secrets. And did we ever get some!

In fact, overall, we were hugely impressed with the honesty, wisdom, humor, creativity and good-naturedness of these guys. (A handful of women responded, but more than 98 percent of the respondents were male.) We liked these people. Many of them were clearly skilled and devoted · lovers, eager to share what they'd learned—some of which

DO WE HAVE DOUBLE STANDARDS?

We certainly do. The questions: "Do you feel men are naturally monogamous?" and "Do you feel women are naturally monogamous?" The variance in the responses is staggering.

	Men	Women
Yes	26.0%	55.5%
No	65.3%	33.8%
No answer	8.7%	10.7%

WHY WE STRIKE OUT.

Forget about pickup lines. They don't work. The question: "Do you know an opening or pickup line that works?"

Yes	10.8%
No	60.8%
No answer	28.4%

we'd never heard of before. In fact, reading through these surveys was depressing at times because so many respondents made us feel like we only thought we had sex lives until we heard what they had to say.

Given the popular picture of males as roving, polygamous, sex-obsessed wolves, ready to bolt from a long-standing relationship at the first sight of a Swedish ski instructor, we were surprised by how many of these guys turned out to be sentimental saps. They gushed with love and adoration for their wives or girlfriends. They called them "my lady love," "my one and only," "my lovely wife" and a few things even cornier. Several mentioned they'd been married to the same woman for 40 or 50 years. They were clearly very concerned about pleasing this one particular woman, had gone to extraordinary lengths to do so and took enormous pleasure in her pleasure. Maybe that's why

YES, BRAINS MATTER MOST.

The question: "What is it about women that attracts you the most?"

Personality	62.2%
Beauty	55.5%
Sense of humor	48.3%
Smile	47.9%
Intelligence	47.8%
Legs	45.0%
Shapeliness	44.3%
Breasts	43.9%
Eyes	43.7%
Butt	42.0%
Hair	37.6%
Sound of voice	34.3%
Height	16.9%

they enjoyed sex so much. (And we're willing to bet she did, too.)

Out of all those responses, we'd have to say there were fewer than a dozen that voiced a bitter or mean-spirited view of women. For all the male-bashing that goes on these days, our guys did not use this opportunity to indulge in female-bashing. In fact, their responses help to shake off an old image of men. There's a tired myth that says a guy who loves sex secretly hates women. He's a playboy. He's a womanizer. A cad. But these men clearly love sex—and they love women. For them sex is the space shuttle to love. They didn't tell us about notches on the bedpost. They told us about true romance.

A Tip of the Hat to History

One final note. While we think we've come up with a terrific book on male sexuality in the 1990s, we don't claim this is the last word on the subject—nor will any book on sex ever be. The sex or marriage manual is as venerable a genre as the cookbook. Every generation reinterprets the riddle of men, women, love and sex, so there's always a need for new books on the subject (even, perhaps, CD-ROMs and virtual reality bodysuits).

In the course of researching this book, we delved into hundreds of sex manuals, ancient and modern, and some of what we found we just couldn't resist sharing—whether for enrichment or amusement. Sometimes we found that older was indeed wiser, and certainly more eloquent. No modern sexologist can top the richness of language and feeling in lines like these, penned by the Tunisian poet Sheikh Nefzawi in *The Perfumed Garden* hundreds of years ago: "And when the cessation of enjoyment puts an end to your amorous frolics, take care not to rise brusquely, but withdraw your member with circumspection. . . . In this way nothing but good will result."

At the same time, we were delighted by the absurdities and Victorian revulsion we found in sex manuals from the early years of this century, so just for your enjoyment we've sprinkled the book with quotes and pictures from some of them, too, under the heading of "The Annals of Ignorance."

Because we never believed it when our high school sex-ed teacher told us sex was always supposed to be serious.

And we hope you didn't either.

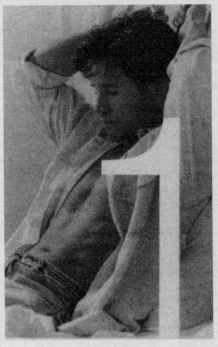

THE MALE BODY

ABSTINENCE

Does It Ever Pay Off to Lay Off?

Coaches should know better.

It's a worldwide myth that athletes will play better if they abstain from sex the previous evening. As if there were some Zen-like logic in not "scoring" in order to score.

Apparently, Roy Hodgson was sold on the myth, because he told his men on the Swiss soccer team that they would have to remain celibate during the entire month of World Cup games that were held in the United States in the summer of 1994. All wives and girlfriends would be barred from the team's hotel.

When the firestorm of criticism did not die down, he finally relented—and his team did so well that they made it to the round of 16 for the first time in 40 years.

Who knows what caused Coach Hodgson to change his mind. Maybe he thought twice after learning that the Italian team's coach also had insisted upon abstinence during the last World Cup games, in 1990. Italy finished third that year; that coach was *finito*. In 1994 a new coach dropped the rule, and the Italians almost won it all. (They lost to Brazil in overtime.)

The great Pele, upon hearing of Hodgson's folly, pooh-poohed the whole idea. In a reaction that could be the anthem for this book, he said: "Generally, I think normal sex is not a problem."

In fact, there is no scientific basis whatsoever to support the notion that abstinence is a winning strategy. The few studies that have been done simply prove that a night of connubial bliss does not sap an athlete's strength the next day. (Indeed, some coaches recommend sex the night before as a way of easing anxiety the next day.)

Why We Abstain

The only thing Coach Hodgson proved is that myths about abstinence won't go away. For at least the last few millennia *not* having sex has been an oddly compelling idea.

Some ancient philosophers thought that semen's grayish froth was a little bit of the gray matter between our ears— and, therefore, not something to be indiscriminately spent. Hippocrates had a slightly different theory: He believed that too many ejaculations sapped the precious fluid inside the spinal cord. (So *this* is Spinal Tap!)

But in Western civilization the chief proponent of abstinence has been the Roman Catholic Church, whose theologians long ago declared pleasurable sex to be sinful, even within marriage. The Church has not been alone in its condemnation; just a century ago, popular marriage manuals were warning that indulging in sex purely for fun "weakens and depraves." Around that time, health fanatic John Harvey Kellogg invented cornflakes because he thought a bowlful was just the ticket for suppressing vile passions.

Abstaining from sex is a personal choice, based on some moral, spiritual or emotional decision. If you choose to abstain, that's that: Other people's arguments really aren't valid, including ours. What we can examine are the effects of abstinence on sex and health. We'll tell you about three times in a man's life when abstinence is a terrible idea—and the one time when it's still a good idea.

Gentlemen, Start Your Engines

First, abstinence can be harmful for men who plan to start families (big surprise?). That is particularly true for men with low sperm counts. "Saving up your sperm" through abstinence doesn't work. In fact, men with low sperm counts ought to try more sex, not less, at the time of their partners' ovulations. For some still-mysterious reason some men need a second ejaculation to overcome whatever inner anatomical hurdles bedevil their output. An American study in the mid-1980s took 20 men with low sperm counts and had them ejaculate twice within an hour after abstaining from sex for three days. Fourteen of them thereupon improved their sperm concentration to the low-normal range. A more recent Israeli study of 576 men came to the same basic conclusion: Men with low sperm counts

> Number of sexual encounters seen on TV by the average teenager per year: 14,000

would be well-advised to have intercourse every day, or better yet twice a day, at the time of ovulation.

Fertility counseling is a highly individualized matter. Some exceptional men who climax several times a day, for instance, ought to slow down to every other day or so if they find themselves having trouble conceiving. They need to give their sperm production a chance to build inventory.

Most of us don't have that problem. Most of us need to make sure we get in the *schwing* of things at least once a week; after ten days, abstinence starts to take its toll on sperm vigor. (By the way, sperm that aren't ejaculated eventually undergo autolysis, which is a fancy way of saying they break apart, dissolve and are reabsorbed by the body. We don't care what your grandmother told you, they don't swim back up to your brain.)

Second, abstinence can be harmful to men with an infected prostate. It is an accepted medical fact that an infection of the prostate, known as prostatitis, is successfully

---

THE ANNALS OF IGNORANCE: 1909

Young men should know the truth about the penalties that follow in the wake of the unchaste. The slightest departure from the continent life out of wedlock may bring physical torments, racking pain, mental anguish and a self-accusing conscience, besides a long list of ills too numerous and horrible to mention.

—From *Clean and Strong: A Book for Young Men* by
E. A. King and F. B. Meyer

overcome only with a combination of antibiotics and frequent ejaculation. Some doctors further infer that regular ejaculation is good preventive medicine because this keeps the prostate well-drained. An infection often presents no symptoms other than an increased white-cell count in the semen, but nonetheless can't be doing a man's body any good.

Finally, there's "widower's syndrome," a disability of the older single gentleman. What happens is he becomes impotent simply because he's been abstinent. All body parts need oxygen in order to be healthy, and the flaccid penis is probably the most oxygen-deprived organ in the body. Luckily for most of us, our manhood gets enough oxygen from our nightly erections to keep us prepared for love, even when we're sidelined. But if our blood vessels clog up with cholesterol as we age, there will be less blood flow—and even less oxygen. The ultimate result is total erectile failure, says Irwin Goldstein, M.D., professor of urology at Boston University School of Medicine. "Bad things happen to tissues that are deprived of oxygen," he says, "and the penis is no exception."

Who's Abstaining—And Who's Not

Given the sexual revolution of the last three decades, abstinence in the 1990s would be merely a quaint notion—but for AIDS. Suddenly, the single guy who's abstinent is hip, not wimpy. Public health officials are fond of calling abstinence the safest sex of all. (The second safest sex, of course, is masturbation.)

Most men regularly complain to sex surveyers that they'd like to be getting it *more*, not less. Small wonder. As the University of Chicago *Sex in America* survey revealed, Americans are not the randy bunch we think we are. Of men ages 18 to 59, one in ten has not touched a woman in a year. Most of these guys are single.

Just about the only group in our society that is enjoying sex more often is teenagers. As recently as 1970, only 4.6 percent of 15-year-old girls reported having had sex; by

1988 it had risen to 25.6 percent. By that age a third of all boys are active. Part of the problem is that puberty is eroding into childhood: The average age of menarche (a girl's first period) is 12½, having dropped three months every decade since the turn of the century. Boys hit puberty, on average, by age 14. Yet neither sex marries until the midtwenties, on average, leaving a dozen years in which biology and propriety are at loggerheads.

> If the Catholic Church wants celibate men, why don't they just recruit guys who've been married for 30 years?
>
> —Mark Russell

And the trend is worrisome. About one-quarter of all sexually active adolescents contract a sexually transmitted disease each year, and the incidence of HIV infection is growing faster among teenagers than any other age group. Statistically at least, once teens embark upon full sexual activity, they are at increased risk not only for disease but for poorer educational attainment as well. In that light, men should become champions of abstinence—not for themselves but for their kids.

Not all societies have this problem. In Japan, men and women experience their first intercourses, on average, at ages 21 and 22, respectively. Here in America the response to our rampant teenage sexuality is to push sex education in the schools—it's now required or recommended in 47 states. But a huge fight has developed over instructional materials. If you have children in school, you may have heard about an "abstinence-based curriculum." Favored by some conservative religious groups, programs such as Teen Aid and Sex Respect inveigh against premarital sex and its advocates pass out bumper stickers that read, Control your urgin'/Be a virgin. Critics call it a fear-based curriculum, claiming it distorts facts and preaches rather than teaches. But those same critics often favor something called Comprehensive Sexuality Education that, at its extreme, teaches first graders to say "uterus" instead of "tummy" and expects a hormone-crazed 14-year-old to make a rational decision about when to start having sex, as if he were ordering a Happy Meal at McDonald's.

For all the infighting, none of these programs has proven itself a stellar success.

When talking about sex with your kids, we have one minor recommendation. Do not repeat the adage we heard in our youth, "Sex is like a savings account—the longer you wait, the more interest you accumulate." There's not a lick of evidence to support it. Plus, they'll only look at you and say, "What's a savings account?"

AGING
It Just Gets Better

It is *never* too late!

Remember when Dr. Ruth burst upon the scene in the early 1980s with that frank advice about sex in the Social Security years? As shocking as she seemed then, she's almost passé now. But you have to give her credit: She didn't merely open the door on the topic, she blew the door off its hinges.

Dr. Ruth is still writing books and speaking to huge audiences of beaming silver-haired fans. She still sticks to the essential message: Yes, age brings change to your bodies— so make a few changes in your lovemaking, and you'll experience pleasures like you've never known.

She talks about oral sex and masturbation. She tells people to buy vibrators, rent X-rated videos and make love in the morning because that's when a man is refreshed. ("Get up, have a light breakfast—and go back to bed.") And if, tra la, he gets an erection, why not add to the fun by tossing a few onion rings around it? If he doesn't achieve an erection, says Dr. Ruth, he can still pleasure his partner. "He can use his finger, he can use his tongue, and guess what: He can use his big toe!"

Is Dr. Ruth trying too hard? Does her incessant cheerfulness seem like too much rouge on a wrinkled cheek? That would be the stereotype of sex in old age. And it's totally off-base. In survey after survey the elderly report that they enjoy sex as much as they ever did. In fact, some enjoy it more than ever.

What Can You Expect?

"There is no question of the fact," wrote William H. Masters, M.D., and Virginia E. Johnson, of the former Masters and Johnson Institute in St. Louis, back in 1966, "that the human male's sexual responsiveness wanes as he ages." Whereas a young stud can get a full erection in three to five seconds, a man in his fifties takes at least twice as long, and a man in his seventies will take three times as long to become erect. And for the first time in his life, he'll need physical stimulation to get erect. No longer will the mere sight of a woman, the whiff of her perfume or the daydream of unzipping her dress be enough to generate a salute as it did when he was young.

For some men erections will be fewer, softer and more fleeting; they may not achieve full erections until just prior to orgasm. And when orgasm comes at last, it's less intense. There's no involuntary toe curl, no anal contractions and fewer ejaculatory contractions. One or two at most.

Masters and Johnson, who measured just about everything, actually took a tape measure to the question of how far a man squirts his stuff. They found that young men's semen can travel one or two feet, while the graying guys are down to 6 to 12 inches. No longer do you feel like you're firing a howitzer: Masters and Johnson use the word "seepage" to describe the usual sensation of orgasm in older men.

And then it'll be a day or two before they can even consider trying to get it back up.

These changes occur slowly across the years, although after age 60 the downhill slope is a little steeper. It occurs in tandem with other indignities—decline in muscle power, dimmed senses, lengthened response times, diminished sex drive, bigger breasts and—merciful heavens!—ear hair.

All that would be enough to make a young man crawl into

a monastery. Yet older men aren't complaining. Though their sexual performances may have slackened, their interest has not. Neither has their satisfaction with their sex lives, which quite possibly are as exciting as their sons' or grandsons', although you won't see them bragging all over town about it. (One study found that 37 percent of married couples over age 60 have sex at least once a week. One in five do it in the great outdoors.)

What's their secret? They've adjusted their attitudes. They're able to slow down, lower their expectations and engage in less urgent lovemaking. If it's a little harder to achieve orgasm each and every time, well, at least premature ejaculation is a thing of the past. They can set a mood, they can introduce novelty, they can enjoy foreplay for its own sake.

A 54-year-old hospital worker who answered our survey says the best sex he ever had started happening all the time once he reached age 40. "I was able to have intercourse for 15 minutes before climax. Age makes sex better," he claims, "because it takes longer and I have more control."

The most in-depth study of sex and aging remains the *Consumer Reports* survey of 4,246 men and women over age 50. The responses paint a detailed picture of a rich and varied sex life: Half the men were receiving oral sex, for instance, and 56 percent were performing cunnilingus on their partners. (In fact, the men were enjoying cunnilingus more than the women, who said they'd enjoy it more if the men were slower, gentler and didn't give them beard burns with their stubbly faces.) Among those men who had passed the milestone of age 70, 43 percent were still masturbating, 17 percent were having orgasms in their sleep and 70 percent were consistently reaching orgasm during coitus. This despite the fact that 44 percent of all the men surveyed said their erections were less stiff and 32 percent said that they frequently lost an erection during sex.

All in all, these men who were born before the Hoover administration were enjoying a gamut of sexual practices including nipple and anus stimulation, sex fantasies and what sex therapists call stuffing, that is, literally stuffing the unerect penis inside the vagina with the aid of lubricants, which sometimes is enough to trigger a full-blown erection.

In our own surveys of *Men's Health* readers we noticed that aging is a gradual process—at least in terms of attitudes. Guys start out wanting to know all about multiple orgasms—his 'n' hers. As the years go by, men become less focused on how to get greater personal pleasure, less concerned about catching a disease and more worried about staying sexually active. Among men age 55 and beyond over half say their greatest sexual fear is impotence.

Old Age Is No Excuse

Erectile failure is a nonevent that threatens to negate our entire masculinity. Traditionally, impotence has been common in old age, and with good reason. There is very little about old age that is conducive to good erections. The usual debilities—high blood pressure, hardening of the arteries, diabetes and other diseases—score a direct hit on erectile response, to which may be added the cumulative effect of years of bad health habits. But here's some good news. Erection problems, although common, are not inevitable. Not by any means.

Most cases of impotence are considered to be treatable, if not curable. For more information, see Erection Problems on page 408. Those men who struggle with impotence are most often beset by other problems. In other words, it's poor health, not old age per se, that's usually the culprit. In one study of 225 older men the guys who were in poor health were six times more likely to be having sexual difficulty.

So if you're experiencing more than the normal "waning responsiveness," stop blaming it on getting old. John C. Beck, M.D., a gerontologist at the University of California at Los Angeles, goes so far as to say, "erection problems are not a natural part of aging. If an older man develops impotence, there almost always is a disease process of some kind—or a reversible cause, such as a reaction to a drug."

If you're having problems, see a urologist. If you're not having problems, the best advice for maintaining sexuality with age is to heed the poet Dylan Thomas . . . and do not go gently into that good night. In other words, don't become a sedentary blob. Get regular exercise, stay trim, don't smoke, don't drink too much and stick to a low-fat diet, because blood vessels that aren't clogged up with fat can clog up with blood—that's what an erection is all about. In fact, there's only one problem with keeping yourself in shape: all the widows out there. You'll have to beat 'em off with a stick.

We'll end with a friendly reminder: George Foreman became heavyweight boxing champ at age 45, Jack Nicklaus won the Masters at 46, George Blanda was still kicking field goals at 48 and Gordie Howe finally stopped playing hockey at 51. They've smashed the stereotypes of age and sports; maybe it's time to rethink your preconceptions about age and sex.

AROUSAL
Where to Find the Key to Glee

You know what arousal is. Or haven't you ever sung *Light My Fire?* Played air guitar along with *Start Me Up?* Watched a woman dance to *Hot Hot Hot?*

Arousal is the spark that starts the sexual interlude. It's everything that comes between desire and orgasm. In the scientific literature about sex, arousal is a broad-brush word signifying the entire constellation of sexual responses in both body and soul.

In men those responses are reflected in an erection, but don't end there. Sexologists, having spent decades watching couples coupling in the laboratory, know that the whole body gets into the act. During the buildup leading to orgasm, our breathing gets heavier, our hearts beat like a drum, our blood pressure soars. Most men get erect nipples; some get a sex flush on their chests. And in case you've never looked, the top of your penis turns deep purple while your testicles swell as they move up tightly against your body.

Moreover, all kinds of muscles involuntarily tense up—or, as William H. Masters, M.D., and Virginia E. Johnson, of the former Masters and Johnson Institute in St. Louis, put it, there are "semi-spastic contractions of facial, abdominal and intercostal (between the ribs) musculature."

That's what happens physically. But arousal, we now know, is not just a physical reaction. Arousal also involves that great big sex organ between your ears. Scientists are still trying to figure out the mind/body interplay, and of course it's terribly complicated, but basically the brain has to make a "hmmm response." The brain's involvement is behind much of what goes wrong with sex. It's also at the heart of whatever goes right.

You can have physical arousal without your brain's involvement—boys begin getting erections while they're still in the womb, after all. And you can be sexually aroused upstairs without the cooperation of your maypole. But ideally, both mind and body are engaged. "You can have one without the other," says David H. Barlow, Ph.D., a psychologist at the State University of New York at Albany. "But then, obviously, you have a problem."

Sex and the Strain Gauge

Among his many credits, Dr. Barlow is known worldwide as the eponymous inventor of the Barlow Penile Strain Gauge. In his work he has spent three decades strapping this wired steel collar onto men's penises, then observing what turns 'em on and what turns 'em off. The device has become a standard tool for assessing sexual arousal.

Over the course of those 30 years he has uncovered some pathbreaking patterns. For instance, we all know that "performance anxiety" can ruin a close encounter, right? Conventional wisdom tells us that anxiety will keep us from getting and keeping an erection. Yet there is evidence that anxiety actually can increase sexual arousal. In the few documented cases of reverse rape, for instance, when gangs of women held men at knifepoint and demanded sex, the men not only got it up, but performed repeatedly.

Dr. Barlow has expanded on this idea. In one experiment, subjects were shown erotic videos—and told they'd receive an electric shock if they did not get at least as hard as the average guy there. They obliged. They got more aroused, as a group, than the guys who simply were shown erotic videos, or who were shown videos and told they might get a shock, but it wasn't tied to their degree of arousal. (Nobody really got a shock.)

Dr. Barlow has theorized that, in normal men, anxiety can focus our attention and wonderfully concentrate the mind—in the same way that precurtain "butterflies" can pump up a comedian for his act. In other words, most men are able to deal with the generalized (nonsexual) arousal that comes with anxiety, and transfer it into sexual arousal—or performance of any kind.

> Sex is one of the nine reasons for reincarnation. The other eight are unimportant.
>
> —Henry Miller

But what the mind can heighten, it can also take away. Dr. Barlow demonstrated that by giving subjects a task to perform at the same time they were watching erotic videos. The task was something fairly simple, like reading a passage from a popular novel, but it was enough to distract them. As Dr. Barlow says, "It took up enough cognitive capacity to interfere with their arousal."

By the way, want to know what really turns us on? When guys were shown videos of aroused women, they got much more aroused than when they viewed videos of women who weren't excited. Nothing arouses like an aroused mate.

The Best and Worst of Sex

For good sex to happen, both the mind and body need to be in sync. Negative emotions, for instance, make people much less arousable. If you're angry, anxious or depressed, if you're worrying about your job—stuff like that will affect your performance, and you shouldn't be surprised if things don't go well under the circumstances.

But while anger dampens arousal in most people, it heightens arousal in others. Sexologists have noted that, physiologically, anger and arousal are a lot alike. Maybe that's why 22 percent of the respondents to our survey told us they've had sex to resolve an argument. Frankly, it's not unheard-of for some couples to have sex during an argument. What's that all about? Donald Strassberg, Ph.D., a sex therapist and psychology professor at the University of Utah in Salt Lake City, has a theory: "Seeing their partner with that much intensity turns them on."

Exactly what is a turn-on varies greatly from person to person. It all depends on what has erotic meaning for you. And if you've ever watched Geraldo, you know that people attach erotic meaning to some pretty strange things—anything from lacy panties to smelly socks. What's that all about? "We know something about what turns people off," says Dr. Strassberg. "We know very little about what turns people on."

We do know this: Arousal makes love fun. It's the really delicious part of sex. It's built up by foreplay, by fantasies, by dirty dancing and diaphanous lingerie. "More than anything else, arousal is what drives good sex," writes Oakland, California, sex therapist Bernie Zilbergeld, Ph.D., in *The New Male Sexuality*. It's what you feel when you stop thinking about your performance and start appreciating your partner's sexiness.

Arousal has been described as a "gradual crescendo" on the way to orgasm. That's probably the healthiest way to think of it. By all means forget the notion that it is, with everyone at all times, a straight uphill march to the peak. You're not on a stair-climber. Nor is she: Women, especially, tend to experience little hills and valleys on the way to the top.

Back in the late 1950s and early 1960s, Masters and Johnson spent 11 years watching hundreds of men and women achieve more than 10,000 orgasms. Their measurements of physical reactions form the basis for what we know today about sexual arousal. They were struck by the similarity between the sexes, and emphasized that. At the time, that was all to the good—society barely acknowledged women as sexual beings. Sex research since then, however, has shaded in some of the differences between men and women. The differences can be summed up this way: Men are *genitally* aroused, whereas women are *generally* aroused. Guys are so simple. Stroke their penises and they have orgasms. Women are much more complicated. A woman's arousal typically is slower and gentler, requiring greater emotional buy-in and increased physical stimulus (that is, lots of caressing and touching). Visual or mental stimulus alone rarely works to trigger a woman, and a crude or stupid comment can instantly shut her down. They need more time to reach orgasms, more in the way of foreplay, and more in the way of "mood." Stimulation to their genitals is just not enough—they can be stimulated to the point of vaginal lubrication, but they won't "feel" aroused if something else is wrong. Everything matters—from the way your tongue touches her earlobe to the tenor of your relationship at that moment. And furthermore, what turned her on last Tuesday may not excite her tonight. That's the way they are. No, it's not a plot to drive us crazy.

But in both sexes arousal is a response, and responses tend to wane when presented with the same old stimulus time after time. Scientists call it habituation. You call it boring. Arousal thrives on novelty. That's why the sex is *so* good when the relationship is new, and why in a long-term relationship we have to work a little to keep it feeling new.

The link between novelty and arousal is known as the Coolidge Effect. If you've never heard the germinal anecdote, here it is.

One day President and Mrs. Coolidge were touring a farm. When Mrs. Coolidge was shown the chicken coop, she asked if the rooster engages a hen in sex more than once a day. "Dozens of times," she was told. "Please tell that to the President," she said.

When President Coolidge passed by the chicken coop, he was promptly told about the rooster's habits. "Same hen every time?" he asked. "Oh, no, Mr. President, a different one each time." Coolidge nodded slowly and replied, "Tell that to Mrs. Coolidge."

CIRCUMCISION
We're Still Debating the Foreskin

It's a boy! Congratulations! Now, before you take him home from the hospital, there's just one decision to make: Will he be having surgery today?

If you decide to have him circumcised, he'll need to be put on a "papoose board" and tied down, his upper half swaddled in a blanket, his bare legs fastened with Velcro straps. The pediatrician or obstetrician cleanses your baby's genital area with iodine, then gets to the task at hand, cutting away the foreskin and then clamping or stitching together what remains. Afterward a waterproof dressing is applied. The whole operation takes about five minutes.

Meanwhile, you're out in the hall, holding yourself.

Circumcision can be done without much pain; some babies even sleep through the procedure. But still, should it be done? Its supporters point to thousands of years of tradition and potential health benefits. Opponents say it's a barbaric custom and the cause of male rage. The American Academy of Pediatrics takes a neutral position. They say: You decide. Hey, moms and dads, it's totally up to you. Just how are you supposed to know?

The Arguments in Favor

Each year in America about 60 percent of all newborn males are circumcised. That fact alone is enough for many parents to give the go-ahead; they want their kid to look like other kids and not get razzed in the locker room. What started out, eons ago, as a religious rite for Jews and Muslims has become, at the end of the twentieth century, a social custom.

Customary though it is, it's also favored by many doctors because of its medical advantages. Edgar J. Schoen, M.D., professor of clinical pediatrics at the University of California at San Francisco, was the chairman of the American Academy of Pediatrics Task Force on Circumcision when it last examined the issue in the 1980s. Since that time, he says, even more information favorable to circumcision has come to light. He calls the procedure "a significant preventive health measure with benefits throughout life."

Let's start with infancy. In the 1980s, studies done at U.S. Army hospitals involving more than 200,000 infants showed that the uncircumcised boys got urinary tract infections at a rate 10 to 20 times that of circumcised boys. In adults such infections happen mostly in women, for whom the usual prescription is vast quantities of cranberry juice. But in babies it's more serious, and the younger the infant, the more devastating the infection. A severe infection during the first month of life will result in a high fever, a bloodstream infection in one-third of infants, meningitis in 3 percent and death in 2 percent of all cases. Dr. Schoen says widespread circumcision in America prevents 20,000 severe urinary tract infections each year.

> The fact that we do not know the long-term impact of this surgery and have not asked to know tells us about our attitude toward males.
>
> —Warren Farrell,
> Why Men Are the Way They Are

Here's another reason infection is more serious for infants, says Dr. Schoen. Often in young babies the foreskin hasn't fully separated itself from the tip of the penis. (The foreskin is fully retractable in 80 to 90 percent of uncircumcised boys by the time they reach age three.) The kinds of bacteria that cause severe urinary tract infections find a home in the warm, moist environment under the baby's foreskin. From there they ascend the urethra. If they climb all the way up to the kidneys, permanent kidney damage can result—very rare but with the consequence later in life of high blood pressure and decreased kidney function.

Next stage: preschool (ages three to five). In uncircumcised boys these are the peak years for balanoposthitis, an infection of the foreskin and glans marked by soreness and inflammation. It occurs most often at this time of life either because boys aren't vigilant in retracting their foreskins to

PERCENTAGE OF MALE NEWBORN INFANTS CIRCUMCISED, BY REGION, 1990	
Northeast:	62.8
Midwest:	75.9
South:	57.1
West:	42.3

wash themselves daily or their foreskins still haven't separated fully yet. Circumcised children obviously don't face this problem.

Nor do they need to worry about phimosis, a condition that afflicts, at most, 1 percent of uncircumcised men. It simply means that the opening of the foreskin is too small and causes erections to be painful, usually starting around puberty. The French king Louis XIV suffered from phimosis; he was circumcised at age 22, causing circumcision to become fashionable among European aristocracy for generations afterward.

Whether uncircumcised men are more prone to catching sexually transmitted diseases is a matter of fierce debate, but Dr. Schoen says that some 50 scientific reports have established a connection. Studies ranging from the patrons of Nairobi prostitutes to gay men in Seattle show that uncircumcised men are at least twice as likely as circumcised men to catch syphilis, herpes, papillomavirus and HIV during unsafe sex.

Finally, says Dr. Schoen, cancer of the penis strikes men of middle age and older. Although comparatively rare—only 1,000 cases a year nationwide—it is almost exclusively a disease of uncircumcised men. In fact, he says the ratio of uncircumcised to circumcised men getting cancer of the penis is 6,000 to 1.

But what about sexual satisfaction? Male mythology decrees that a foreskin allows greater ejaculatory control—i.e., makes a man less of a Quick-Draw McGraw. That's just a phallic fallacy, say William H. Masters, M.D., and Virginia

E. Johnson, of the former Masters and Johnson Institute in St. Louis: 35 of the 312 men in their classic study were uncircumcised, and they enjoyed no special edge. In 29 of those 35 the foreskin retracted fully during intercourse (as it should), revealing the tip of the penis in all of its exquisite sensitivity. "Thus," they concluded, "a retained foreskin probably contributes little, if anything, to the individual male's ejaculatory control."

The Arguments Against

Phooey, say opponents of circumcision. They argue that, in removing the foreskin, you are tearing off 15 square inches of nerve-rich, highly erogenous tissue that contributes to a man's sexual pleasure. Nature put it there. It belongs there.

Opponents argue, with some validity, that foreskin-related infections and diseases are very rare among men who perform a little basic hygiene (pulling it back and washing with soap whenever in the shower or bath). In other words, keep it clean and all the medical scare talk is just that—talk.

Circumcision is surgery, they add, and as with any surgical procedure, things sometimes go wrong. Although the rate of complications after surgery is less than 1 percent and the complications are almost always minor, the things that can go wrong are the kinds of things that make a strong man blanch: hemorrhage, infection and deformities caused by a botched job. Although there is no convincing evidence, opponents claim that later in life such complications

> You shall be circumcised in the flesh of your foreskins, and it shall be a sign of the covenant between me and you. He that is eight days old among you shall be circumcised; every male throughout your generations, whether born in your house or bought with your money from any foreigner who is not of your offspring . . .
>
> —Genesis 17:11–12

can lead to impotence, painful erections and bleeding during sex.

Because pediatric circumcision is considered to be nonessential, private health insurance sometimes does not cover its cost (usually $100). Publicly funded health programs are moving away from it as well: The Oregon Health Plan, for instance, no longer covers routine circumcision for its residents who are uninsured or covered under Medicaid.

Circumcision has its roots in primitive sacrifices meant to appease the gods or desensitize young men to pain. Those opposed to the procedure—men's movement gurus Warren Farrell and Sam Kean among them—consider it to be an inhumane act of genital mutilation. Because it is such a profound violation of personal boundaries, they argue, it could even contribute to the unexplainable anger and violence that is particularly endemic among American males.

If you don't buy that theory, it is at least worth noting that 80 percent of the planet's males are, as they say, "intact." Most of them seem to be getting along just fine.

Last Words of Advice

If you decide upon a medical circumcision for your child, hopefully your physician will perform it in conjunction with something called a dorsal penile nerve block. The doctor injects one-tenth cc of solution containing 1 percent lidocaine (better known as novocaine) into the base of the penis a few minutes before the cutting. A little Tylenol afterward will ease the lingering pain.

If you decide not to have it done, watch your baby when he urinates to make sure the hole in the foreskin is large enough to let him "go" in peace. As noted above, an infant's foreskin is usually not retractable for months or years. Once separation occurs, be sure to retract it to clean the area underneath with soap and water. Then teach him how to do this himself. That will prevent the chronic inflammation that may lead to bigger problems.

DURATION
The Long-Lasting Truth

It's impossible to determine the length of the average roll in the hay. A survey done by researchers at the University of Chicago showed that 69 percent of men think they spent 15 minutes to an hour at their last "sexual event," and another 20 percent said it lasted longer than an hour. But as psychologists know, most people overestimate the time that activities take; as *we* all know, men are incurable braggarts. All men want to last and last and last inside a woman; most men don't.

The hard truth: For most men the clocked dash from vaginal penetration to Big Bang is two to seven minutes, say researchers.

Well, at least we men of the 1990s are doing better than our fathers and grandfathers. Having interviewed thousands of men in the 1940s, the late Dr. Alfred C. Kinsey declared that 75 percent of them ejaculate within 2 minutes; William H. Masters, M.D., and Virginia E. Johnson, of the former Masters and Johnson Institute in St. Louis, conducted a monumental 11-year study in the 1950s and 1960s that found that, on average, a man will hold out for $2^1/_2$ to $3^1/_2$ minutes.

If you're reading this because you think you might suffer from something called premature ejaculation, please sit back and breathe a sigh of relief. Now you know: When it comes to ejaculatory control, the average Joe is no marathon man. Too-rapid ejaculation is endemic in young men, especially young men who haven't had anybody since who knows when. Giving the problem a fancy name may make it more of a sexual disorder than it needs to be, considering that sexologists cannot even agree on its definition.

But we'll borrow parts of two well-established definitions for you to try out on yourself, namely: (1) Do you feel you simply have no control over your ejaculation and (2) do both you and your partner agree that it's a problem in your love life? If so, then you owe it to yourself to look into the matter. For more information, see Premature Ejaculation on page 460. It's very fixable. Furthermore, not doing anything about it can lead to bigger problems if it becomes an increasingly worrisome distraction.

Over on the opposite end of the male-performance spectrum there's something called retarded ejaculation, or delayed ejaculation. It's a much less common problem. It may afflict older men whose reactions are dampened by age; it can be brought on by alcohol abuse or medications. But it can also be rooted in personal problems such as stress, anger, lack of trust in one's partner or some deep-seated aversion to intercourse. If you're having a problem, you need to ask yourself what else is going on in your life? Then get the appropriate help.

ERECTION
How to Be on the Up-and-Up

You need a new muffler. You drive to the shop and park in front of a bay. The mechanic takes over. He drives your car onto the tracks of the hydraulic lift, gets out and pushes a button on the wall. Suddenly, your three-ton Cherokee floats off the floor like a ballerina. Up, up, up it rises, pushed skyward by a big, gleaming steel column, a glistening, foot-thick, triumphant metal pole. When it's done rising, your car is over your head.

A good description of your erection, yes?

Actually, a hydraulic lift is similar to an erection in one way: for both, everything depends on the flow of fluids. But beyond that, sorry, we really can't compare the two, other than to stroke our male egos.

Instead, let us use a more humbling metaphor to explain how an erection works. We've all tooted on noisemakers at New Year's. You know the kind that's coiled up until you put it to your mouth and blow, whereupon it pops up and out? Don't let the ladies know, but that's us.

In a nutshell an erection goes like this: A stimulus, coming from your brain or your genitals or both, zings along nerve pathways to widen the arteries that lead into your penis. Blood floods into all the tiny caverns in the corpora cavernosa—two main tubes of tissue that make up the core of your penis. This flood quickly increases by nearly tenfold the amount of blood in the penis, expanding it like a little noisemaker. The inflowing blood strains against the sheath surrounding each of the cavernosa, creating rigidity—just as mere air can make a basketball rock-hard. The flow of blood out through the penile veins is virtually squeezed off by the expanded erectile tissue. So the erection continues until the nerve messages stop.

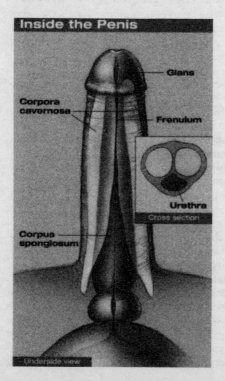

Inside the Penis

Glans

Corpora
cavernosa

Frenulum

Urethra

Cross section

Corpus
spongiosum

Underside view

The most complicated part of an erection is its connection with the nervous system. There are two nerve pathways involved. If your penis is touched erotically or happens to be enveloped by a vagina at the moment, the erection is being ordered up (or sustained) by that part of your wiring that controls stuff like digestion. In other words, it happens without you having to think about it. It's a reflex.

The other path to hardness is for you to contemplate a vision of Sharon Stone or engage in

THE ANNALS OF IGNORANCE: 1919

Copulation is ... dangerous immediately after a meal and during the two and three hours which the first digestion needs, or having finished a rapid walk or any other violent exercise. In the same way if the mental faculties are excited by some mental effort, by a theater party or a dance, rest if necessary, and it is advisable to defer amatory experience till the next morning.

—From *Love: A Treatise on the Science of Sex-Attraction* by Bernard S. Talmey

a steamy late-night telephone conversation. That's the other erectile pathway at work: the one leading from your brain. The best erections (and the most satisfying sex) are the result of the synergy created when both sets of synapses are firing away.

As you might guess, there are different nerve pathways for erection and ejaculation. That's why ejaculation can occur without erection, just as an erection can occur without ejaculation.

Just as all men's penises are slightly different, so, too, are their erections. There is no one proper "angle of the dangle." It's typically neither straight out nor straight up, but rather somewhere between 90 and 180 degrees (with 0 degrees being pointed at the ground), like the northeasterly arrow on the circle in the symbol for the male gender.

Sometimes we get erections when we don't want them and sometimes we don't get them when we do want them. Or they come and go at will—their will, not ours. During long lovemaking sessions, for instance, an erection may rise and fall like ancient empires if the stimulation needed to produce full erectile response is momentarily interrupted. The only important point about that is to not make it an important point. Don't get anxious about it. Emotions like hostility and guilt can subvert an erection; so can a lack of emotion. Anxiety is a well-known wet blanket. "If the anxiety is strong enough, the penis won't be," quips Oakland,

California, sex therapist Bernie Zilbergeld, Ph.D., in his book *The New Male Sexuality*.

Erectile failure can also be caused by physical problems, like hardening of the arteries. And it's frequently the side effect of medications. For more information, see Erection Problems on page 408.

Care and Feeding of Erections

Hey that's real swell, you might say, but what about *my* erections? What can I do to improve them?

We hate to sound like nags, but all the usual advice about a low-fat diet, plenty of exercise and maintaining your proper weight is especially vital to the health of the intricate vascular maze that lies just beneath the surface of your spear.

Above all, don't smoke: A study by the Centers for Disease Control in Atlanta found that men who smoke are nearly twice as likely as nonsmokers to develop erectile difficulties.

Okay, here's one more piece of advice any guy can live with: To have better erections, have more erections. "Having an erection is good for an erection," says Irwin Goldstein, M.D., professor of urology at Boston University School of Medicine.

Let's say you chopped off your penis, says Dr. Goldstein with a twinkle in his eye, and threw it in a blender. Having analyzed the contents thereof, you'd find that more than 50 percent consists of muscle. Not striated muscle like your biceps; smooth muscle like the walls of your blood vessels or your gut. Much of this muscle is located in the tiny blood vessels that are the end points of the major penile arteries. Think of them as exit ramps. When this muscle tissue is signaled to relax, blood floods the penis. These muscles work involuntarily and cannot be bulked up by exercise. So don't start attaching free weights to your diddler.

Like all other tissue in the body, this smooth-muscle tissue needs oxygen to survive. It snatches that oxygen from red blood cells passing by in the blood. Alas, the unaroused male member doesn't get much blood: only ten milliliters or less per minute, which is less than 0.2 percent of what's circulating. Apparently, that isn't enough, because the body has a terrific mechanism to recharge your erection system even when your love life stinks. That is, the erections you get in your sleep—about four per night on average.

Here's the point: As we age and our penile arteries clog up with cholesterol, even less oxygen is circulating. That causes the muscle tissue in the penis to be slowly replaced by collagen. By the time 70 percent of it is collagen, you have complete erectile failure. The way to reverse this process—or prevent its occurrence in the first place—is to keep the muscle tissue in the penis properly oxygenated.

With an erection.

"That's my excuse to my wife," says Dr. Goldstein.

EROGENOUS ZONES
Where It's Good for You

In the Woody Allen movie *Love and Death* a maritally frustrated Diane Keaton encourages the advances of an ugly, buck-toothed twerp.

"Your skin," he says. "It is so beautiful!"

"Yes, I know!" she replies breathlessly. "It covers my whole body!"

Discussions of erogenous zones sometimes sink to a narrow, rather mechanical level—that good sex is merely a matter of pushing the right buttons. Maybe it's time to rediscover that the whole body is covered with erogenous zones, and that the skin itself is one great big erogenous zone. All the pleasures of sex come through the nerve endings within the skin. We're the naked ape, remember. That's partly why we're so sex-crazed.

Erogenous zones are those parts of the body that are particularly sensitive to sexual stimulation. There's no denying that some spots on the skin are "hotter" than others, for an undisputable physiological reason: They have more of the sensory endings that allow you to feel pleasure when touched the right way.

We're pretty sure you've already noticed this, based on your experience with your own penis. The most sensitive parts are the skin at the tip of the penis (glans), its outer rim (corona) and something called the frenulum, which is a strip of skin just below the glans on the underside.

The penis is the center stage of man's sexual pleasure. But other sensations are waiting in the wings. The other erogenous zones common to most men are the mouth and tongue, ears, nipples, prostate (the so-called male G-spot), anus, scrotum, the spot between the anus and scrotum called the perineum and, yes, the toes.

When men become too fixated on sexual performance, when they seem to have gotten trapped in some vision of coital perfection, they may end up at a sex therapist. Often what they'll be told, as a treatment, is to keep engaging in sex, but refrain from doing the "Big It"—intercourse. And one of the things that may be suggested to them, as an alternative, is toe-sucking. The point: There's plenty of good sex to be had merely exploring erogenous zones.

Yes, They Do Get Weary

But remember: Erogenous zones are a map, not a Michelin Guide. They tell you where to go, not what to do when you get there. Each person is slightly different: Some zones are more highly arousable than others. And for each person "just the right touch" is for her to know and you to find out. It might range from a tender bite to a lick or a kiss or merely the tickle of a feather. Which is why, of course, sex with a new person can consist of endless hours of exploration.

Once that relationship is no longer new and you've learned her most reliable excitements, she may well grow weary of having you go straight to those places—yes, even though she begged you to touch her there. But since the body is full of potentially erotic spots, you can renew her arousal by seeking out brand new places.

Judging from our *Men's Health* magazine survey, most

men make it a practice to explore female erogenous zones. Most know, for instance, that stimulating the clitoris will almost guarantee her an orgasm. So will stimulating the labia minora, the inner lips of her genitals. You probably also know that the entrance to her vagina is nerve-rich. And several sex manuals describe coital positions designed to stimulate that magical area on the roof of her vagina a few inches in, the place that some researchers call the G-spot.

Some of you lucky ones have mates who are real explorers, too. "With most men and women, one nipple is usually more sensitive than the other," writes a 46-year-old warehouse worker, in response to our survey. "In my case, it's the left one. Another area is the testicles. Still another is the man's anus. In fact, if a woman can go so far as to have his penis in her mouth, with one hand stroking his sensitive nipple and the other tickling his anus (with a finger or even a feather), she can probably bring him to orgasm very quickly. If not, there's something wrong with him."

EVOLUTION OF SEX
Why We Are as We Are

Are men and women basically the same inside?

That's a question every generation tries to answer for itself. Being baby boomers, the authors know all too well what answer their big, jerky, know-it-all generation came up with. Back around the early 1970s it became an accepted fact that women were not only our equals in some figurative sense, but the same as us. Oh, there were a few small plumbing differences, but that's it. There were no innate differences. If only we could strip away the culturally imposed stereotypes, we were exactly alike.

Ah ha! we said. That will be our job, to throw out all those tired, wornout traditional sex roles that a patriarchal society had foisted upon us. We would stop saying *viva la différence*, because there was no difference. And to prove it, we'd make it evaporate in a single generation. When we had kids, we'd give the little girls tool belts, we'd make the little boys play with dolls and we'd put them all in the same uni-sex outfits.

All well and good—but that wasn't soon enough. Women began hectoring men to remodel themselves in the new, androgynous, Alan Alda mode. We would define the New Male. As for those men who did not, well, they were sexist pigs. They got the Glare. All their comments, all their actions (ours, too, unfortunately) were screened for any hint of the reactionary idea that men and women might be innately different.

It has made our love lives extremely confusing.

After nearly three decades of role-smashing, men and women are at each other's throats more than anyone thought possible. And despite some very determined efforts at non-sexist child rearing, today's little boys tend to be a bit rowdy and girls a bit prissy. Many a baby boomer, having endured parenthood, has come to the secret conclusion that our zeit-geist got it exactly wrong. Instead of men and women being born the same and socialized to be different, maybe we're different at birth and socialized to be more alike.

Science has shifted feet as well. Whereas 25 years ago the predominant assumption was that biology doesn't much matter, there is now accumulating evidence that men and women are indeed different at their cores. Blame it on evo-lution.

And while a few feminists belittle these exciting new the-ories as the last gasp of male dunderheads out to prove that women are naturally better at taking out the garbage, the rest of us can gain fresh insights into why we are the way we are.

Was Sex an Accident?

Even though each new generation of teenagers thinks it invented sex, we can safely dispense with that illusion. Sex has been around for a lot longer than humans. In fact, it probably began three billion years ago when the earliest bac-teria found a new way to mix up their genes. As methods of reproduction go, sex is not very efficient. Remember your biology lesson from high school, the one about one-celled amoebas duplicating their DNA and simply splitting in two? That's cloning, the no-muss, no-fuss way to reproduce. Some species, like the whiptail lizard, still clone themselves. Since sex is not the only reproductive option, botanist Lynn Margulis from the University of Massachusetts in Amherst has called it "a beautiful accident."

It seems to have been an accident waiting to happen. Over 99 percent of higher organisms reproduce sexually. For whatever reason sex got started, it proved to be immensely valuable as a way to mix up genetic traits and create more diversity in a given species, thereby allowing a species to evolve with changing environments. It was, in other words, the booster rocket for evolution.

Since Charles Darwin first proposed the notion of natural selection nearly 150 years ago, virtually all life on this planet has been examined in terms of its evolutionary fitness—how certain traits may have helped some organisms within a species survive and thrive and so get passed along (via sex) to the succeeding generations in greater and greater numbers, as if some unseen hand were "selecting" that trait. (If you're a creationist, you may believe an Unseen Hand did indeed select that trait.)

The human species has been evolving for some 100,000 to 200,000 generations. A lot can happen over the course of all those generations—it took only 5,000 generations, for example, for a wolf to be turned into a Chihuahua. Well, as each human generation creates the next, some of us are more successful in the mating game and have more offspring. Maybe we have bigger biceps, stronger hearts, bigger brains. And if some aspects of our brains can develop over evolutionary time—the ability to learn language, for example—why can't reproductive aspects evolve, too? If we can look at men and women worldwide and find universal differences between the sexes, maybe those differences can be explained in terms of evolution—i.e., those differences are part of our brains because at some point they helped our ancestors mate more prolifically. That's what the emerging field of evolutionary psychology is all about.

Its advocates claim that if you buy the theory of evolution, you have to go along with the idea that gender attitudes evolved, too. You may not like what's evolved, but you cannot deny the innateness of it. Robert Wright, in his book *The Moral Animal*, puts it this way: "The idea that natural selection, acutely attentive to the most subtle elements of design in the lowliest animals, should build huge, exquisitely pliable brains (that's you, dummy) and not make them highly sensitive to environmental cues regarding sex, status and various other things known to figure centrally in our reproductive prospects—that idea is literally incredible."

Your Cheatin' Brain

The Moral Animal made the cover of *Time* magazine when it appeared in the summer of 1994, not because it contained new research but because it was the first book attempting to summarize the work of evolutionary psychology for a mass audience. ("Infidelity" read the cover headline below a broken wedding band, "It May Be in Our Genes.")

The book examines the age-old characteristics about men, or at least some men, that women despise the most—we're always eager to have sex, we'll get drunk and do it with strangers, we care more about beauty than brains and once we get successful in middle age, we dump the women who have stood by our sides for 20 years in favor of hot, young "trophy wives." He also examines the age-old characteristics about some women that men hate—they're gold diggers, they try to trap us into marriage and once we're married, they suddenly lose interest in sex but can spend hours perusing the want ads in search of the jobs they think we should apply for. Wright urges us to think about these characteristics in terms of evolution. Why would they have mattered to all those eons of hunter-gatherers in our past?

All our differences are rooted in the fact that men can have more offspring than women. Theoretically, men can spread their seed far and wide—and so the men who liked to do that got to be, disproportionately, the ancestors of the men walking around today. According to records, the winner of the all-time paternity award was Moulay Ismail the Bloodthirsty, emperor of Morocco; he sired 888 children. "It's a little chilling to think that the genes of a man nick-named Bloodthirsty found their way into nearly 1,000 off-spring," Wright notes. "But that's the way natural selection works: The most chilling genes often win."

Since a man can always opt for genetic quantity, evolu-tionary psychology predicts that he will be more open to casual sex and that he will tire of monogamy if he sees a chance to get more of his genes into the next generation. That will always be our siren song. So it's hardly a surprise that many men feel restless with their wives at midlife. Her fertility may be on the wane, but his isn't. Most societies deal with this innate urge by allowing polygamy—980 of the 1,154 societies, past or present, for which anthropolo-gists have data have permitted a man to have more than one wife. Not just any man, mind you, but the wealthy man, the high-status, alpha man with the resources to support more offspring. Those oh-so-primitive tribes may have had a bet-ter solution than our practice of serial monogamy and skipped child support. At least it dealt with the urge to pro-create while saying, much more effectively, "You're not wiggling out of your previous obligations here."

But since the middle-age hotshot will be taking on some new obligations, of course he'll find some cutie-pie. Beauty is not in the eye of the beholder; it is, universally, a signal of maximum baby-making ability. "The generic 'beautiful woman'—yes, she has actually been assembled, in a study that collated the seemingly diverse tastes of different men—has large eyes and a small nose," says Wright. "Since her eyes will look smaller and her nose larger as she ages, these components of 'beauty' are also marks of youth, and thus of fertility."

Thus, nose jobs.

What motivates women? The evolutionary key to females is they can't have 888 kids. They don't do quantity—but they can do quality. They invest more in each offspring, making sure each child is, come its time, genetically suc-cessful. As Wright writes, "It makes Darwinian sense for a woman to be selective about the man who is going to help her build each gene machine." And so her coyness is no crime.

Since women are choosy by nature, men will always be competitive by nature, hoping to be the guy who gains the main chance. Scientists starting with Darwin call this male-male competition. You may know it by other names: war, football, one-upmanship, office politics, the salesman-of-the-month award.

As for children, then and now, they were better off with two parents than one. The kids who received fatherly resources and attention—evolutionary psychologists call it male parental investment—had a better shot at survival. That's why, in every human culture on record, marriage is the norm. That's also why women still tend to seek out mates who seem to be better providers—those with not only strength but brains and status and the willingness to commit these resources to their offspring.

Status is a touchy subject in America—we're supposed to be a classless society after all. But the desire for status, whether in small groups or in the larger society, is part of our brains. As Wright notes, group hierarchies are found in all of our closest relatives (the apes), in every human society ever studied and even among groups of children too young to talk. High status means more resources. But most of all, it means more access to sex. You don't have to be Wilt Chamberlain to know that.

Our feelings of ambition and pride, our stinging sense of shame when we've messed up, all are designed to help us climb the status ladder. All were felt keenly by our distant forefathers who earned reproductive payoffs once they climbed that status ladder. Are men naturally self-centered? Do we suffer from just a wee bit too much self-esteem? Well, no kidding. It's all part of our attempts to outmaneuver the competition.

"The man-sized ego," says Wright, "was produced by the same forces that created the peacock's tail: sexual competition among males."

Because men and women seek different qualities in each

other, they are often at odds. Marriage, for example, contains its own cross-purposes. "Whereas the woman's natural fear is the withdrawal of his investment," says Wright, "his natural fear is that the investment is misplaced." That he's providing for some other man's child, in other words. In some past societies men resorted to chastity belts to keep their most basic fear regarding their wives in check.

A drastic measure, to be sure. But studies have shown that, even today, men are most upset by the thought of their partners engaged in sex with someone else, while women are most upset by their partners' emotional attachments elsewhere.

Somewhere along the evolutionary line insane male jealousy must have paid off, however. It's behind the classic double standard, that traditional desire to bed whores but marry a virgin. And just maybe it's behind the lack of sex drive that plagues so many women. Given their mates' touchiness, hypothesizes Wright, "it could be adaptive for a married woman to not feel chronically concerned with sex."

It's the Same All Over

The Moral Animal refers frequently to the work of David M. Buss, psychology professor at the University of Michigan in Ann Arbor and author of *The Evolution of Desire*. Buss has coordinated the largest-ever survey of the human condition. In the 1980s he canvased the mating preferences of more than 10,000 people in 37 countries—and found that some of our sexual traits are truly universal.

In essence, he discovered that men everywhere tend to view women as sex objects and that women everywhere tend to view men as success objects. No one said Darwinism was pretty: Some of our most shallow, stereotypical behavior makes the most evolutionary sense.

Worldwide, it turns out, men are more promiscuous than women. Like the character Sam on *Cheers*, they spend an inordinate amount of energy pursuing short-term sexual encounters. But they also want to marry a chaste woman to avoid, if at all possible, spending their resources on another man's genes. In no cultures do women desire virginity in a mate more than do men.

Men the world over also place a greater premium on looks. In every one of the 37 cultures surveyed, physical attractiveness is more important to men than to women when choosing a mate. Moreover, the standard of beauty is everywhere tied to youthfulness—i.e., a woman who will provide a man with a great number of fertile years.

Women everywhere place a premium on brains, status, ambition and money. In seeking short-term mates, they will look for, shall we say, generous men, men who "are willing to impart immediate resources," as Buss puts it. But when seeking long-term mates, they will consider factors such as ambitiousness and potential earning power.

"We found that sex differences in the attitudes of men and women were strikingly consistent around the world," wrote Buss in the journal *American Scientist*. "In 36 of the 37 cultures women placed significantly greater value on financial prospects than did men."

Life is oddly like the fairy tales. Cinderella gets the Prince. Marla gets The Donald.

Why All This Is Good News

Let's not get carried away. First of all, evolutionary theory acknowledges that it is only part of what influences our daily sexual behavior. It is intermingled with early childhood experience, the messages we receive from religion, society and culture and the "live and learn" kinds of events throughout adulthood that sometimes leave us wiser.

Also, evolutionary psychology is careful not to say that all men are simply programmed to brag, fight and get caught in the gazebo with their neighbor's wives. Nor, having done all these things, can a guy throw up his hands and blame it on his genes. We're not robots. We're men with, hopefully, some free will.

But we can accept the fact that a part of our brains want to get us into trouble. That a part of the male mind will, when placed in a crowded cocktail party, cause his gaze to act like a heat-seeking missile in pursuit of the prettiest young woman in the room. That part of our brain will urge us to invent all kinds of reasons not to get married or all kinds of reasons to divorce our menopausal wives.

Of course we'll catch hell for being the way we are. That's just part of the game. But we don't have to beat up on ourselves. Let women argue with a couple million years of our evolution if they want to. It won't do them a lot of good. Women cannot change us.

We know a mother who was determined to raise her son in such a way that he would not turn out to be one more violent, testosterone-poisoned male roaming the earth. She barred toy guns from her house. No pistols, no swords, no pretending that sticks are swords. One day at lunch she placed a peanut-butter-and-jelly sandwich before him at the kitchen table. He carved it into the shape of a gun, pointed it at her and said, "Bang, bang!"

Evolution does not fully explain any one individual. But it does explain the broader averages and sheds light on—rather than denying—those universal human tendencies. Like why she circles the want ads. And why, when you get lost, you refuse to ask someone for directions.

> On lying about the number of lifetime sex partners people claim to have had: "The possibility that fantasy partners . . . made up a considerable portion of some lifetime lists was borne out when subjects agreed to further conversations in this delicate area. 'I counted Elvis, Mookie Wilson, Brad Pitt, Seiji Ozawa, Anthony Hopkins—but not in that hockey mask—and, go figure it, Senator Moynihan when I filled out that part,' Mrs. Phyllis K., a Sun Belt restaurant hostess, said cheerfully. 'It's who I'm thinking about then that matters with me.'"
>
> —Roger Angell, making fun of sex surveys in *New Yorker* magazine

FORESKIN
The Great Disappearing Act

The foreskin is a thin sheath of skin that's attached to the skin covering the shaft of the penis. It's a little like the hood of a sweatshirt—it can cover the head (glans) of the penis, or it can be retracted to expose it. Actually, it's more like an oversized turtleneck.

If you need to be told this, it's because you're like most American men: You don't have one. The doctor cut it off right before you left the hospital after being born.

Does that mean you're missing out on something? That's the big debate. Circumcision has no effect on penis size, but some men claim it adds greatly to sensitivity.

The foreskin consists of an outer layer of skin plus an inner layer of mucosal tissue similar to the skin inside the eyelid. A band of tissue called the frenulum holds the fore-skin in place: During intercourse the foreskin slides back so that about an inch and a half of that soft inner foreskin is exposed to the vaginal walls, along with an equal amount of outer foreskin. During masturbation the foreskin can glide back and forth—highly stimulating say those in the know. Friends of the foreskin also claim that it keeps the glans moist and protected throughout life, extending full sexual enjoyment into our last decades, when a man needs more physical stimulation to get and keep an erection. Some men of advanced age find that their circumcision-exposed glans are so toughened up they might as well be kneecaps.

Problems of the Foreskin

A very small percentage of uncircumcised men wind up with a condition called phimosis. That simply means the foreskin does not develop properly and cannot be fully retracted to reveal the head of the penis. The solution is sur-gical—either circumcision or a dorsal slit to widen the fore-skin's opening so it will slide back and forth.

THE FORESKIN

The foreskin is a sheath of skin that covers the head of the penis. The majority of American men had their foreskins removed shortly after being born, but the practice is beginning to decline as research shows the health benefits of removing the foreskin are less than once thought.

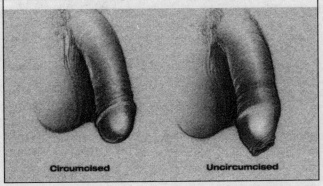

Circumcised   Uncircumcised

A bigger problem is chronic infection underneath the foreskin. Its complications are many, but it's easily headed off by a simple daily washing with a mild soap and water. "Good hygiene is the best preventive medicine for uncircumcised men," says Marc Goldstein, M.D., of New York Hospital—Cornell Medical Center in New York City. If you do get a common fungal infection, marked by swelling and redness, Dr. Goldstein advises treating it three times a day with an over-the-counter cream containing 1 percent clotrimazole (Gyne-Lotrimin). If the problem persists after a week, see a urologist or dermatologist. Infections under the foreskin, although rare, are not to be taken lightly. Left untreated, they can cause penile scarring, painful erections and phimosis.

The Restoration Movement

Some men who feel they were shortchanged by circumcision are attempting to re-create a foreskin by stretching the skin remaining on the penile shaft.

Jim Bigelow is a California psychologist in his sixties and author of *The Joy of Uncircumcising*. He uncircumcised himself over a period of five years—and wrote about the results. Why would anyone bother to do this? "When we lost our foreskins," he says, "we lost the most delightful aspect of our sexuality." He guesses that more than 5,000 men have joined the movement.

"Restoration" is perhaps a misleading word to use; Bigelow acknowledges having built a "replica." Results vary, depending upon how much of the original tissue is left and how much elasticity it has. (Chances are, if your circumcision scar—a brown band of skin where the doctor cut and stitched—is close to the corona, the outer rim of the penis near the tip, you have less of the mucosal inner lining remaining than if the scar is higher up on the penile shaft.) Men who had their foreskins fully removed will tend to have thicker replicas because they're using the more leathery shaft skin. But men who have a fair amount of original tissue left say their restored foreskins are good enough to fool a doctor.

The skin stretching is done in three phases. In the first phase Band-Aid-like tape straps hold the shaft skin as far down over the glans as possible. In the second phase rings of tape are used; in phase three a small weight is used to further stretch the skin until it resembles a normal foreskin.

And what would this movement be without some entrepreneur to fill the new demands? No less than five different manufacturers have come up with products, including one weight called the P.U.D. Tugger. Bigelow, in his book, reviews them and provides ordering information. He also provides enough information to make this a completely do-it-yourself project. But we strongly advise you to consult with a doctor before doing science experiments on your penis.

A network of men who are attempting this has sprung up in more than a dozen cities. For more information on joining a foreskin restoration support group, write to R. Wayne Griffiths, 3205 Northwood Drive, Suite 209, Concord, CA 94520.

FREQUENCY
Bad News: It's Infrequent

Discussing sexual frequency is like discussing salaries: We all want to know what everyone else is getting. A little of that is envy, but mostly we want to know because we think we deserve to get more.

It has been an item of faith in the sexology world that individual sexual activity is spread out over an enormous range. Among the 12,000 men that the late Dr. Alfred C. Kinsey and his colleagues interviewed in the 1940s, one man had exactly one orgasm in the previous 30 years. Others had four or five a day. With a range like that, who's to say what is "normal"?

Fair enough. But we also know, as a matter of common sense, that despite the extremes out there, most ordinary mortals fall into a tighter, more predictable range of behavior. Which is what? Now we know, thanks to the definitive 1994 University of Chicago sex survey.

In their book *Sex in America* the researchers reported, "Those people who are supposed to have the most sexual intercourse are having it less often than those who are supposed to be having intercourse the least."

Truths about the Church Lady

American heterosexuals fall into roughly three groups. About a third of us have sex with a partner twice a week or more. Another third of us have sex a few times a month. And a third of us get it a few times a year, if at all.

Does that strike you as being a little tepid, a little boring?

After all, these are people ages 18 to 59 in a nation that invented the Pill and went on to give the world *Melrose Place*. The entire planet thinks we're doing it 15 hours a day here!

Sex in America's researchers were as surprised as a bunch of newly arrived refugees. "Americans do not have a secret life of abundant sex," they announced.

Leave your racist stereotypes at the door: It doesn't matter whether you're Black or White. Neither group does it more often. Educational level is no predictor. Nor is religion: You might think the devout would be more inhibited than their heathen counterparts, but no. In fact, 9 percent of conservative Protestant women reported engaging in sex four or more times per week. So did—hey, only 7 percent of conservative Protestant men. Uh-oh!

Who does engage in sex most frequently? Married people. Yes, those very people who are assumed to have dull-as-dust sex lives and who need books such as *Hot Monogamy* to get things cooking again. The researchers say the "critical factor" in sexual frequency is being part of a couple. If you're single, you're statistically likelier to have less sex. So much for the swinging playboy image. Having more partners does not lead to more actual sex, say the researchers, unless you belong to that 5 percent of men who claim to

---

THE ANNALS OF IGNORANCE: 1834

... It were better for you not to exceed in the frequency of your indulgences (intercourse) the number of months in the year; and you cannot exceed the number of weeks in the year without impairing your constitutional powers, shortening your lives and increasing your liability to disease and suffering; if indeed, you do not thereby actually induce disease of the worst and most painful kind.

—Advice to married men, from "A Lecture to Young Men" by Sylvester Graham, inventor of the Graham cracker

have five or more sex partners per year. These wild-and-crazy guys do outperform the married men.

The other, more obvious factor is age. Sex is most abundant for couples in their mid-to late twenties who are living together but are not married yet. It is, alas, a distant dream to the average single woman in her fifties. The falling-off in frequency starts early, at age 30. Even though by this age three-fourths of us are married, we're also married . . . with children. We've started to work, commute, mow the lawn, build a deck, shovel the driveway, drive the kids to and from soccer practice and fix our dumb brother-in-law's car. We still have loads of sex drive, but we're starved for time.

Strange Disparities

After age 30 a curious thing happens in the data. Men begin reporting more sexual activity than women of the same age group. By the time they reach their fifties, 11 percent of men—but 30 percent of women—report no partnered sex in the last year. And among women in their late fifties, more than four in ten are completely out of the game. Other surveys confirm this disparity into old age.

What's the deal? Higher mortality rates for men mean that there are more older women left mateless; there may also be higher bragging rates among those men remaining alive. There's also the tendency for some older married men to find younger women as their "constant companions." Finally, older women do report a loss of interest in sex—at least the loss of interest in sex with the men they married so many years ago. The *Sex in America* survey found that one in three older women felt a lack of interest in sex during the last 12 months.

But here's the strangest disparity of all: How much time we spend engaged in sex (very little) as compared with how much time we spend thinking and dreaming and daydreaming about it (all the time). Thoughts about sex help determine what clothes we put on in the morning, what car we drive, what jobs we like, which gym we join, what beer we drink and what food we eat. Without it, Madison Avenue and

Hollywood would both disappear. Pretty good for an activity that takes up less than 1 percent of most people's waking hours.

MASTURBATION
Why It's Still Considered Bad

If there's one thing many doctors and therapists wish they could convince you of about masturbation, it is not to feel guilty about doing it.

There. You've been told. Of course you can tell yourself that a thousand times. It just doesn't do much good. The fact of the matter is most people masturbate (that is, self-stimulate yourself sexually, usually to the point of orgasm), and most people feel at least a little guilty about it.

The *Janus Report on Sexual Behavior* came out in 1993 with the statistic that just 13 percent of Protestants think masturbation is a natural part of adult life. The authors of this book, having grown up in heartland Protestant homes, nod and say, "That sounds about right."

More definitive figures come from the 1994 University of Chicago survey that was the basis for the book *Sex in America*. About half of all men and women who masturbate say they feel at least a little guilty at least some of the time. Furthermore, guilt doesn't seem to ease or worsen with frequency. If you divvy up the people who masturbate once a year, once a month or once a week, roughly half of each camp experiences some guilt, despite the fact that this is the 1990s, and medical and scholarly attitudes have changed.

After two centuries of anti-masturbation hysteria the pendulum has swung so far in the other direction that, in some quarters, it's actually encouraged. Beginning 20 years ago, the new forward-thinking message coming from society's experts was that masturbation is "okay," especially for young women since, for their gender, it's a more reliable

SPANKING THE MONKEY

Here is a partial list of slang terms for male masturbation as taken from various books, magazines and computer bulletin boards.

Bashing the candle
Bleeding the weasel
Bleeding the weed
Bludgeoning the
    beef-steak
Bluffing the banana
Bopping the baloney
Burping the worm
Choking the chicken
Cleaning your rifle
Corking the bat
Cranking the shank
Cuffing the carrot
Dating Rosie Redpalm
    and her five sisters
Fisting your mister
Five-knuckle shuffle
Flogging the dog
Flogging the frog
Flogging the hog
Flogging the log
Flute solo
Jerkin' the gherkin
Hacking the hog

Looping the mule
Manual override
Painting the pickle
Pocket pinball
Pocket pool
Polishing the banister
Polishing the rocket
Pounding your flounder
Pumping the python
"The Rattlesnake Shake"
    (Fleetwood Mac song)
Roping the pony
Shaking hands with the
    unemployed
Slamming the hammer
Slappin' pappy
Spanking the frank
Spanking the monkey
Teasing the weasel
Tossing the turkey
Walking the dog
Whipping the willy
Wonking your conker
Yanking the crank

ALONE TOGETHER

A newsletter all about masturbation, *Celebrate the Self*, carries very explicit news, advice and reader experiences. It caters to surprisingly equal numbers of gay, straight and bisexual male readers. Write to Celebrate the Self, P.O. Box 8888, Mobile, AL 36689.

---

road to orgasm than intercourse. (It also had strong support from extreme feminists—masturbating women have one less reason to depend on men.) Today's college texts on sex education carry how-to drawings and step-by-step instructions. A sexual practice that was once called self-abuse now goes by the code words self-stimulation. Or autoeroticism. Or self-pleasuring.

> Of all the various kinds of sexual intercourse this has the least to recommend it. As an amusement it is too fleeting. As an occupation it is too wearing. As a public exhibition there is no money in it. It is unsuited to the drawing room.
>
> —Mark Twain

Even Ann Landers has given it her blessing. The only "sin" about masturbation is, in her words, "making people feel guilty about responding to this fundamental human drive.

The Underrated Sex Act

So why all the guilt? "It still isn't widely acknowledged as a valid form of sexual expression," says Betty Dodson, Ph.D., author of *Sex for One*, who was dubbed the Mother of Masturbation when she began teaching women how to masturbate back in the early 1970s. She continues to conduct masturbation workshops for women—and continues to be the nation's leading spokeswoman for what Victorians used to call the solitary sin.

"We need to celebrate masturbation," says Dr. Dodson. "We've way overrated partnered sex in this country and way underrated masturbation. Partnered sex is so complicated. It's always got processes going on. It's really not what comes naturally." Yet masturbation, while technically more successful, has the aura of failure. "It's an interesting kind of guilt we feel about masturbation," she says. "Not so much 'I'm a bad person' as 'This isn't what I really want. I'm set-tling.' It lowers our self-esteem." When doing it, many people feel a teeny bit like losers.

For some people the guilt feelings come more from a vague sense of sin and evil than any sense of personal defeat. For that, Dr. Dodson blames religion. "It really is organized religion that does the most damage," she says. "We all have some degree of repression because of that. Some people just overcome it better than other." Overcoming the guilt is especially diffi-cult, she acknowledges, because it's instilled in us in early childhood—"when Mommy removes the hand." Having taught women the how-tos for a quarter-century, Dr. Dodson is one of the few people in America who agreed with former U.S. surgeon general Joycelyn Elders, M.D.: Masturbation should be taught. Literally. "It's practicing for sex," she says, and people need to practice sex just as a ballerina needs to practice before pirouetting onstage. "Sex is an art form. It's pathetic what goes on out there in the name of sex. Most people are just groping."

> "Come, Big Boy, come," screamed the maddened piece of liver that, in my own insanity, I bought one afternoon at a butcher shop and, believe it or not, violated behind a billboard on my way to a bar mitzvah les-son.
>
> —Philip Roth, *Portnoy's Complaint*

The Benefits—Besides the Obvious

In 1994 Dr. Elders lost her job as U.S. surgeon general after telling reporters at a United Nations conference on AIDS

that masturbation is "something that is a part of human sexuality and it's a part of something that, perhaps, should be
taught." Most of us would agree that no harm is done teaching teens that it's not a health hazard. But most men, at least,
sneer at the thought of formal instruction. In the normal
process of adolescent exploration they stumble upon the
same handful (sorry) of techniques that makes them feel
good: rolling it against the body or between the palms like
pastry; stroking the penis, especially at the sensitive part
below the head, called the frenulum; and aided by a lubricant, varying the rhythm and grip in the process. Some gay
men learn from each other at masturbation parties.

More to the point is what masturbation teaches. It teaches
you about your own sexual response. It helps you tell your
partner what really pleases you. It often is a part of professional sex therapy. It can help young men gain more ejaculatory control. And men of all ages can use it to learn
advanced techniques like multiple male orgasm. Basically,
what you use is the stop-start technique, taking yourself to

THE ANNALS OF IGNORANCE: 1916

Some young men, having heard of the injuriousness or sinfulness
of masturbation, give up the habit; that is, they give it up as it is
usually practiced, but they do not give it up altogether. They practice what we call mental, abstract or psychic masturbation; that is,
they concentrate their minds on the opposite sex, upon lascivi-
ous pictures, imagine all sorts of things, until ejaculation takes
place.

They think that as long as they do not do anything manually,
everything is all right. There is no greater error. For of all the kinds
of masturbation, this sort of psychic masturbation is the most
baneful, most injurious and most likely to lead to neurasthenia
(nervous breakdown) and impotence.

—From *Sex Knowledge for Men* by William J. Robinson, M.D.

the point of impending orgasm, stopping (or squeezing the penis at the frenulum) until the pre-ejaculatory sensations subside, then starting up again and continuing for several cycles to an explosive finish.

If nothing else, it makes men less needy—a twerpy quality in us that always manages to repel the opposite sex.

As for women, masturbation can teach them how to have an orgasm. For 29 percent of sexually active women in this country orgasm during partnered sex is at best a sometime thing. Perhaps as many as one in ten younger women has never experienced an orgasm—a problem that you probably haven't run into yourself. But for them masturbation can put them on the right arousal curve. They can learn exactly what sorts of moves will bring them to a peak, and they can get comfortable with those sensations.

It's What Men Do

Despite its potentially greater benefits for women, more men do it, and they do it more often. Among male respondents to the *Sex in America* survey nearly one-third masturbate once a week and roughly another third say they perform it anywhere from a few times a year to a couple times a month.

This confirms previous, more limited surveys, such as one carried out by Harold Leitenberg, Ph.D., psychology professor at the University of Vermont in Burlington. In a survey done among 280 students at his school, 81 percent of the males but only 45 percent of the females said they'd ever masturbated, and the men who did

> Don't knock masturbation—it's sex with someone I love.
>
> —Woody Allen

engaged in this pastime at a rate nearly three times that of the women.

The gender gap may be universal. Among German teenagers interviewed in 1990, 87 percent of the boys but only 41 percent of the girls had masturbated. To our knowledge, no one has ever surveyed a culture in which the women out-masturbated the men.

Our self-pleasuring is not confined to the Boy Scout years. Though the practice is more prevalent in the teenage years among both sexes, men continue to do it into middle age. Not until their fifties did a majority of men tell the *Sex in America* researchers they were no longer masturbating—and then only a slight majority.

Notably, solo sex doesn't live up to its "loser" image as the sexual outlet of last resort, say the researchers. "Married people were significantly more likely to masturbate than people who were living alone." The practice is what they call "a component of a sexually active lifestyle."

> We all have to do it. It's part of our lifestyle, like shaving.
>
> —Jerry Seinfeld

Among the blind.

No, no, no, that's just a joke. Luckily, we can joke about it now, but two centuries ago medical science became seriously convinced that masturbation was the cause of virtually every disgusting debility known to man. Maybe it was a mixup of cause and effect—after all, you could walk into any insane asylum of the era and witness poor souls with, unfortunately, too much time on their hands, if you catch our drift. At any rate, the connection spread far and wide following the 1741 publication of *Onanism, or a Treatise on the Disorders of Masturbation* by the Swiss doctor S. A. D. Tissot. (Apparently, he's the guy who started the rumor that it makes you go blind.) By the 1800s Sylvester Graham was inventing the Graham cracker in the hopes that it would be the sort of nourishment that would help prevent the average young boy from becoming a "confirmed and degraded idiot." And Dickens readers of the age knew that the character Uriah Heep was a masturbator by his description: a pale man without eyebrows who rubbed his clammy palms together. By the end of the Victorian era 14 patents had been granted for devices that restrained masturbation in young boys.

We're so much smarter now.

On the other hand, you don't hear much these days about Pee-Wee Herman, do you?

NIPPLES
Why Do Men Have Them?

No discussion of a man's erogenous zones would be complete without a special mention regarding his nipples. When William H. Masters, M.D., and Virginia E. Johnson, of the former Masters and Johnson Institute in St. Louis, observed hundreds of men reach orgasm during their classic 11-year study, they noticed that, in most of us, the nipples get erect and often swell late in the game. Sometimes the swelling doesn't go away until hours later. Masters and Johnson also made note of the fact that foreplay with the nipples is a big part of male homosexual activity.

All of which makes some heterosexual men uncomfortable about having their breasts stimulated. After all, if they enjoy it, does that mean they're . . . girls?

Regardless of how sexually self-assured you are, you've undoubtedly wondered—as we have—why we have what we have. Join the club. Stephen Jay Gould, Harvard zoology professor, National Book Award winner and *Nova* adviser, confessed that it was the most-often-asked question sent along by the readers of his regular column in the magazine *Natural History*. As one troubled librarian put it: "Why do men have nipples? This question nags at me whenever I see a man's bare chest!"

The biggest mistake people make, Gould wrote by way of a long and elegant reply, is that people automatically assume male nipples must be there for a reason; they must have some purpose past or present. Even Plato made that mistake, speculating that men have nipples because humans were all hermaphrodites once upon a time. Others have suggested that men have nipples because in primitive societies they sometimes nursed babies when food supplies grew scarce.

Gould says phooey.

The short answer is men have nipples because women have nipples, and biology is very frugal with its templates. Women's larger breasts are the product of evolutionary development; that the professor doesn't doubt for a moment.

They did (and still do) fulfill a purpose. But these wonderful milk-producing machines are in turn produced by the female's own particular hormonal bath. Different hormones shape our sex differences. But we're not two different species after all (even though it often seems so). We're both built from the same genetic DNA. And that DNA creates the same raw material. It's nature's way of economizing.

The same is true with our sex organs, says Gould. "The clitoris and the penis are one and the same organ, identical in early form, but later enlarged in male fetuses by the action of testosterone. Similarly, the labia majora of women (the hair-covered outer lips of the vulva) and the scrotal sac of men are the same structure, indistinguishable in young embryos, but later enlarged, folded over and fused along the midline in male fetuses."

By the way, the fact that the clitoris and penis emerge from the same fetal tissue tells you a lot about what a woman really needs to reach orgasm.

"The two sexes," Gould goes on to write, "are variants upon the same ground plan. Males have nipples because females need them—and the embryonic pathway to their development builds precursors in all mammalian fetuses, enlarging the breasts later in females but leaving them small (and without evident function) in males."

Now you know.

ORGASM
All about the Big Bang Theory

It is the Big O—the moment we replay in our heads, the book passage that gets dog-eared, the scene that brings on the R rating. It is the subject of endless self-help sex manuals and the target of laboratory research. It is, as the poet e. e. cummings said, "Muscles better and nerves more." It's a bodily response that somehow relieves pain, boosts the immune system and leads to all sorts of commitments.

And yet most of us are not nearly living up to our potentials.

Like many things regarding men and women, their orgasms are both the same and different. Back in the late 1950s and early 1960s William H. Masters, M.D., and Virginia E. Johnson, of the former Masters and Johnson Institute in St. Louis, watched hundreds of men and women reach orgasm—more than 10,000 orgasms, all told. And they were struck by the amazing similarities. In both sexes, orgasm is

> Give me chastity—but not yet.
>
> —St. Augustine's prayer

the peak of a long process of progressive arousal, for which it is the explosive release. The nipples get erect, a flush spreads over the stomach, chest and neck, and heart races, blood pressure soars, one breaks a sweat and all kinds of muscles involuntarily contract. (Look down at your feet the next time you break the sound barrier and you'll see your toes do a wacky curl, the big toe jutting out and the others bending over backward.)

Our sex organs fill up with so much blood, parts of them turn purple. The man's ejaculatory contractions occur at an interval of 0.8 second; in the woman contractions of the uterus and the muscles in the outer third of the vagina occur at precisely the same frequency. Also in both sexes the sphincter muscle in the anus—the one we close to keep from passing gas—contracts involuntarily two to four times at 0.8-second intervals.

That's what goes on behind closed doors.

The biggest difference between the sexes is that the man cools down right away. Men—most men anyway—go through a refractory period that lasts anywhere from a few minutes in young studs to a couple of days in the older male. During it, he is inert to arousal's charms. She, on the other hand, "generally maintains higher levels of stimulative susceptibility," as Masters and Johnson put it so clinically. She can go on to experience wave after orgasmic wave—as many as 134 in a laboratory setting, according to one report.

Men can have multiple orgasms, too, although it's more often a bit of a circus trick. What you can do is override the refractory period; you bring yourself to orgasm but screech on the brakes in that second when you feel you're about to come but just before you actually ejaculate. For more information, see Multiple Orgasms on page 300. Some men do this because they're obsessively goal-oriented and would like nothing more than to turn sex into yet another competitive sport. Other men might learn this to prolong a delightful afternoon, to please their partners or simply to gain more control over their own love rhythms.

Where That "Coming" Feeling Comes From

In men ejaculation and orgasm are really two separate bodily events; you can have either without the other. But don't let the science fool you; our really satisfying orgasms include both. Masters and Johnson noted that among the few men who were multiejaculatory in their laboratory, those guys reported that the first time felt the best. And among all 312 males they studied, the larger the fluid volume being shot off, the more pleasurable the orgasm was, subjectively.

Ejaculation is a two-stage process. In the first stage the sex accessory organs—the prostate gland, the seminal vesicles, the epididymis and vas deferens—all squeeze their stuff, the various ingredients of semen, into the urethra, which is the tube leading out to the end of the penis. Also at this time, a sphincter muscle between the prostate and the bladder clamps down so when we move on to stage two, semen doesn't go up into the bladder and urine doesn't come out in the semen. All this activity produces a feeling of inevitability, a sense that the semen is quite literally "coming." It lasts only two or three seconds.

Then comes stage two, when all sorts of pelvic muscles you had no idea you had begin their contractions. They occur in unison to the rock-steady beat of 0.8 second, forcing the seminal fluid out of the penis with that rhythmic squirt we live for.

Better Sex for Both Sexes

Some people claim that men must have invented intercourse because they're the only ones who get any fun out of it. We won't touch that one, but the irrefutable truth is that, indeed, men reach orgasm more reliably from coitus than do women. Three-fourths of us, but less than a third of women, always have orgasm while having intercourse, according to the 1994 *Sex in America* survey conducted by University of Chicago researchers.

Since men usually come out on top, it's almost piggish to talk about further enhancing our experiences, but . . . so what. Basically, orgasms are more intense if the arousal leading up to it is more intense. And that can be fulfilled by noting the advice in numerous chapters of this book—everything from lingerie to lubricants. In particular, many men report more powerful orgasms after doing something called a Kegel exercise for a few weeks. For more information, see Kegels on page 171.

Women reach orgasm more reliably from masturbation than from coitus. Part of that is pure physiology: the clitoris, which is a woman's most surefire route to getting all fired up, is not directly stimulated by vaginal intercourse. And part of it is timing: Some (not all) women take longer to reach orgasm via vaginal penetration than the men they're mated with.

No wonder we're always at cross-purposes.

The inherent differences between the sexes could be neatly overcome, it was once thought, by achieving the ideal of the simultaneous orgasm. We say it was thought because it's not thought about so much anymore. Oh, it still takes center stage in steamy romance novels (the "bodice-rippers"), but in real life it gives many people the performance jitters. "It's falling out of favor," says J. Kenneth Davidson, Ph.D., a sociologist at the University of Wisconsin in Madison. Dr. Davidson conducted a study of 805 nurses in 15 states and, man, oh, man, we don't want to stereotype anybody but this turned out to be a group of highly sexed women. About half reported having more than one current sex partner, 43 percent were usually multiorgasmic and during a typical sexual encounter virtually all of them did virtually everything. If anyone was likely to achieve that mythical moment, these women were. Yet only 17 percent reported climaxing around the same time as their partners. (Forty percent said they had their first orgasm before their partners, while 31 percent waited—or had to wait—until afterward.)

Given the difficulty of simultaneous orgasm, the new rule, "ladies first," makes sense. It's more than just sexual politeness: Davidson's study of nurses found that the multiorgasmic R.N.s were more likely to have partners who delayed their orgasms until after they had their first ones.

Notes toward a Definition

Odd, isn't it? Men have orgasms more often, yet women can have more orgasms. A 26-year-old escrow secretary who answered our *Men's Health* magazine survey posed the ultimate mystery: "I still don't understand why men are said to be more sexual than women, yet they aren't able to have as many orgasms."

Neither do we.

Further, did you know that some women can actually fantasize their way to climax? Three researchers at Rutgers University in New Brunswick, New Jersey, proved that beyond a doubt by finding ten women ranging in age from 32 to 67 who claimed they could reach orgasm by themselves, without even touching themselves. The researchers—*G Spot* co-authors Beverly Whipple, Ph.D., Gina Ogden, Ph.D., and Barry R. Komisaruk, Ph.D.—brought these ten women into their laboratory, then witnessed the attempts while measuring for certain objective confirmations including blood pressure, heart rate, pupil dilation and pain tolerance. Seven of the ten women passed the tests.

Hey, men can do this, too! In our (wet) dreams.

Their research paper, published in the *Archives of Sexual Behavior*, shook up the scientific world's already-hazy notions of what an orgasm really is. Is it a reflex? An involuntary response? Is it centered in the body, the mind or the groin? "There is no universally accepted definition of orgasm," the paper notes.

But Dr. Komisaruk thinks that, after 30 years of research, he's getting closer.

Dr. Komisaruk is a behavioral neuroscientist, so he tends to look at the human orgasm from the central nervous system's point of view. And he believes an orgasm has close relatives in a few other bodily functions, like the sneeze, the yawn and the stretch. Each of those, he says, involves a repetitive stimulus that builds—in his words, "recruiting more neural activity in the brain that ultimately reaches a peak of excitation, activating, in turn, a new system." Like the tickle that causes the sneeze. Thus, he says, "a genital orgasm is just a special case of a process that is a general property of the nervous system." There's a stimulus, a buildup and a unique motor output as the resolution.

That sounds like a nice, innocuous, arcane theory, but it has a potentially incendiary conclusion. "There are definitely different types of orgasms," he says. This may be politically incorrect to say in some quarters inasmuch as millions of women spent decades being misled by Freudian psychologists. In 1905 Freud distinguished between a clitoral and vaginal orgasm, but went on to speculate that the clitoral orgasm was "clitoral onanism," i.e., was immature and something a healthy woman should outgrow. For half a century thereafter some of his followers insisted that the clitoral orgasm could lead to neurosis and frigidity. Finally, in the 1950s the late Dr. Alfred C. Kinsey declared the Freudian ideal, the vaginal orgasm, to be a "biological impossibility"; in the 1960s Masters and Johnson announced that physically there was no such thing.

But since then we've learned about the G-spot, a highly sensitive area inside the vagina with its own set of nerve pathways that some sex researchers say produces an orgasm all its own. We've learned that women consistently report differing sensations regarding orgasms reached via masturbation versus coitus. And by experience we know not all orgasms feel exactly the same. Not for women or men—who may have an equivalent, the prostate gland.

Komisaruk's theory says, in essence, to trust these feelings. "If you stimulate different places in the body, you'll get different responses and perceive them differently," he says. "They can feel very different, depending on the different parts of the body that are recruited into the climax."

Maybe the notion of a vaginal orgasm will re-emerge—minus the old Freudian finger wagging.

PENIS
Controlling Your Privates

Think of it as a Mercedes SL. Maybe you'll be nicer to it.

Men are incredibly cavalier about their penises. We name it, yell at it, ignore it, insult it, slap it around. Whether we're engaging in sports or the sport of love, we leave it unprotected and vulnerable.

Consider this for a moment: What if you had to replace it tomorrow?

You're looking at close to $50,000 when all's said and done. You'll endure at least a month of pain and suffering, and you'll need professional help in reconciling yourself to the final product.

Yes, doctors can reconstruct a penis. The operation is called a phalloplasty. Different specialists employ different surgical procedures but basically they take skin from your abdomen or forearm and roll it up, creating a sausagelike appendage suitable for urination, but little else. There's no erectile tissue; for something approaching that function, you need a pump, an insert or a special sleeve.

The would-be patients for this operation include men who've had the type of accident we dare not imagine and people who feel they were born accidents—transsexuals who were born with women's bodies but who consider themselves men.

That some people will go through so much to get what you take for granted illustrates two truths.

(1) The penis is the mental and physical center of mas-

culinity; (2) that's one fine piece of machinery hanging between your legs.

Complicated Plumbing

You see, a penis is a lot more complicated than a hunk of rolled-up skin with a hole down the middle. But let's start with the hole. The tube that ends at the tip of your penis is called the urethra and it travels all the way back to the bladder, the storage organ for urine. The urethra is surrounded in the penis by soft tissue called the corpus spongiosum. The tip of the penis, the incredibly sensitive glans, is comprised entirely of this tissue. Glans is Latin for acorn, which is what it looks like, kind of.

As for the rest of the penile shaft, just beneath the skin's surface are two side-by-side canisters of erectile tissue, the corpora cavernosa. A central artery runs down the middle of each. During an erection these cavernosa are the go-to guys. They become engorged with blood, turning your penis into a huge virtual artery. For more information, see Erection on page 23. Each central artery branches off into thousands of tiny endings that, on cue, flood microscopic spaces, causing them to swell and stiffen. It's a marvel of human anatomy that surgery cannot duplicate. And it allows the penis to perform two very different functions: urination and fertilization. Two tools in one. Think of it as the Swiss Army knife of human anatomy.

OTHER PLACES, OTHER NAMES

Ambassador (Chinese)	Lingam (Sanskrit)
Arrow of Love (Tantric)	Mushroom of Immortality
Crimson Bird (Chinese)	(Chinese)
Dart (Arabic)	Phallus (Phoenician/Greek)
Discoverer (Arabic)	Plough (Tantric)
Flute (Chinese)	Searcher (Arabic)
Key of Desire (Persian)	Tortoise (Chinese)

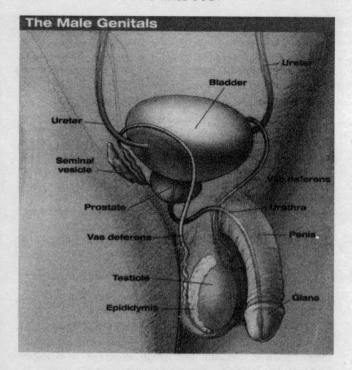

The Male Genitals

Ureter

Bladder

Ureter

Seminal vesicle

Vas deferens

Prostate

Urethra

Vas deferens

Penis

Testicle

Glans

Epididymis

You'll be flattered to know that your penis is bigger than you think. It goes deep inside you, back nearly to your anus. It ducks under your prostate, where it forks in two; these two forks, called the crura, are attached to pelvic bones. (You may be able to feel them during an erection by pressing a finger between your anus and scrotum.) Like any well-built skyscraper, your penis is founded upon these "footers" below the surface; they give it stability. You and the Empire State Building.

All of this is summarized in the accompanying diagram. Some of you will ask, "Where's its brain?" Wise guys. Others may ask, "If it's a 'boner,' where's the bone?" Humans don't have one, although many other mammals do.

WAR IS HELL

In 1300 B.C. King Menephta of Egypt defeated the Libyans and their allies and cut off more than 13,000 of their phalli as souvenirs. On an ancient monument at Karnak an accounting is given.

Phalluses of Libyan generals	6
Libyan phalluses cut off	6,359
Siculian phalluses cut off	222
Etruscan phalluses cut off	542
Greek phalluses presented to king	6,111

No, it's not a bone, or a spear or a cannon or a sword or a power tool or a blunderbuss. We'd like to think it's invincible but it's not. No wonder some women treat it insensitively. One 48-year-old university administrator complained in our survey, "Women think that a man's penis is like a rod or a gear shift and can be handled roughly. They don't appreciate how sensitive it is and that a gentle touch goes a lot further."

Where do you suppose they get that attitude?

If you're having a problem with your penis, it's probably addressed somewhere in this book. If you have bumps or lesions on the skin or there's a white, puslike discharge from the urethra, see part 8. If you've injured your penis during sex—and believe it, you'll know by the cracking sound followed by excruciating pain—see a urologist. If your penis is bending sharply upon erection, see Peyronie's Disease on page 456. This condition, too, requires medical counsel.

> Happiness is a warm gun.
>
> —John Lennon

PHEROMONES
Your Own Love Potion Number Nine?

So far, this is a concept more popular with script writers than with scientists.

The idea is humans have a "sixth sense," with an organ all its own located about half an inch up inside the nose. It has a very fancy name: the vomeronasal organ, or VNO. It detects pheromones, which are chemical signals given off by other humans. Signals that, among other things, say yoo-hoo . . .

Script writers have certainly gotten aroused by this idea.

In an episode of the television show *L.A. Law* the character Douglas mistakenly puts on a pheromone perfume meant for women—and immediately gets mashed by some big, beefy guy. In the show *Northern Exposure* the local disc jockey's pheromones hit their monthly peak and women start hanging around outside his cabin day and night. Get the idea? You've also seen it in movies such as *Boomerang* or *Porky's*. Or you've read about it in Patrick Suskind's best-selling thriller, *Perfume*.

A couple of entrepreneurs have climbed aboard this bandwagon, manufacturing pheromone perfumes with brand names like Athena and Realm. But before you rush out to buy a case, be aware that there are a couple of minor hitches.

First of all, it has not yet been proven that humans produce pheromones.

Second, you could take a bath in that stuff and it still wouldn't help you get a date.

A Kiss Is Just a Kiss?

The rat's VNO has been studied for the better part of two decades by Charles Wysocki, Ph.D., a neuroscientist at the Monell Chemical Senses Center of the University of Pennsylvania in Philadelphia. Pheromones rule the insect world, and the VNO is indeed a sense organ in some advanced amphibians, most reptiles and many mammals. Pheromones are what calls the male moth from miles away. It makes the male rhesus (a monkey) go to pieces. It's what seduces the sow into arching her back and assuming the position. In fact, hog farmers use a product called Boar Mate, an aerosol can of pig pheromone, that they spray under a sow's nose to get her in the mood for a little artificial insemination.

As for us, alas, a human pheromone has yet to be isolated in the laboratory. But we may have been seeing its effects. Supposedly, pheromones are emitted by our skin, our hair, our saliva, our urine and menstrual flow. And Dr. Wysocki says one thing known for sure, so far, is this: "There's something in humans, both male and female, that does affect the female menstrual cycle." Studies have shown that women's menstrual cycles become synchronized when living in close proximity (such as college students on one floor of a dorm). And perhaps you've heard of this bold experiment: When women in one study had the underarm odor of a stranger wiped upon their upper lips, they began menstruating at the same time as that stranger. What some people won't do for science.

> To be sensual is to respect and rejoice in the force of life itself, and to be present in all that one does, from the effort of loving to the breaking of bread.
>
> —Phyl Garland,
> "Sound of Soul"

Dr. Wysocki is studying whether or not that effect works by influencing the woman's hormone levels. If that proves to be the case, science will be one step closer to identifying a human pheromone. This is a particularly daunting task because researchers are trying to identify something that's odorless. The proponents of human pheromone theory maintain that we don't smell pheromones the same way we smell, say, someone's underarms. They work unconsciously to influence our attitudes. James Vaughn Kohl, author of the first nonfiction book about human pheromones, *The Scent of Eros*, says flatly, "Pheromones have played a role in every personal preference I have ever developed."

But that is still in the realm of theory. Here's a fact: "We all have our own unique odor print," says Dr. Wysocki, created in part by specific genes we carry. Intriguingly, the same set of genes regulates our immune system. Thus, our body's weaponry for fighting off microbiological invaders also may clue us in on whose genes are most unlike our own—which is, in the scheme of natural selection, a good thing. And just how would we be clued in? By kisses. "A kiss," Dr. Wysocki hypothesizes, "is a vestigial behavior for an exchange of chemical information" about potential mates. The more different their genes are the better, because the "hybrid" children of such a union will be more resistant to pathogens such as viruses, bacteria and parasites. So, yes, there may be a biological basis to the old expression "opposites attract."

Researchers at the University of Chicago believe they've found proof. Among the Hutterites, a religious sect living in parts of the American Northwest and Canada, men and women tend to choose partners with the biggest difference in their histocompatibility complexes, the scientific name for one's individual immune system.

So there.

Even if the existence of human pheromones is proven one day, Dr. Wysocki doesn't believe it's going to change the dating game. "I don't think we will find an aphrodisiac," he says. "It's not going to be a reflex." If anything, it will be but one component in the eternal mystery of why we fall in love.

As for the perfumes, Wysocki says at least some of them contain animal pheromones. Be careful where you wear it—or you may hear behind you a friendly little "oink, oink."

PROSTATE
The Little Ring of Fire

If you poke your abdomen just above your penis, that's where it is, sort of—deep inside you, in front of the rectum and below the bladder, surrounding the urethra like a doughnut.

Say hello to your prostate.

Not to be confused with pros*trate*, as in lying down, totally exhausted, knocked out by her love. That's what young men talk about.

The pros*tate* is what old men talk about.

For much of your twenties and thirties your prostate keeps in shape, maintaining its trim figure and youthful weight of 20 milligrams. It's a little bigger than a quarter in size. Doctors like to compare it to a walnut. But then, starting in the late forties, it starts growing, at least in some of us. And it keeps growing. And growing. It's the only organ in the human body that keeps growing with age. By age 80 two-thirds of us have enlarged prostates.

Scientists don't know why. They know amazingly little about the prostate, other than the fact that it's one of the sex accessory glands. Girls don't have one. Its primary function, together with its two wing-like attachments, the seminal vesicles, consists of providing the fluid for your semen. In that fluid is sugar to feed the sperm,

> Love is an exploding cigar which we willingly smoke.
>
> —Lynda Barry

alkaline substances to counteract the acidity of your urethra and her vagina and substances to make the fluid thicken at first and then make it clear. For more information, see Semen on page 69. Its product is important. During ejaculation your body is literally throwing your seeds at a woman's cervix. If you were just tossing out sperm cells, you'd be tossing feathers instead of footballs.

The prostate probably has other functions. Scientists don't really know what they may be, but Donald S. Coffey, Ph.D., triple professor of urology, oncology and pharmacology at Johns Hopkins University in Baltimore, hazards a guess. "Here's what I think it does: If you were a bacteria and walked up your urethra into your penis, it would look like the Holland Tunnel," he says. "I think all the orifices of the body are protected by glands so that you don't get infected. The prostate is loaded with zinc, which kills bacteria. Furthermore, it has all these enzymes called proteases, which chew things up. So I think that's its role: to keep the system clean."

Word is slowly getting around about this organ for a different reason—with its bundles of nerve endings it can be the site of sexual pleasure. In some circles it has come to be known as the male G-spot, and in fact, it seems to be the great unexplored sexual center of the human male. For more information, see Male G-spot on page 295. Unfortunately, that tidbit is eclipsed by its wider reputation: the site of agony and cancer in later years.

What Can Go Wrong: A Prostate Primer

The problems with prostates boil down to the fact that as men age their prostates tend to get enlarged or cancerous, or both.

As it grows, it can get as big as a baseball and still not cause any problems. But if it starts to squeeze against your urethra . . . yikes. You have difficulty urinating, despite a constant urgent feeling that you need to. One in four elderly men end up undergoing surgery to correct the problem, which is called benign prostatic hyperplasia, or BPH for short.

BPH comes on slowly. If you're under age 40 and these symptoms appear suddenly, then quite possibly what ails you is a garden-variety bacterial prostate infection. The treatment consists of antibiotics and frequent ejaculation.

If those are the only problems that the prostate presents you with over the course of your life, count yourself among the blessed. Prostate cancer has become the most diagnosed cancer in America. It strikes one in nine men, mostly in their fifties and older. If you're an African-American, your risk is much greater.

Medical science is steadily improving the odds of detecting the disease at earlier stages, which improves the chances of complete recovery. The most monumental advance has been the development of a blood test for PSA (prostate specific antigen). This test first came into use around 1990. It detects elevated levels of PSA in the blood, which could be a

---

THE ANNALS OF IGNORANCE: 1925

. . . very frequently bad cases of sex abuse (masturbation) are set up in children through the pressure of feces upon the sexual nerves. Relieve this condition, cleanse the bloodstream of the poisons set up, by this means directing full nutrition to the nerve centres, and the sexual aggravation ceases, and the child becomes normal.

—From *A Complete Book of Sex Knowledge* by Bernard Bernard, D.Sc., editor, author, philosopher, scientist, idealist and champion athlete

---

signal of cancer in its early stages. The trouble is it could also be a signal of a symptomless prostate infection. But even so, the test has twice the predictive power of a mammogram. And it's still being refined. This test is administered in combination with a digital rectal exam. You drop your trousers, bend over, hear the snap of a rubber glove . . . that one. You'll get over it.

But when should you be tested? And what do you do about it once you find out? There are the chief controversies surrounding prostate health. For more information, see Prostate Problems on page 465.

A Tomato a Day?

Edward L. Giovannucci, M.D., an instructor at Harvard Medical School, is a leading expert on the epidemiology of prostate cancer. Which means? He studies huge groups of people to see who gets it, who doesn't and whether any patterns emerge.

Prostate cancer's risk factors aren't as clear-cut as, say, smoking and lung cancer. Furthermore, the factor that puts you at greatest risk is the one you can't do anything about: your family's history of the disease. If just one of your relatives has gotten the disease, your chances are two to three times greater than the average guy's of getting it. If three or more relatives have gotten the disease, your chances are more than ten times greater. Family history also means the cancer tends to strike earlier: 43 percent of the cases in men younger than age 55 show a family history of the disease.

That said, here's one risk factor you can control: what you eat. The research to date suggests strongly that a diet high in fat, especially fat from red meat, acts as an environmental "trigger," more than doubling your risk of getting the disease. Dr. Giovannucci's own study found that chowing down on steak five days a week increased men's risks by 160 percent. Moreover, it seems to put men at greater risk of having the disease advance to its later, inoperable stages.

Okay, so an overfamiliarity with steak house menus will increase your chances of getting prostate cancer later in life. Nag, nag, nag. But Dr. Giovannucci has some good news: Tomatoes seem to decrease your risk. "We're not yet ready to say, 'A tomato a day keeps your urologist away,'" he says. "But we have some promising preliminary evidence."

The key ingredient may be lycopene, a nutrient similar to beta-carotene, the stuff of carrots. In nature both help protect plants from sunlight damage. Once we eat them, they may keep up the same antioxidant function, performing a little damage control on behalf of our DNA.

"We're just beginning to explore this," he notes. Very little is known on the microbiological level about which components within vegetables are effective against cell mutation. But on the macro level, says Dr. Giovannucci, the picture is much clearer: Some 200 epidemiological studies, worldwide, have shown that a diet high in vegetables and fruits is very likely to reduce your risk of many types of cancers.

So skip the steak house tonight and find a place with marinara sauce on the menu.

SEMEN
The View under a Microscope

The pretty young woman hands you an erotic video—and a clear plastic cup with a blue lid.

Your job is to get your precious seeds of life into the cup. Without her help.

You are about to undergo something called a semen analysis. It's not something you'd have done out of curiosity and, judging by the faces of the men who show up at the laboratory door, it's not done willingly. It's done as part of fertility counseling. It's done because you've been trying to start a family, but nothing's happening. It's done because the doc wants to know if you're shootin' blanks.

Up until now you haven't sat around thinking about your semen. Oh, there was the time an old girlfriend once asked you, as you begged her to perform fellatio, whether it was harmful when swallowed. You, having no idea what the answer really was, told her, "Of course not!" The answer really is: Of course not, unless you are HIV positive or are infected with some other sexually transmitted disease. Barring that, and as long as she's not one of the rare ladies who's allergic to semen, there's no problem. In fact, it's a mere five calories per spoonful.

A semen analysis doesn't analyze semen so much as the sperm in the semen—which is 5 percent of the total at most. The rest of it, the plasma, consists of fluids from the prostate and seminal vesicles, fluids that contain fructose (a sugar), protein, citric acid, alkalines and a host of other substances that will make life hospitable where it's going and give it the energy it needs to make the long swim through the uterus and up a fallopian tube. The sperm is the only cell designed to travel outside the human body. Your little astronauts need a lot of rocket fuel to make the trip.

You are not expected to fill the cup. Most men donate the usual teaspoonful or two. That's enough. Swimming around in there are up to 90 million sperm, sperm that started out in your testicles nearly 100 days ago.

A Physical for Your Sperm

We visited a state-of-the-art andrology lab in suburban Philadelphia. It's part of a large fertility practice run by Jerome H. Check, M.D., and his associates. Andrology is the science of sperm vitality; it's the subject of enough research to support its own scientific journal, *Archives of Andrology*. Dr. Check is a frequent contributor.

If you had come along with us for a semen analysis, you would have trotted down the hall with a video then ambled back after a few minutes with your "sample." One of the andrologists then would place your sample in a body-temperature incubator for 20 minutes or so until it cleared. (Just after ejaculation all semen is a whitish froth the consistency of nearly-set Jell-O, but it eventually becomes clear and runny.) When all was clear, she'd take it out of the incubator and, with the medical technician's version of a turkey baster, she'd begin dribbling portions onto a row of microscope slides and would apply colored dye to some of the specimens.

> Q. What's the difference between a lawyer and a sperm cell?
> A. The sperm cell has a one-in-a-hundred-million chance of becoming a human being.

At this point the smell of semen is still pungent—a unique scent that's been compared to oil of wintergreen and the flowers of the Spanish chestnut tree. But Anita, one of the andrologists on duty today, is unfazed. "I don't notice the smell," she says. "I guess it's like working in a doughnut shop—you don't pay any attention to it anymore."

Your sperm are now ready to undergo a battery of tests to determine their fitness for fertilization. The tests will be performed with the aid of a microscope that magnifies your little tadpoles 100 to 1,000 times, depending upon the particular test. A semen analysis will not determine the cause of every case of "male-factor" infertility, but generally it gives your doctor a pretty clear idea of your odds.

A thorough semen analysis will include the following:

Volume: Just how much precious bodily fluid did you and the erotic video produce together? A normal range is two to five milliliters. A low volume might indicate a problem such as retrograde ejaculation, wherein semen is being forced up into the bladder rather than out the penis.

Liquefaction: After 15 or 20 minutes in the incubator it should be clear. If it takes an hour or longer, that's a problem.

Viability: Quite simply, are your sperm cells dead or alive? The dead ones take up a pinkish stain. If the majority are dead, that's obviously a problem.

Count: The andrologist literally counts the number of sperm within a 100-space grid on the slide—but you can see right away what's going on. Guys with fertility problems have a few goofy-looking sperm swimming around. If there's no problem, peering through the microscope looks exactly like driving into a blizzard.

Motility: How many are swimming? And how well?

Immature sperm: If they're being released from the testicles too soon, they'll be clumped in big, amoebalike blobs with a bunch of wiggly tails sticking out.

Morphology: Their physical appearance is paramount. Under the microscope even the average guy's sperm can look like the Mutant League. Some have no heads, some have two. Up to half of your sperm can be duds and you can still be considered "normal." It's the good-looking sperm that get ahead in this life.

THE ANNALS OF IGNORANCE: 1902

There is a vast amount of vital force used in the production and expenditure of the seminal fluid. Wasted as the incontinence of so many lives allows it to be, and prostituted to the simple gratification of fleshly desire, it weakens and depraves.

—From "What a Young Wife Ought to Know" by Mrs. Emma F. Angell Drake, M.D.

HOS: Short for the hypo-osmotic swelling test. Sperm pass the test if their tails coil up in reaction to a solution of sugar and salt. If they don't, something's wrong with their outer membranes. As a measurement of potential infertility, "It's the one test I'll hang my hat on," says Dr. Check.

No Problems, Just Challenges

That's not all, folks: Andrologists also test for plasma viscosity, the presence of white blood cells, which could indicate an infection, and the presence of antibodies on the surface of the sperm, which would prevent it from fertilizing the egg. For some tests a computer is used. Computer-aided semen analysis is more than just a backup to double-check the work of the technicians. It measures such factors as sperm velocity and linearity to give the fertility specialist an even clearer picture of semen health. (Linearity is a measurement of whether the sperm can swim ahead in a straight line; some just keep going around in circles.)

How does the doctor use all of this information? It depends on what's wrong. Some guys cannot be helped easily. Perhaps they've flunked the morphology test because their sperm heads have no acrosome, a kind of microbiological football helmet. Their sperm cannot penetrate an egg without some very expensive medical assistance. Other guys just need a little hormonal adjustment, a change of medication or an IUI—short for intrauterine insemination. In this procedure the andrology lab spends an hour concentrating your speediest, most gung ho sperm via a "sperm wash" and places them in a catheter. Meanwhile, the doctor has given your wife an ultrasound to see if her ovaries have released an egg yet this month. If so, the doctor injects your sperm (via the catheter) right into your wife's uterus, bypassing the often-troublesome mucus that clogs the cervix (the narrow passageway between the vagina and uterus). All for only $125 at this office.

Even if you get bad news from a semen analysis, it's really all to the good; your fertility treatment can now be tailored to your situation. And these days, there's a treatment for just about every situation. Even if the sperm in your semen are all dead, for example, doctors can retrieve viable sperm directly from your testicles. For more information, see Male Infertility on page 365.

SEX DREAMS
How Your Brain Works Out the Kinks

Let's see. You had sex with your son. Or your son's wife. Or was that your mother-in-law? Wait a minute, now you remember: You were having sex with your minister's wife and that dumb dog of hers. You were in a taxi and it went off a bridge, and you were plunging down and down and down . . .

Then you woke up.

Someone once said dreams are what we wake up from; that's about the only surefooted comment we can pass along. Man has been trying to interpret his dreams, sifting their contents for prophecies and omens, ever since Adam. The poet and journalist A. Alvarez, in his book *Night*, writes,

> Dreams are an involuntary kind of poetry.
>
> —Jean Paul Richter, German writer

"Over the centuries the craziness of dreams has been a persistent source of uneasiness for everyone who has ever woken in a sweat and thought about where he has just been in his dreams and what he has been doing."

In the second century A.D. Artemidorus compiled the popular wisdom of his day into *The Interpretation of Dreams*, and this is how he read the meaning of your dreams about sex with your son: "To possess a son who is not yet five years old signifies, I have observed, the child's death. . . . But if the son is more than a child, it has the following meaning. If the father is poor, he will send his son away to school and pay his expenses, and will strain off his resources into him in this way. . . . To have sexual intercourse with one's son, if he is already a grown man and living abroad, is auspicious. But if the son is not far away and is living with his father, it is inauspicious. For they must separate because intercourse generally takes place between men when they are not face to face . . . "

Two millennia later we still don't take dreams at face value. The people nowadays who engage in the art of interpreting dreams abide by the notion that our dreams are mostly metaphors and symbols, that they're a form of consciousness radically different from our walking thoughts. Alvarez says they are a great game of charades—"inner dramas in which mental activity expresses itself physically in signs and gestures. They are ideas in dumb show, thinking in mime." Think of it: For 100 minutes a night you're Marcel Marceau.

> For the waking there is one common world only; but when asleep each man turns to his own private world.
>
> —Heraclitus, Greek philosopher

If dreams are metaphors, then at least some dreams about sex aren't necessarily about sex. And some dreams that aren't about sex really are. Freud believed this to a fault. Never mind the manifest content, he said, you have to discover the latent content, the true, hidden meaning, and that is probably about sex. Thus, tunnels in the dream world represent vaginas, umbrellas represent penises and walking up stairs means coitus. This got pretty silly. Freud theorized that a dream about dentistry, for example, was really a dream about masturbation. (Because you'd get your teeth pulled. Get it?)

It's been established, by scientists in sleep laboratories, that men have more sex dreams than women. It's also known that men's dreams tend to be populated by more men than women—so it's not terribly surprising if men occasionally show up in the sex dreams of men who are confirmed heterosexuals by day. But are they really having a homosexual dream? When male subjects in sleep laboratories have been awakened while they were having erections (and we all have erections every night, sometimes for hours on end), only rarely did they report having erotic dreams at the time. It's too bad we can't see when a sleeper is having a sex dream—for then we would know if such dreams and erections often happen together.

It helps to know that a dream is rarely what it seems, but still, it's highly disturbing to have a dream about, say, incest with your children. Robert L. Van de Castle, Ph.D., a behavioral psychologist and dream researcher for 30 years, says most dreams are unpleasant. Perhaps we shouldn't shy away from that. "Checking in with our dreams for an assessment of our emotional welfare is similar to checking in with a doctor for an assessment of our physical welfare," he writes in his latest book, *Our Dreaming Mind*. As for an incest dream in particular he tells us there could be many interpretations, depending upon the dreamer's situation. "These dreams can occur when we're not doing well in our dating relationships," he says. By seeking out a family member, we're finding comfort in something known and in someone with whom we don't fear rejection.

If you're interested in dreams, scads of books offer ways to interpret them. One popular volume is Gayle Delaney's *Living Your Dreams*. She tells you how to remember your dreams and how to dream about problems you'd like to solve. She also describes a way of interpreting dreams by way of interviewing yourself. You are, after all, the producer and director of these "movies of your mind."

SEX DRIVE
Why It's So Variable

Hundreds of men who answered our *Men's Health* magazine survey complained that women don't comprehend the awesome power of the male sex drive.

"Men's sexuality is a beast," says one respondent, a 39-year-old television researcher, "with all the beauty and ferocity you'd ascribe to a predator. It takes a great deal of concentrated effort to focus that sexuality, put limits on it and make it work within the confines of a monogamous relationship. I don't think women realize the work it takes for men to keep that beast penned without it going stir-crazy."

It's not true that *every* man has more sex drive than *every* woman, of course. There are millions of highly sexed women in this world. But our sex does seem to have gotten the lion's share. Twice as many of us masturbate, and we masturbate more frequently. We think about sex more (much more). According to the 1994 *Sex in America* survey conducted by University of Chicago researchers, 54 percent of men think about sex every day or several times a day; two-thirds of women say they think about sex only a few times a month or, at most, a few times a week. And when asked about sexual difficulties, about 15 percent of men reported lacking interest in sex at some point in the last 12 months—whereas one in three women couldn't be bothered.

If your relationship does not mirror the general imbalance out there, you are one lucky man. The discrepancy between sex drives mars millions of marriages. It eats away at long-term relationships, robs us of feelings of attractiveness and

---

THE ANNALS OF IGNORANCE: 1812

. . . allow me, my good sir, to remark that reading and observation have concurred to convince me that promiscuous intercourse pollutes the mind much more than the society of one unchaste woman would do. For when a man is in the habit of visiting a diversity of lewd women, he soon acquires such an unconquerable thirst for variety that he is perpetually longing for some untried individual, with whom he hopes to meet with a fresh allurement, to give a new zest to his impure pleasures.

—From "Letters on Marriage, on the Causes of Matrimonial Indelity and on the Reciprocal Relations of the Sexes" by Henry Thomas Kitchener

leads us to assume all the "fizz" has gone out of a bond. It makes our wives wonder, too, "Why am I not craving this man's love? What's wrong?" It's not far-fetched for her to come to this conclusion: "I'm with the wrong man."

The difference in sex drive drives many couples into counseling. "In my practice it's by far the most common sexual problem," says Donald Strassberg, Ph.D., a sex therapist and psychology professor at the University of Utah in Salt Lake City. "And it's the most difficult to treat."

How to Deal with Differences

Sex drive is now generally accepted to be an appetite, like hunger or thirst. It tends to establish its own level and stay there, defining your sexuality for much of your adult life. It is thrown off-track only by major changes, like alcoholism, depression, the side effects of medication or the onset of certain illnesses, like diabetes or Parkinson's disease. Many of us cruise right into old age with the fires still burning. But others don't. That's because of the decline in testosterone levels that sometimes accompanies our later years. Some therapists treat such deficiencies with small amounts of what we're missing. But treating so-called male menopause is controversial and not without risk. For more information, see Male Menopause on page 440.

Experiments of the last several years have shown testosterone to greatly affect sex drive in both men and women, believe it or not. "The fact that men have from 10 to 20 times more testosterone than women is one of the primary reasons they experience more desire," writes Patricia Love, Ed.D., in her book, *Hot Monogamy*.

Dr. Love, a marriage and family therapist in Austin, Texas, can make a singular claim—she's one of the few people who know what it's like to have both the high sex drive of many men and the low sex drive of many women. You might say she's looked at sex from both sides now. The reason is that she took testosterone supplements for three months under a doctor's care. What a difference. "It was like night and day," she says. "I thought about sex constantly. It was easy to get aroused and easy to come to orgasm. I *wanted* to have sex."

But she didn't want facial hair. And she didn't want acne. Unfortunately, she was getting both, so it was time to stop the treatments. She returned to her old self, a "low-t person," as she puts it. These days "the needle on my sex meter points to zero most of the time."

Being a low-t person means she needs more inducements to get aroused. She needs things to be "right." Stress, lack of time and daily distractions—those things get in the way. You have to have the time, the mood, the "Do Not Disturb" sign hanging on the hotel room door. And foreplay is a must. "Otherwise," she says, "it's just a mechanical act." Whereas, for the person with moderate or high sex drive, "it doesn't matter if you're stressed. Sex is relaxing," she says. "You can go and go all day, get into bed late and still be ready. Your low-t partner will say, 'Aren't you exhausted?' And you'll say, in effect, 'That's the point.' "

As Dr. Love discovered, you can't fool with your basic level of sex drive without potentially disastrous consequences. So if it's a problem in a relationship, a couple needs to work it out with negotiation, not with a magic pill. Dr. Love's book lists nine suggestions for "the partner with greater desire." In other words, men, mostly.

1. Be more direct in asking for sex. Her response will greatly depend on whether you're being romantic and loving, or terse and demanding. It's all in the delivery.
2. Initiate sex out of love and desire, not out of habit. Are you sure *you're* all that interested every time you bring it up?
3. Become an expert in creating desire in your partner. Exactly what is it that floats her boat?
4. Accept the fact that your partner may need extra stimulation. Hey, whatever it takes: food, a video, soft music, a fantasy, a toy. Are you rushing her?
5. Don't deliberately heighten your level of desire.
6. Honor your partner's sexual preconditions. If she doesn't want to do it on the hood of your car when it's 17 below, respect that.

7. Consider masturbation.
8. Redirect some of your sexual energy. This sounds like the old "do a few push-ups" advice from the 1950s. But it could mean: Realign your lives. Is she a lot busier than you? Do you basically come home from work without a care in the world and get aroused watching her bend down to empty the dryer?
9. Do not confuse lust with love. When she blows you off, try not to take her total, flat-out rejection to heart. "That's easier said than done," admits Dr. Love, "but the facts help. When one of my patients realized that the discrepancy is biological, she said, 'I think it's freeing. I don't have to take my libido or my partner's libido so personally.'"

It doesn't free you from finding a solution, of course. Both partners need to take more responsibility for a discrepancy in sex drives. If they're committed to staying together and making their marriage happier, they need to take ownership of the problem.

But once they create more room for sex and make it work for both of them, the discrepancy can disappear. "When each of us gets aroused," says Dr. Love, "then it's anybody's game."

SEXUAL PREFERENCE
The Science of Homosexuality

A 66-year-old college professor who answered our *Men's Health* magazine survey says he knew before he got married many decades earlier that he was gay—but he loved his wife and still does. "Our marriage has yielded two children and four grandchildren and many blessed years together," he writes. "And some fair to good sex. Honestly."

He does note, however, that "it has never dulled my other attraction to men." Marital sex "has almost never attained the same kind and amount of arousal. I have had several attractions and 'crushes' almost past my point of self-control. But I have really remained faithful. At a price."

Here is a man who, strictly in terms of sex, would have preferred being gay. He made his choice in life. He says any man who shares his feelings will need to make a choice. "Some today feel freer to come out and live that natural inclination, some are forced into lives of hidden satisfaction and/or celibacy and some of us manage to make relatively good husbands and fathers."

Note that he refers to his homoerotic feelings as "that natural inclination." Some would dispute the word "natural," but our professor has the evidence on his side. Contrary to our birds-and-bees image of nature, it exists in virtually every species of mammal ever studied for gender preference. The late Dr. Alfred C. Kinsey noted that males have been seen mounting other males—and ejaculating—in monkeys, goats, dogs, rats and baboons, among other creatures. "Every farmer knows that cows quite regularly mount cows," he wrote in his 1953 work, *Sexual Behavior in the Human Female*. "He may be less familiar with the fact that bulls mount bulls, but this is because cows are commonly kept together while bulls are not so often kept together in the same pasture."

> Contempt of sexuality is a crime against life.
>
> —Friedrich Nietzsche

It's a bad, old joke that all Greeks were homosexuals, but Plato did exalt boy-love. Considering what we know about classical Athens, he was preaching to the choir. Ancient Rome was much the same: Julius Caesar, in his youth, was nicknamed the Queen of Bithynia while visiting the King of Bithynia. Romans joked about him being "the husband of every woman and the wife of every man." And halfway around the world at that time, same-sex love was simply part of Chinese court life. According to some sources, it was regarded as just another lustful urge rather than a sexual orientation. It was called the passion of the cut sleeve because of the devotion shown by Emperor Ai, who cut off his sleeve rather than disturb the sleep of his beloved boy lover named Dong.

Many Americans feel that homosexuality is now as prevalent in this culture as it was in ancient Athens—especially right after they watch newscasts of AIDS activists shouting at politicians and chanting, "We're here, we're queer, get used to it!" It's safe to say many are not too darn pleased. For their part, gay rights activists find it fits their agendas to have us believe as many as one in five of us have homosexual tendencies.

So what's the truth? How many people are gay? The *Sex in America* folks set out to find the answer. In 1994 University of Chicago researchers asked the question in three different ways because, conceivably, "gayness" could be defined by some combination of behavior, attraction and self-identity.

Same-sex behavior provides the least definite measurement: 9 percent of men ages 18 to 59 said they had ever had sex with another man, 5 percent said they'd had sex with another man since age 18, but only about 2 percent said they'd had sex with a man in the past 12 months. Phrased in terms of attraction: About 6 percent said the idea of sex with other men was appealing. Phrased in terms of self-identity: Only 2.8 percent thought of themselves as homosexual or bisexual.

Here's where the perception of prevalence may come from: 9 percent of the men in America's 12 largest cities identify themselves as gay, compared with 1 percent of men in rural areas.

The researchers felt their own data didn't begin to answer the most perplexing questions about homosexuality. Is it properly defined by what someone's doing now or by what he's ever done? Should it be based more on what he wants to do? In short, is it an attitude or a behavior? Is it a "lifestyle choice," as some religious conservatives claim or are people born gay? Is it an "us" and "them" thing—you're either gay or straight? Or is sexual preference more of a continuum? That is, are we all pretty much pansexual in our bones? Freud thought so; in a coinage that has since become famous, he said that as children we are "polymorphously perverse." To put it crudely: But for the effects of upbringing and the inhibitions of our culture, we'd jump on anything that walks or whinnies.

Discovering Some Innate Differences

Dr. Kinsey thought so, too. He was a believer in an innate continuum of male sexuality. To measure that continuum, he devised the Kinsey Scale, a seven-point spectrum ranging from exclusive homosexuality to exclusive heterosexuality.

Do you buy it? Do men's sexual leanings seem to be that richly diverse to you? Personally, we would have guessed that most guys clump up at either end of the scale rather than in the middle. And in fact that's exactly what happened when Dean Hamer, Ph.D., a Harvard-trained molecular geneticist at the National Cancer Institute, queried a group of men.

Dr. Hamer had been slaving away for ten years studying the regulation of genes in yeast cells when he switched to a topic that tickled his personal curiosity: What makes people gay?

He got a grant and gathered a "sample" group of 114 gay men and 99 of their male relatives. He asked them to rate themselves on the 0-to-6 Kinsey scale according to four distinct aspects: self-identification (how you think of yourself), attraction (who you want to be with), behavior (who you end up with) and fantasy (who you daydream about). The four aspects correlated well—nobody, luckily, considered himself straight but fantasized about other guys. But they also left remarkably little in the way of a middle ground; almost all were easily categorized as either gay or straight. And what categorized them most of all was their fantasies: More than 80 percent of the men fantasized entirely about either men or women. Dr. Hamer and his associates concluded that sexual orientation was even more of an attraction than it was an "action." Which is what our college professor seems to be telling us.

Notably, there was very little change over time. The gay

men commenced their love lives being gay; their first crush was on a boy or man in 96 percent of the cases. Out of guilt or a desire to conform they may have dated girls while in school, but they were aware of their real attractions. On the other side of the scale some straight guys did experiment with some same-sex behavior in early adolescence—but their first crush nonetheless was on a girl, and their fantasies were always about women. "Most of the men we studied," concluded Dr. Hamer, "have always had the same sexual orientation and expect that it never will change."

In his book, *The Science of Desire*, Dr. Hamer displays these findings, then goes on to recount the part of the research that made him famous: the discovery of a possible genetic basis for homosexuality. He zeroed in on 40 of the 114 gay men in his sample, the 40 who had gay brothers. Given the latest genetic techniques, he was able to look directly at the brothers' DNA, the molecules that carry each person's genetic information. And he writes, "We found that a small region of the X chromosome, Xq28, appeared to be the same in an unexpectedly high proportion of gay brothers." To be exact, 33 of the 40 brothers, a far higher number than chance alone would predict. "This finding provided the first concrete evidence that 'gay genes' really do exist."

That's not all. In tracing the family trees, Dr. Hamer found far more gays on the mother's side of each man's family than on the father's side. This finding fits in neatly with his X-chromosome discovery. Gayness, he theorizes, is a recessive X-linked trait, like color blindness and hemophilia. Without getting into a short course on genetics here, let's just say X-linked traits appear more frequently in men than in women and are passed on to men through the maternal side.

Dr. Hamer was not the first to show that homosexuality runs in families. Previous work on this had been done by J. Michael Bailey, a psychologist at Northwestern University in Evanston, Illinois, who showed that the identical twin brothers of gay men had a 50 percent likelihood of also being gay, but fraternal twin brothers had only a 20 percent chance. Dr. Hamer's work added new depth to these statistics so that we now know, for example, that 14 percent of the brothers of gay men are likely to be gay as well as 7 percent of their maternal uncles and 8 percent of their cousins through an aunt on their mother's side.

We also know, because of research conducted in 1991 by Simon LeVay, Ph.D., that there may be physical differences in the brains of gay men. Dr. LeVay, at the time a neuroanatomist at the Salk Institute in San Diego, performed autopsies on men and women and zeroed in on the anterior hypothalamus, a region that plays a key role in our basic drives, like hunger, thirst and sex. He focused on four small groups of cells called the interstitial nuclei and found that one of them, INAH-3, was, on average, the same size in women and gay men, but two to three times larger in heterosexual men. Other scientists have found that a region called the anterior commissure, which connects the left and right halves of the brain, is larger in gay men and women than in straight men.

A New Direction

So, is biology at the heart of sexual preference? Everyone agrees that the evidence to date is slender. We don't know whether there is a gay gene or set of genes. If there are, we don't know whether they might strictly determine our sexual nature or only nudge it a little. We don't know how to explain bisexuality, or even heterosexuality. We don't have a clue as to what's up with transsexuals, those people who feel they are men trapped in women's bodies or vice versa. Their sex does not match their gender.

And if homosexuality turns out to be genetic, i.e., inherited, why hasn't it died out? Could it be that sex is not just about reproduction and that same-sex behavior has been a survival strategy in the past—much as it is today in many prisons in America? Oh, there's a lot to be learned.

What's important is that the latest research reflects a new direction—and a refreshing change it is. Finally, the medical and scientific communities have abandoned their shame-and-blame approach to sexual preference. Youngsters have to realize: Just a generation or two ago homosexuality was thought to be a mental illness. Only in 1973 did the American Psychiatric Association remove homosexuality from the therapist's bible, the *Diagnostic and Statistical Manual*. When many of us were growing up, progressive people firmly believed it was caused by a smothering mother and distant father.

And growing up in the 1950s, there were more than a few of us who had distant fathers.

SIZE
The Truth about Big

Are you man enough to take the ultimate test? Then go get a ruler, right now, and drop your drawers—away from the window, please. We don't want the neighbors talking about you again.

You're going to find out whether your pen name should be Biggus Diccus or Tiny Tim.

First, the ruler. Hopefully it will have inches along one side, centimeters along the other. Also, it should have no sharp edges because you're going to:

1. Place it over your penis.
2. Push that ruler back into your abdomen about as far as it will go without injuring yourself.
3. Stretch your limp noodle along the ruler and note the mark where you've landed. No cheating!

That's the method used by two doctors a few years ago when they rounded up 63 Canadian men and tugged their molsons. What's more, they measured height and shoe sizes to see if there's any truth to the folklore that you can estimate a man's most intimate dimensions by appraising his overall body size or the size of his feet. The folklore goes both ways: It's said to be either directly or inversely proportional, depending upon which street corner you heard it on.

The doctors found only the weakest of correlations. "This puts to rest some mythologies," says the study's co-author, Jerald Bain, M.D., associate professor of medicine at the University of Toronto and the medical director of that city's Health Institute for Men.

But to get to the point: The men ranged in size from 6 centimeters (2⅜ inches) to 13.5 centimeters (5¼ inches), with 9.4 centimeters (3¾ inches) being the average "stretched penile length."

So. How'd you compare?

And the Short Shall Grow Long

But it's not that simple. Three decades ago the sex researchers William H. Masters, M.D., and Virginia E. Johnson, of the former Masters and Johnson Institute in St. Louis, found that smaller penises tended to add more length with an erection than the well-endowed among us. They took a group of 40 guys whose little Richards measured roughly 3 to 3½ inches when flaccid. These guys nearly doubled in size, by another full 3 inches, by the time they were fully erect and heading toward orgasm. Another group of 40 guys, whose penises averaged 4 to 4½ inches when unaroused, increased in size by slightly less than 3 inches when fully erect. One guy with a 3-inch penis added 3½ inches; another guy with a 4¼-inch penis added only a bit more than 2 inches.

The upshot being? The small fry strain to hit the six-inch mark, the real big boys top the seven-inch mark.

The rare exceptions to this rule include those poor souls who did not receive enough masculinizing hormones during fetal development; they suffer from a condition called micropenis. Their manhood may be a fraction of an inch in length.

There. Do you feel better?

On the other hand, some men have been measured at 10 inches when standing at attention. The porn star Long Dong Silver is reputed to pack an 18-inch pistol.

There. Do you feel worse?

The point is that debates over penis size are all about the size of egos, not anatomy. If you really want to measure something, measure the pleasure.

Because what matters is not the size of your boat but the commotion of the ocean.

SMEGMA
It's Not a Nice Nickname

Smegma is a white paste that forms under the foreskin of uncircumcised men. It's the product of sloughed-off skin cells and the foreskin's natural lubricants. It has been described as a "cheesy substance." If allowed to build up, it can irritate your skin and give off a funky smell.

But you would never let it get to that point, because if you're uncircumcised, you are retracting your foreskin to rinse yourself in the shower every morning. And if you are circumcised, you lost the ability to produce smegma a long time ago.

What you didn't lose is the ability to use the word smegma as part of a withering insult. It also makes a good name for a frat house mutt or a cat that will never, ever get any respect.

Real men don't actually say the word smegma. But they know what it means.

TESTICLES
Why You Hang So Low

How are they hanging?

It's a flip question, but men ask it because it gets at the essence of male health. For many, healthy testicles is a metaphor for general well-being. And yet, not much can be said about our testicles without foreheads wrinkling and legs getting crossed.

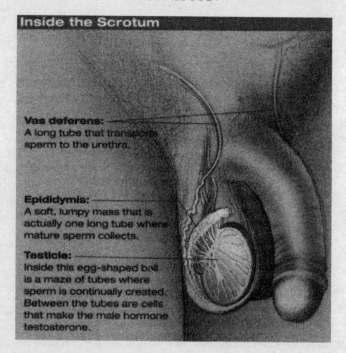

Inside the Scrotum

Vas deferens: A long tube that transports sperm to the urethra.

Epididymis: A soft, lumpy mass that is actually one long tube where mature sperm collects.

Testicle: Inside this egg-shaped ball is a maze of tubes where sperm is continually created. Between the tubes are cells that make the male hormone testosterone.

So we'll start this off gently. First, we'll give you a quick tour of the engineering marvels down there. Then, we'll get around to mentioning a few potential problems.

The word testes comes from the Latin word for "to testify" or "to witness" (hence testimonial). The early Romans placed their hands over their testicles when taking an oath. Obviously, they, too, held the notion that a man's welfare was deeply centered there. For there in the testicles is where we produce our half of our kids' genetic makeups; that we all know. But we also produce there 95 percent of the male hormone testosterone that gets shipped out into our bloodstream, affecting all points of the body.

Beginning in the womb, the testicles pump out testosterone to shape our brains and sculpt our genitalia. At puberty this activity resumes with a vengeance, affecting everything from our brains to our body hair, endowing us with upper-body strength but plaguing us with acne. The testicles keep pumping out testosterone all our adult lives, affecting our sex drive, our aggressiveness and our performance on math tests.

Within each egg-shaped testicle you would find, were you to crack it open, a maze of tubes that has been compared to a ball of yarn or a hunk of spaghetti. Between the tubes, special cells called Leydig's cells produce testosterone. And within the tubes, sperm are born and raised. The sperm travel out the testicles into the epididymis, a soft, lumpy mass at the back and top of the testicles that you can feel when you examine yourself for testicular cancer. It's actually one long, continuous tube that, if stretched out, would be longer than a bowling alley.

The sperm exit the scrotal sac via a long, thin cannon of a tube called the vas deferens. This name is always good for one weak joke in every high school biology class—it's part of the vas deferens between boys and girls, yuk yuk. During the emission stage of orgasm the vas quickly moves millions of sperm from the epididymis to the urethra.

By the way, just because one testicle hangs slightly below the other does not mean you're a freak of nature. It does that on all of us. On 85 percent of us the left one hangs down.

Your testicles are contained in that wrinkled, hairy bandanna of skin called the scrotal sac, or scrotum. This, too, is not as simple as it seems. The skin here is thinner and contains less fat than your skin elsewhere. Its chief feature, that wrinkled-prune look, is actually nature's clever way of varying the exterior area of the skin available for heat loss. It's all part of the amazing ability of the scrotum to keep the testicles slightly lower than body temperature—5.6°F below it, to be exact. Your testicles go up and down like a yo-yo thanks to a special muscle, the cremaster, which contracts when they get too cold (or when you're about to ejaculate) and relaxes when they get too warm. It's been shown that the testicles need a slightly lower temperature to produce their vast quantities of sperm. If that ability is affected—if your testicles do not descend in your youth, if you hang out in a hot tub or even if you wear tight underwear—your sperm count will drop.

Boxer shorts: the revenge of the nerds.

Ball Troubles

"A real kick in the balls" is a phrase men use all the time to describe an insult or a setback. Yet we don't seem to have enough respect for the lasting damage that can arise from a real kick in the balls. Listen to this.

Wolfram E. Nolten, M.D., an endocrinologist at the University of Wisconsin in Madison, conducted a study of 179 infertile men. He found that 30 of them had incurred "blunt testicular trauma," which, translated from medical journalese, means a major hit to the groin, including bruises, swelling and pain lasting longer than 24 hours. The 30 guys were injured back in high school or middle school, years and years ago. Mostly, their injuries were the result of playing contact sports—especially football, wrestling and karate—without an athletic supporter. Now here they were, a decade or two later, unable to start families.

In this study at least, a kick in the balls seems to account for nearly 17 percent of male infertility problems. Traditionally, it has been difficult to identify a cause in the majority of cases of so-called male factor infertility, so this study is something of a breakthrough. The link to testicular injury, remote in time as it may be, nonetheless makes sense, claims Dr. Nolten. "Once a testicle is injured, a whole series of hormonal processes are triggered with the end result being a substantial increase in testicular estrogen production," he says. "And estrogen, especially when generated by the testicles, inhibits sperm production."

The take-home message is pretty clear. If you haven't found a good, comfortable athletic cup, find one. One top source is the BIKE Athletic Company, whose catalog carries a variety of soft and hard cups for youths and adults that are claimed to be "the official protective cups of major league baseball." For a free catalog, call 1-800-251-9230.

The most common cause of testicular pain results not from injury but from a condition called epididymitis, a bacterial infection of the epididymis. In addition to the pain, you'll be able to feel a swelling or lump on your epididymis. Get to a doctor; you'll most likely be put on an oral antibiotic until it clears up.

A swelling or lump down there immediately engenders fears of testicular cancer. True, it's the number one cancer in young men, but it does not strike many of us. In 1994 only 6,800 new cases were detected. And thanks to improvements in treatment, it has the highest cure rate of any cancer—when detected early, it is 97 percent curable. If you perform a monthly exam in the shower you'll probably be able to catch it in time. Slowly roll each testicle between your thumb and fingers. You're looking for a hard, irregular lump the size of a pea that doesn't feel anything like the surrounding tissue.

That said, you may be greatly relieved to know that lumps and bumps on the testicles are usually benign. The sac around one of the testicles can fill with fluid, forming a hydrocele. Or the veins will dilate, causing a varicocele. (It may look like a varicose vein.) Hydroceles may require treatment; varicoceles generally do not unless discomfort or fertility problems arise.

Okay, enough talk about pain and disease. Let's end this discussion on a cheery note by reminding ourselves of the tremendous pleasure that can be derived from testicular stimulation. A respondent to our *Men's Health* magazine survey sent us a poem—self-penned, we're quite sure—entitled "Ode to Ball Savvy." We'll skip right to the good part.

To women, words come to mind like "neglect" and
*   "ignore."*
To men, there is but one word: more, more, more.
Be gentle, but grasp firm,
the sweetness of Ball Savvy is watching him squirm.
Why now does Ball Savvy attract so much attention?
Because women have always focused on the
*   Erection.*

For years, "the boys" were thought to like juggling.
In fact, the Tao of Ball Savvy is all about snuggling.
And so to wrap up our first lesson, suffice it to say,
be enthused, be excited and keep "the boys" in play.

TESTOSTERONE
Making a Man out of You

What makes a man a man? Testosterone.

Maybe you thought it was your Y chromosome that makes you such a stud muffin, but that's not the half of it. You can be born with a Y chromosome in every cell in your body—genetically, you're *un macho completo*. But if for some reason your male hormones haven't kicked in and done their work, you will be born with a vagina, labia and something that looks more like a clitoris than a penis.

Testosterone is only one of the male hormones, but it's the most important one. (Male hormones are known as androgens, which is Greek for man maker.) It begins to assert its complete control over you in the womb. In week eight, to be exact, when you are roughly an inch long. Theoretically, you could still go either way at this point—you have sex structures with bizarre names, like the labioscrotal swelling. But your Y chromosome has already caused you to form a protein called H-Y antigen, which has caused your gonads to become testicles. And with the development of testicles comes the creation of Leydig's cells, which pump out testosterone.

From here on out, testosterone calls the shots. In the next several weeks, it will make sure that the labioscrotal swelling becomes a scrotum, not the labia majora. It makes sure you get a penis, not a clitoris, out of the same swag of embryonic tissue. Likewise with all the internal sex organs, like the prostate. This is when you get the whole nine yards. And the amount of testosterone coursing through you, small as you are, nearly equals the amount found in an adult male.

Now comes the real mystery. After the plumbing work is

over and done with, testosterone levels in male fetuses rise for a second time. It happens toward the end of pregnancy and continues for the first two months after birth, before dropping back down again until puberty. "Testosterone rides a roller coaster until birth," is how University of California, Los Angeles (UCLA), brain researcher Laura Allen, Ph.D., describes it. "We don't know what the second rise does. I suspect it makes the male brain different."

Dr. Allen, her colleague Roger Gorski, Ph.D., and others at the UCLA School of Medicine have spent the last couple of decades examining both human and animal gray matter in an attempt to determine the differences between male and female brains, and the extent to which those differences can be matched with sexual orientation. They and others have been discovering parts of the brain that are different in men

THE ANIMAL HOUSE EFFECT

Most college campuses have a fraternity similar to the one made famous by the movie *Animal House*—a civilization-free zone known for great kegger parties, lousy grades and the house-keeping skills of a neutron bomb.

To test the theory that testosterone might have something to do with frat boys' beasty-boy behavior, psychologists Marian Hargrove, Ph.D., and James Dabbs, Jr., Ph.D., of Georgia State University in Atlanta, extracted information from 98 members of five different fraternities at universities in the Southeast.

Result: Yup, high testosterone levels were definitely linked to the most rambunctious frat houses, where there were more parties, worse academic performances and community service awards were virtually nonexistent. What's more, even attempting to do research involving these dudes was difficult, explained Dr. Dabbs: "High testosterone fraternities did not respond to letters, their houses were not neat and they were far more interested in money to buy a keg than in any contribution to science."

and women—and alike in women and gay men. They openly talk of a "male brain" and a "female brain" the way we would talk of other body parts. And they expect that one day science will be able to correlate the differences in brain structure with larger differences in behavior—the way they can, right now, correlate hormones and behavior in laboratory rats.

Imagine tinkering endlessly with hormone levels, watching the resulting behavior, then dispatching with the subject, freezing the brain and slicing off wafer-thin samples for viewing under your microscope. You don't get to do that with humans, but no one will stop you from doing that with rats. So scientists at the UCLA lab know a lot about rats. In one of Dr. Gorski's experiments a male rat, Mork, was deprived of testosterone and dosed with female hormones, while at the same time a female rat, Mindy, was dosed with testosterone. When placed together, they acted out the flip side of the usual romantic scenario: Mindy meets Mork, Mindy mounts Mork, Mindy leaves Mork. Not only that, but Mork's brain was female. An area called the SDN—sexually dimorphic nucleus—was smaller than in normal males. If he had ovaries implanted in him, he would be able to ovulate; his brain was that ready for femininity.

> The whole subject is as yet hidden in darkness.
>
> —Charles Darwin, writing about why there is sexual intercourse at all

You don't even have to castrate Mork to get roughly the same results, says Dr. Allen. Had they simply "stressed" the mother rat during Mork's 21-day stay in the womb, researchers could have delayed the testosterone surge that gave him a male brain. "Delay that surge by one day and you feminize the brain," she says.

You begin to see the gender-bending possibilities of testosterone.

Rats are not humans, but every so often nature conducts an experiment of sorts, dosing a genetically female fetus with androgens. This is what happens during a condition called congenital adrenal hyperplasia (CAH). The adrenal gland, which gives every woman a little dose of testosterone, in this case goes overboard, secreting an excess such that her external genitalia may be nearly masculine in appearance at birth. If it goes undetected, this condition will continue to make a man of her right through puberty. But even if the condition is corrected after birth, the behavioral effects can be lasting throughout childhood—and beyond. CAH girls are more likely to be described as tomboys. Though they may marry in adulthood, they'll still spend their leisure hours splitting wood, tinkering with cars and shooting beer cans off the tops of fence posts with their rifles.

Why do men score higher than women on the math section of standardized tests? Why do we have a stronger sense of direction? Why do we have better "visuospatial ability"— skillfulness in reading maps and blueprints and imagining things in 3-D? It may all come down to how much testosterone we got when we were minus 30 days and counting.

Of course, that was then. This is now.

Are You Missing Something?

Beginning at age 50 or so, testosterone levels in some men begin a gradual decline, although the decline often doesn't amount to much until the seventh decade of life. Not all men experience the decline, and since there's enough of a range of "normal" testosterone levels in the blood, not all declines make themselves disagreeably evident. Nonetheless, if you're an older man whose life is now marred by reduced sex drive, fatigue, weakness and muscle loss, thinning hair everywhere, and perhaps a sudden change in your voice or the girth of your gut, you may be suffering from a deficiency of testosterone.

In women, production of the female hormone estrogen drops off precipitously after menopause, causing hot flashes and a number of other, fairly dramatic symptoms. In men, by contrast, the drop-off in our hormones is so gradual that it doesn't receive as much medical attention. But it's enough that some researchers refer to this phenomenon as male menopause or andropause. For more information, see Male Menopause on page 440.

In both men and women there's no sex drive without testosterone. Women who've had their ovaries or uteri removed in surgery are sometimes given testosterone supplements (in combination with estrogen). Otherwise, their sex drives vanish. Some physicians even prescribe testosterone supplementation for women who experience menopause the normal, nonsurgical way and whose libidos inexplicably begin to flag in the process. Two problems: The side effects can include a lower voice, more body hair and a more manly, muscular body shape, and no studies have been done to determine long-term effects.

With all the male-bashing that's been occurring, testosterone has been getting a bad rap. When mentioned in the context of the gender wars, it's usually followed by the word "poisoning," as if the male hormone were responsible for war, rape, wife abuse and the glass ceiling. In point of fact, testosterone does not appear to be the cause of violent behavior. But it does appear to be the cause of many good things, among them:

Healthy hearts: Contrary to earlier medical belief, it now seems that testosterone may help prevent heart attacks, or at least lessen the damage to coronary arteries when they occur. It may be that testosterone raises the level of high-density lipoprotein ("good") cholesterol in the blood, which helps keep our arteries clear.

Tighter guts: A Swedish study of 23 men with major spare tires were put on testosterone supplements for eight months. It shrank their lard.

Stronger muscles and bones: Testosterone is the reason we don't suffer from osteoporosis to the extent women do, later in life. It also enables us to add mass to our muscles when we exercise them. (That's why bodybuilders use steroids, a synthetic form of testosterone, to exaggerate the hormone's normal effect.)

All indications point out that normal levels of testosterone, circulating in our blood every day, are what help us maintain an optimistic, can-do mood, a sharp memory and a range of cognitive skills.

Are we terrific or what?

TONGUE
Mastering the Mouth

There's an old joke about the world's best lover. The joke's answer is a guy with a ten-inch tongue who can breathe through his ears. Our answer is any guy who uses his tongue.

The tongue is your most versatile sex organ. You can touch with it, taste with it, lick with it. You can lick her; you can lick whipped cream or warmed-up butterscotch sauce off her. Unlike your penis, it is equally effective when hard or soft. And you know something, you never have to worry about it getting too excited. Men think their penises are so essential to lovemaking, but if women were actually forced to choose between the two, we wonder: How many would take the tongue?

The typical tongue is four inches long and weighs a mere two ounces. It's essentially an array of muscles and nerves held together by a membrane covered with thousands of taste buds. Ask a typical doctor what the tongue is for and he probably won't say sex. Rather, he'll talk about its role in moving food around the mouth and down the throat, in shaping air so you can speak and in detecting flavors. Taste is actually a chemical reaction: Your taste buds—filled with tiny receptors—interact with the many liquid substances in food and send the sensations to the brain via nerves.

Can the tongue "feel good"? That's more a function of your brain than anything else. No one goes around stroking their own tongues for pleasure, but who would deny the enticing feeling of a soft French kiss? Which puts the tongue in the same category with many other parts of the body: Merely rubbing it isn't sexually gratifying on its own; your brain has to be aroused before touch becomes erotic.

As the chief instrument of foreplay, the tongue is put to inventive use in both kissing and oral sex. Here's another technique: Alex Comfort, M.D., D.Sc., in *The New Joy of Sex*, recommends something called a tongue bath when you want to indulge in a slow, drive-her-crazy pace of arousal. He describes it as "going systematically over every square inch of a partner, tied if they like, with long, slow, broad tongue strokes." Also available in mini-versions for Type A couples.

> The Bedroom Arts (lovemaking techniques) comprise the entire Supreme Way and can themselves suffice to help one achieve the goal of Immortality. These arts are said to enable a person to avert calamities and become freed from misdeeds, even to change bad luck into good fortune.
>
> —Taoist scholar Ko Hung, 284–364 A.D.

The men who responded to our *Men's Health* magazine survey know all about the tongue's ability to enhance their sex lives and consistently bring their partners to orgasm. Yes, that's in the way you're thinking, but also not. They need their tongues to chat her up, to whisper sweet nothings or to talk dirty to her, whatever the mood calls for. The world's oldest, most famous sex manual, the *Kama Sutra*, declared, "Though a man loves a girl ever so much, he never succeeds in winning her over without a great deal of talking." Two thousand years later nothing has changed.

WET DREAMS
Nothing to Be Ashamed Of

Infants only days old can have erections. Little boys can have orgasms. But it takes a young man to have a wet dream. Wet dreams—also known as nocturnal emissions—are physically impossible until puberty, until about a year after the testosterone-flamed growth spurt has begun. Its occurrence depends upon the development of the entire sperm machine—the testicles, the prostate and its seminal vesicles. When those sex organs are up and running, a wet dream is your first clue that they are "good to go."

In that way, wet dreams are a lot like menarche, a young lady's first period. Like menarche, there is no "right age" for it to begin. A Belgian study found that among a group of boys, the average age of first ejaculation was 13 years, 2 months. But that can easily vary by a year or two. (If it occurs significantly earlier than 2 years before that, see a doctor; your child could have a rare endocrine problem). Once they commence, they come on like gangbusters; the late Dr. Alfred C. Kinsey found that boys under age 15 could have as many as 12 a week. They usually decrease in frequency with age, although Dr. Kinsey was able to document its occasional incidence in men in their seventies.

Virtually all young men have wet dreams. They're perfectly normal. But if a young man grows up in a house where sex is embarrassing, shushed up or frowned upon, then his first wet dream can make him feel very much alone and confused. Like a girl's first period in such a house, a wet dream will be cause for shame. Our Western heritage has not always handled this event with understanding and aplomb. In a sixth-century penitential, *Book of David*, nocturnal emissions were regarded as a kind of bush-league sin, requiring penance. Boys were instructed to sing seven psalms in the morning and live on bread and water for one day. Now that is a sin—because there's absolutely nothing you can do to prevent yourself from having them.

Nonetheless, as recently as a few generations ago, supposedly logical people had some really, really weird ideas about wet dreams. In 1916 William J. Robinson, M.D., wrote a book very much like this one entitled *Sex Knowledge for Men*. This section in *his* book was called Pollutions or Wet Dreams. The good doctor notes that quacks of the era frightened people into believing that wet dreams led to impotence, insanity and early death. Tut tut, he says. If they happen every now and again, no problem. "But if the pollutions occur more than once a week, then they are abnormal or pathologic and you must lose no time in consulting a reputable physician." Alas, that would have led you to someone like this guy. He would have told you to give yourself an enema every evening, tie a towel around yourself with the knot to the rear so you'll wake up if you roll onto your back and—above all—keep your feet warm. "Cold feet," he wrote, italicizing for emphasis, "are not infrequently a cause of pollutions."

Naturally, "the modern dances" were to be avoided as well.

You have far more erections during sleep than wet dreams. Wet dreams may simply be your reproductive system running a check on itself, but nocturnal erections are your penis's way of "breathing." Medical science now believes it may not get all the oxygen it needs from blood flow during the day, so it compensates with up to three hours of pumped-up flow at night. For more information, see Erection on page 23. If what concerns you is the content of your

---

THE ANNALS OF IGNORANCE: 1834

… let him sleep on a hard bed and rise early in the morning and take a shower-bath of cold water; or plunge into cold water or sponge his body all over with it—and, in either case, rub himself off briskly and freely with a coarse towel, and follow that freely with a good, stiff flesh-brush, and then exercise vigorously in the open air or in the gymnasium for an hour before breakfast … and let him exhilarate himself by free and copious draughts of the pure air of heaven!

—Advice on how to prevent nocturnal emissions—a loathsome disease also known as nocturnal self-pollution—from Sylvester Graham's "A Lecture to Young Men"

dreams rather than its spillage on your sheets, see Sex
Dreams on page 73.

ZIPPER
When You're Caught on the Fly

This may be the best argument for circumcision we've ever
heard.

One night several years ago doctors at the Naval Hospital in San Diego had to deal with a screaming four-year-old
in sleeper pajamas. The boy had pulled up the zipper on his
pj's and caught his foreskin between the zipper teeth and
the fastener casing. Yeow. Since the boy had been in this
nightmarish state for three hours, the first thing the doctors
did was anesthetize him. Then they grabbed a bone cutter
(a decent pair of wire snips would also do the trick) and
broke what is called the median bar of the zipper. Go
ahead, look at your zipper. Yes, right now. Looking down
on it, you'll see that the only thing connecting the inner
face to the outer face is a piece of metal on top. That's what
the doctors cut. The zipper fell apart. The boy was free at
last.

Now you know how to be the hero in case this ever happens in your neighborhood.

The doctors in the San Diego caper wrote a report for the
Journal of Emergency Medicine. They offer a few words of
advice.

Wear underwear. Something should get between you
and your Calvins.

Watch the downstroke. Surprisingly, opening your zipper is more dangerous than closing it. (Hmmm, that applies
to all sorts of situations.)

Don't panic. "Extraction by vigorous manipulation,
including attempts at unzipping the skin or prying the zipper
are usually unsuccessful, painful and can lead to further
injury," the doctors reported.

Use an oil can. In some cases a liberal application of mineral oil could be enough to unsnag the penis, according to another report in a medical journal.

If these helpful hints aren't working, don't hesitate to visit a doctor or an emergency room. By that point, you'll be needing an M.D. to prescribe a sedative anyway.

We don't know where that four-year-old San Diego boy is today. But you can bet he's wearing button-fly jeans.

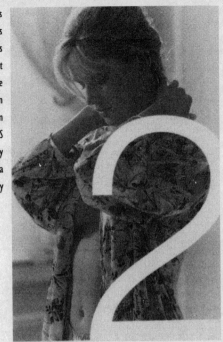

THE FEMALE BODY

BREASTS
Why Men Love Them So

It's hard to imagine anything more entrancing than a woman's breast, especially a breast swollen with sexual excitement, firmly pendulous as a sun-ripened mango, a succulent melon raised to your hungry lips, nipple erect, pert and uplifted, aflame with . . .

Oh—sorry.

But, hey, maybe we can be forgiven, since that's one of men's absolute favorite sexual daydreams. In fact, in one University of Missouri study of male sex fantasies, kissing a pair of monumental breasts was the second-most frequently mentioned fantasy (outranked only by the thought of getting turned on by a pair of terrific legs).

The really interesting news is that when women in the same study were asked their favorite fantasies, the one they mentioned most often was . . . having a man kiss their breasts.

A Distinctively Human Act

The late Dr. Alfred C. Kinsey, a former zoology professor, pointed out that while the desire to kiss and fondle a woman's breasts may seem about as natural to you as anything can possibly be, it's actually fairly uncommon among other animals. "Mouth-breast contact," he reported, "constitutes the one technique in human petting behavior that is most distinctively human."

We must all be pretty human: Various sex surveys have shown that over 90 percent of men enjoy stimulating their lover's breasts during sex, whether by mouth, hand or otherwise. Oddly, women don't enjoy it quite as much as men do, some evidence suggests. In fact, if you think of female masturbation techniques as the key to understanding what actually turns women on most, it's interesting to note that only

11 percent of the nearly 8,000 women Dr. Kinsey studied said they liked to stroke their own breasts during masturbation (compared to 84 percent who stroked their clitoris or labia minora, the soft inner lips that surround it). Only a very small percentage of women can reach orgasm purely through stimulation of their breasts, other sex surveys have shown.

It seems a contradiction: Many women fantasize about having their breasts kissed, but when it really happens, many don't seem to enjoy it that much. "Women do report taking pleasure in watching their partners having pleasure," says Shirley Zussman, Ed.D., a certified sex therapist and co-director of the Association for Male Sexual Dysfunction in New York City. "She may be aroused, indirectly, by watching him kissing her breasts. That's what excites her."

The Pleasure of Breasts

American males are often accused of being obsessed with big breasts, and it's probably true. The French, by contrast, maintain that the ideal breast should fit inside a champagne glass. Don't forget, though, that the size of a woman's breasts has no more to do with a woman's sex drive than the size of your penis has to do with your sex drive, says Judith Seifer, R. N., Ph.D., president of the American Association of Sex Educators, Counselors and Therapists. A flat-chested woman is as likely to be sexually charged as a woman who is very well-endowed.

And breast size has nothing to do with breast sensitivity, either. Jolan Chang, writing in *The Tao of Love and Sex*, a book about ancient Chinese sexual techniques, observes that "strange as it may seem, the size or beauty of a woman's breasts is irrelevant to whether she enjoys them being kissed, sucked or licked." But he goes on to say: "With many women there is a direct connection between nipples and vulva. Stimulating these two delicate buttons either by kissing, sucking or caressing will . . . quickly result in the vagina overflowing with lubricant."

You may have discovered on your adventures that a

woman's breasts may occasionally exude a few dewdrops of sweet-tasting liquid that isn't milk. This exotic exudate has been described in erotic literature as witch's milk, white snow or sometimes even the peach juice of immortality.

"The mammary glands can express sweet-tasting, plasmalike fluids when a woman is not lactating (producing milk)," Dr. Seifer explains. "We don't know why, but we've noticed that some women using Norplant (an implantable contraceptive) will drip from the breast. This also occurs when women have elevated blood levels of prolactin (a hormone that induces milk production), which is sometimes caused by a lesion on the anterior pituitary gland."

Interestingly, women with pituitary lesions also have difficulty reaching orgasm until the lesion is surgically removed, Dr. Seifer says. So if your woman is having trouble reaching orgasm and she's got the peach juice of immortality on her blouse, consider suggesting that she see a doctor.

What Happens during Arousal

The sex researchers William H. Masters, M.D., and Virginia E. Johnson, of the former Masters and Johnson Institute in St. Louis, spent a lot of time carefully observing what happens to people's bodies when they get sexually aroused. (You've probably noticed a few things yourself, but you probably didn't take notes.)

One of the key things Masters and Johnson noticed about the female breast was that the "virgin" breasts of a young woman who has never suckled a baby undergo quite different changes than the breasts of a woman who has breastfed.

The first visible evidence of sexual excitement in an unsuckled breast, they found, is nipple erection. This usually occurs very shortly after any sort of stimulation. Often her nipples don't become erect simultaneously—one may get erect very rapidly while the other lags behind. This is especially true if her breasts are markedly different sizes or one of the nipples is slightly inverted (nipples can be "innies," too, just like belly buttons).

At the same time, the areola (that beautiful dark disk around the nipple) also begins to swell. In fact, because the areola tends to swell faster than the nipple, there's often a momentary impression that the nipple has disappeared, or that she's lost her nipple erection. Well, that's not so; it's just that everything is swelling with the vasocongestion (damming up of blood) that's one of the essential elements of arousal. Her whole breast may swell as much as 20 to 25 percent; at the same time, a fine tracery of veins appears on her breast, sometimes standing out in bold relief. You'll also probably notice a pink mottling of her skin called the sex flush, spreading like an ocean sunset from her upper belly to the top, sides and then undersides of her breasts.

After she's reached orgasm (or after she begins cooling off—the "resolution phase" of the sexual response cycle), the sex flush rapidly fades away. Her swollen areolas quickly return to their pre-aroused state. Because they shrink more rapidly than her nipples do, you may have the momentary impression that she's having a new nipple erection (sometimes called a false erection), but that's just nature trying to fool you.

The Suckled Breast

In women who've suckled babies (especially more than one), this sexual swelling is much less dramatic. In fact, women who have breastfed "frequently show little or no increase in breast size" when they're aroused, Masters and Johnson reported (partly because milk production increases the venous drainage of the breast). Older women's breasts don't swell during arousal so much either. And as a general thing, the more slack and pendulous the breasts of a woman of any age (otherwise known as the National Geographic effect), the less likely they are to swell during sexual stimulation.

You may not have noticed it, but your own nipples probably also got erect the last time you were aroused. In fact, Masters and Johnson reported, "few men under 60 years of age ejaculate without an obvious turgidity (swelling), if not full erection, of the nipples." This other, tinier erection, which tends to fade away as a guy gets older—just like your other one—often persists for a long time, sometimes even hours, after ejaculation.

A Word about Technique

One of the most important things to remember about ravishing a woman's breasts is that you need to get feedback from her about what she likes and doesn't like, Dr. Zussman says. Breast sensitivity varies greatly from woman to woman, and at different times in the same woman. Especially during the few days before her period and during the first few months of pregnancy, her nipples and breasts may be so sensitive that she doesn't want to be touched at all. Be gentle, go slow. Don't knead them like bread. Adore them.

If She's Had Implants

What about women who've had breast implants—do they have any less feeling in there?

"Well, some do, some don't—the more surgery involved, the less feeling they have," Dr. Seifer says. "Actually, there's usually a more profound loss of feeling in breast reduction surgery than implant surgery because sometimes they move the nipple around and really reconstruct it."

Women who've had breast reconstruction surgery after a mastectomy for breast cancer often are struggling with their sexual self-esteem as well. In fact, "women with breast cancer are often more afraid of losing their husbands or lovers . . . than they are about the possibility of facing a cruel and untimely death," observed the late Helen Singer Kaplan, M.D., Ph.D., former director of the human sexuality program at New York Hospital-Cornell Medical Center in New York City. The great majority of husbands and lovers don't lose sexual interest in their mates after mastectomy—provided they were turned on by her before the surgery, Dr. Kaplan said. But latent marital and sexual problems are likely to be stirred up by the mastectomy, and therapy may be useful. The most important thing is to keep the lines of communication open.

"The man may be grieving also, especially if he's a 'breast man,' " says Dr. Seifer. "It's important to be able to say, 'Damn right I'm gonna miss those things!' and not pretend that you don't."

> I think I made his back feel better.
>
> —Marilyn Monroe after a private meeting with John F. Kennedy

Occasionally, a man who has ravished his wife's breasts for years will be filled with dread and guilt when she develops breast cancer—especially if the breast he tends to favor is the one that develops a tumor, observes Jude Cotter, Ph.D., a psychologist and sex therapist in private practice in Farmington Hills, Michigan. He'll harbor the terrible fear that it was he who caused the cancer. But there's no known connection between breast stimulation and breast cancer, so this is not really anything to worry about.

So enjoy yourself.

Welcome to the human race.

CLITORIS
It Exists Purely for Pleasure

"How do I feel about the clitoris?" one guy responded to the questionnaire for the *Hite Report on Male Sexuality*. "I feel in awe of the little bugger. It's gotten so much publicity and become the focal point of so much rancor that I have the urge to salute it when I see it."

Sheesh. That little pink pea, tidily tucked away under the layers of her labia, has become so tangled up in sexual politics it's easy to forget what it's for. It has nothing to do with political correctness, political incorrectness or political anything. It's there for one purpose only: to make her gasp with pleasure.

Because it has no other known purpose than sexual joy,

wrote William H. Masters, M.D., and Virginia E. Johnson, of the former Masters and Johnson Institute in St. Louis, "the clitoris is a unique organ in the total of human anatomy." Even the male penis, well-known for its own capacity to produce pleasure, has other functions, such as serving as a conduit for urine. But in women the urethral opening through which urine escapes the body is located elsewhere. The clitoris is there, apparently, simply because nature wanted women to be happy.

With a little help from you, of course.

The Basic Problem

Still, despite all the hoopla about it, many men apparently do not grasp the essential thing about the clitoris: Many women need direct clitoral stimulation in addition to intercourse in order to reach orgasm. Because of its odd, aloof location at the top of the vaginal opening, it's often a bystander to the main event, nearly untouched by all the commotion.

More than half of all women (some say as many as three-quarters) need additional clitoral stimulation to climax, according to June Reinisch, Ph.D., former director of the Kinsey Institute for Research in Sex, Gender and Reproduction in Bloomington, Indiana. In sex researcher Shere Hite's study group of several thousand women, 30 percent said they could regularly reach orgasm through intercourse alone, but 44 percent said they could orgasm easily if their lovers devoted some additional time to direct stimulation of the clitoris.

Which is why using a hand, a tongue or something else before and during intercourse usually helps a great deal. The position you choose for intercourse is also important. Most experts say that the female-superior position (woman on top) is the best one for maximizing contact with her clitoris. For more information, see Positions on page 317.

Anatomy 101

If she'll let you, it's a fun at-home science project to gently explore her genitals, lifting back those pink layers of skin to

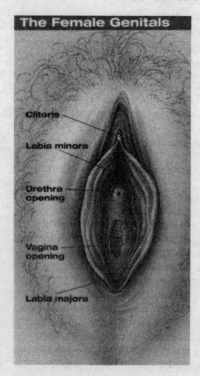

The Female Genitals

Clitoris

Labia minora

Urethra opening

Vagina opening

Labia majora

find the clitoris. (You'll find it above the vaginal opening, where the top of the inner lips meet, beneath a fold of skin.)

Actually, though, all you'll really find is the glans, or head of the clitoris (what we earlier described as a little pink pea); the rest is tucked away inside her body and largely invisible to the eye. If you look at a cutaway drawing of its internal structure, though, you'll see something that looks quite a bit like . . . er . . . a penis. (No, no, we're not saying that the clitoris is less or more than the penis, just that they're homologous, meaning similar in structure and origin but not in function. This is not surprising, since both clitoris and penis are formed from the same embryonic tissue.)

The glans is mounted atop a shaft, like the shaft of a penis. And like a penis, the shaft has two corpora cavernosa—a pair of spongy cylinders lying side by side that fill with blood during erection. Yup, when she gets hot, her clitoris produces a sort of erection, though its extent varies a good bit from woman to woman. Masters and Johnson found that in some women this swelling, or tumescence, is barely noticeable; in other women the clitoris doubles in size. Also, they note, it's not precisely accurate to say this swelling is a teensy erection, because it's only the glans that swells, not the whole shaft.

They also discovered an amazing variation in the size and appearance of clitorides: "The shaft may be quite long and thin and surmounted by a relatively small-size glans, or short and thick with an enlarged glans." The late Dr. Alfred C. Kinsey found that black women often had bigger clitorides than Whites: "Clitorides measuring more than an inch are apparently very rare among Whites, but may occur in 2 or 3 percent of Blacks, or at least they did so in the limited number of black histories we took," he reported.

The important thing, though, is that none of this seems to make much difference.

"In terms of sexual sensitivity, it makes no difference what size a woman's clitoris is, since it still has the same number of nerve endings no matter how big or small it may be," says Beverly Whipple, Ph.D., an authority on female sexuality and associate professor in the College of Nursing at Rutgers University in New Brunswick, New Jersey.

Does its position—whether or not her clitoris is high or low—make a difference? No, Masters and Johnson reported, since the penis rarely comes into contact with the clitoris during intercourse anyhow. Does it matter whether a woman's clitoris swells a lot during arousal? No again, they say. They observed "obvious tumescence" in women capable of having multiple orgasms and also in women who couldn't climax at all.

The Aroused Clitoris

What does matter then? Direct stimulation. Masters and Johnson reported that the clitoris responds more slowly than the penis, reaching full tumescence long after the guy is fully aroused and chomping at the bit. But it responds much more rapidly and intensely, they found, if it or the mons (the soft mound above the vaginal opening) is stimulated directly rather than indirectly (say, by licking her nipples).

Weirdly enough, they also reported that in the plateau phase (when her excitement peaks, but before she climaxes) the clitoris rather abruptly retreats beneath its hood of skin. Often, they say, the whole length of the clitoral body shortens by 50 percent or more, so that just when you're most ardently searching for it, it disappears. If you (her lover) slack off during the plateau phase, the clitoris will peep out again, but heat up the action, and it retreats. Again, direct stimulation has a more pronounced effect: The clitoris shrinks back more quickly and earlier than if you're only stimulating her breasts or vagina, they say.

More recent researchers have voiced some skepticism about this scenario, though. "I'm not convinced the clitoris does retract during the plateau phase; I think the engorgement of other tissues, like the labia, may only make it appear that way," Dr. Whipple says. And Masters and Johnson do admit that it's hard to see exactly what's going on in there during the climactic moments.

As a practical matter, though, much can be learned about clitoral technique from observations of the way women masturbate. (Studies have shown that among women who masturbate, over 90 percent can reach orgasm easily this way.) Masters and Johnson, after observing hundreds of women doing it, concluded that none did it quite the same way. But most women focused on the clitoral glans only during the excitement phase, and then only with lubricant because it's so sensitive. Right after orgasm it often becomes so sensitive they avoid touching it directly. Instead, they tend to focus on the shaft of the clitoris, the mons and the inner labia, or lips, which Masters and Johnson believe to be "fully as important as the clitoris or mons as a source of erotic arousal."

She Said, He Said

When Shere Hite asked women about their men's clitoral techniques, they produced a regular Greek chorus of complaints about men's selfishness, clumsiness and ignorance of female anatomy. They complained that guys were too rough, too impatient, too fast, too slow, too off-target or that they changed rhythm at the wrong time. "It seems like he is trying to erase my clitoris!" one woman groused.

Well, in our *Men's Health* magazine survey we got an answering chorus of complaints—about women's reluctance to tell us how they like their clitorides to be touched. "We are not mind readers!" one guy exploded. "Talk to us and tell us how you feel, and what's going on for you!" Said another, "If you don't like our recipe for lovemaking, then give us some ingredients that will satisfy you!" Many said they'd love it if their lovers were more articulate about what they wanted. "A guy tends to believe that if a woman does not complain, he's not doing anything wrong," said one. "But women who are verbal in bed make me hornier!"

The only way to resolve this clitoral conflict (which we reckon will still be in progress the day the world ends) is for both women and men to learn to ask for what they want and say what they mean.

"The most important thing is simply to talk to her, to find out what types of stimulation pleasure her, to feel comfortable communicating sexually," says Dr. Whipple. "It's also important for her to be aware of what's pleasurable to her and feel comfortable saying this to her partner." In other words, it goes both ways.

Not only do women differ in the kinds of clitoral stimulation they prefer but hormonal fluctuations change the way the same woman likes to be touched at different times, Dr. Whipple says. (When Hite's group was asked what sort of clitoral touch they craved, their answers were all over the map: "firm, quick, constant movements . . . rapid side-to-side massaging . . . a light, teasing, tentative touch . . . soft then hard.")

Considering all this, how on earth is a guy supposed to know how to please her? Well, there's no way you could possibly know unless you ask. Or, best of all, get her to show you what she likes. If you're comfortable enough with each other to try this, just lay beside your lady and watch her masturbate while you gently caress her body, suggests San Francisco sex therapist and author Lonnie Barbach, Ph.D. Then after four or five minutes of watching, you take over the job while she guides your hand. Don't worry about her having an orgasm. Just try to learn how to pleasure her. One of Dr. Barbach's clients, a very religious woman, was at first very reluctant to try this. Finally, though, when she timidly asked her husband if he'd like to watch, she discovered he loved watching, and "she reported that his technique had improved a thousand percent when they made love afterward."

EROGENOUS ZONES
Finding Her Sexual Hot Spots

Women are amazing (as if you didn't already know that). Consider this: The late Dr. Alfred C. Kinsey, in his interviews with thousands of females, found a handful who were capable of reaching orgasm simply by having their eyebrows stroked, their earlobes kissed or a bit of pressure applied to their teeth. More recent researchers have found women capable of bringing themselves to climax simply by thinking about sex, without any physical stimulation at all.

Which suggests something about women's erogenous zones (places on the body that are especially responsive to erotic touch): Women tend to be less narrowly focused on the genitals and more sensitive to the entire body's potential for sensuous pleasure than men are.

"For most women, being touched and stroked all over is an essential prelude to arousal, perhaps because it takes them longer to become aroused than men," says Shirley Zussman, Ed.D., a certified sex therapist and co-director of the Association for Male Sexual Dysfunction in New York City.

Some men know this secret of female sexuality only too well—like the 55-year-old metallurgist, a respondent to our *Men's Health* magazine survey, who mentioned that after his first year of marriage (at age 28) he and his wife had decided to cut back to having sex four to six times a week. Clearly a devoted and accomplished lover, he loved to linger over foreplay, he told us, "stroking her body, legs, stomach, breasts, neck, brow. Just soft, gentle strokes on her naked flesh gradually working my way to her opening. . . . I like the feel of her body beneath my fingertips. The smoothness of her thighs. The way she giggles when I draw circles."

We're willing to bet that woman loves this guy!

Top Spots

The most sexually sensitive part of a woman's body, of course, is the clitoris. The budlike head—often the only part that's visible—can be so sensitive, in fact, that it's painful to her if you stimulate it too roughly, or without lubrication. In a series of famous experiments Dr. Kinsey had five gynecologists using glass, metal or cotton-tipped probes explore the genitals of almost 900 women to find out which areas were most sensitive. When the probe gently touched their clitorides, 98 percent of the women were aware of it—some of them exquisitely so. (Of course, this also suggests that a very few women have no feeling there at all; women really are different from each other!)

> . . . for three days they went at it without repose, showing the way the millrace flows and how the industrious spindle goes. They gave the lamb suck, they startled the buck, they tried on the finger ring for luck. They cradled the child, they kissed the twins, they polished the sword till it had not a speck, they taught the sparrow how to peck, they made the camel show his neck.
>
> —The Arabian Nights

The delicate inner lips that surround the clitoris, the labia minora, are also highly sensitive—98 percent of the women in Dr. Kinsey's study were sensitive here also. "As sources of erotic arousal, the labia minora seem to be fully as important as the clitoris," he wrote. One revealing proof of this is that he also discovered 84 percent of the women who masturbated did so by stroking both the labia and the clitoris. The labia majora, a pair of outer lips, tend to be much less erotically sensitive than the inner ones. (Interestingly enough, during early development in the womb the genitals of males and females start out as the same embryonic tissue; only gradually do they differentiate into clitorides and penises. And a woman's labia develops out of the same embryonic tissue that turned into your scrotal sac when you were a tiny tot.)

The entrance to the vagina is another terrifically erogenous zone for most women. It's really only the outer couple of inches that are richly supplied with nerve endings, though. The deep, interior walls of the vagina really have few nerve endings and are quite insensitive when stroked or lightly pressed, Dr. Kinsey reported. (Modern-day advocates of the G-spot, allegedly located on the interior top front wall of the vagina, say Dr. Kinsey's discreet 1950s gynecologists didn't discover it back then because it's only responsive to deep pressure; they just gently probed, fearful of arousing Mrs. Cleaver in the examining room.)

A Little Farther Afield

The mouth, lips and tongue are among a woman's most erogenous zones, according to Miriam Stoppard, M.D., who says in *The Magic of Sex* that "stimulating a woman's mouth . . . can set her whole body alight, and has a direct effect on arousing her genital organs. On the other hand, erogenous stimulation of any other part of a woman's body often produces a reaction in her mouth."

There's a similar connection, well-known to gynecologists, between a woman's breasts and nipples and her genitals. When a pregnant woman is nearly ready to give birth, stimulating her nipples can often induce the uterine contractions of labor. During sex play a man's gentle dalliance over a woman's breasts can also send sexual signals that tingle all the way down to her vagina. Still, not all women like it as much as guys do—Dr. Kinsey found that only 11 percent of women said they frequently stimulated their own breasts during masturbation. Be gentle, because her nipples may be highly sensitive, especially before her period.

The span of skin between her genitals and anus, the perineum (the place she'd make contact if she straddled a fence), is also "highly sensitive to touch, and tactile stimulation of the area may provide considerable erotic arousal," Dr. Kinsey found. Deep penetration of the vagina or the rectum may stimulate deep-seated nerves in this area.

Many women also are erotically responsive in all sorts of other, less obvious locations, like the area around their navels and lower abdomens, the inner sides of their thighs, buttocks, throats and armpits. Those women who can be brought to orgasm by earlobe kissing apparently can do so partly because during arousal the earlobes become engorged with blood and become increasingly sensitive during that time.

The only way to find out what other parts of her body become deliciously eroticized when she's aroused, is, as lazily as possible, to go in search of them with your tongue.

G-SPOT
Does It Really Exist?

Back in the early 1980s, after the publication of a book called *The G Spot and Other Recent Discoveries about Human Sexuality*, hunting for the G-spot became a national pastime on a par with throwing stuff at the TV on Super Bowl Sunday.

The Grafenberg spot, so named after a German obstetrician who described it back in the 1940s, was supposed to be a tiny, bean-shaped area lying just behind the front upper wall of a woman's vagina, about 1 to 2 inches inside the vaginal opening, that upon stimulation produced terrific orgasms for some women that seemed to be quite different from those triggered by clitoral stimulation. Many of these women reported that before or during their climax they also "ejaculated" a fluid that did not appear to be urine.

Naturally, the discovery of something about female sexuality that appeared to be genuinely new (after all these years) got everybody talking. But more than a decade after the book appeared, the experts are still talking—and there's still no agreement among them about whether the G-spot and/or female ejaculation actually exist, and if they do, what they're for.

In one comment typical of the doubters, Domeena Renshaw, M.D., professor of psychiatry at Loyola University Stritch School of Medicine in Chicago and a prominent sex authority, sniffed that "in our hurried, mechanistic culture," the whole idea of a G-spot has "an instant public appeal. Press a button and get a magic climax in 60 seconds." The G-spot, she concluded, "must remain unacceptable as a scientific fact for the gynecology textbooks."

Yet many other authorities disagree. "From the medical data we've seen, as well as anecdotal data, we are absolutely convinced that the phenomena (G-spot and female ejaculation) exist—and that virtually all women have this biological potential," says J. Kenneth Davidson, Sr., Ph.D., professor of sociology at the University of Wisconsin-Eau Claire, who with two colleagues polled over 1,200 professional women in the United States and Canada about their own experiences. The study concluded that "while many professionals are still debating the existence of a sensitive area in the vaginal barrel, the majority of women in this study believe that such an area exists and have experienced the pleasurable sensations associated with its stimulation."

To be precise, 66 percent of these women said they knew of "an especially sensitive area in their vaginas that if stimulated, produced pleasurable feelings." And 40 percent said they'd ejaculated at the moment of orgasm (though not every time).

Some of the guys who responded to our *Men's Health* magazine survey were also aware of all this, if only vaguely. One 20-year-old student told us that one of his preferred methods for helping his lover reach orgasm was to "stimulate her G-spot (if that's what it is). Whether it is actually a G-spot or whatever, she finds it very pleasurable to have the top of her vagina stimulated. If I reach in with a finger and hook it upwards and apply pressure to that area, she finds it very pleasurable."

The Evidence in Favor

The G-spot—or whatever it is—is not really a new discovery at all, observed Alice Ladas, Ed.D., Beverly Whipple, Ph.D., and John Perry, Ph.D., in the 1982 book that touched off the ruckus. In 1944 Dr. Ernst Grafenberg and prominent American gynecologist R. L. Dickinson, M.D., had described a "zone of erogenous feeling . . . located along the suburethral surface of the anterior (top) vaginal wall." This erotic hotspot, they said, "seems to be surrounded by erectile tissue like the corpora cavernosa (of the penis) . . . in the course of sexual stimulation the female urethra begins to enlarge and can be easily felt."

Though its size and location vary considerably from woman to woman, when stimulated, it often swells to the size of a dime or even a half-dollar, they said. With proper stimulation it becomes, in effect, a tiny, half-hidden, female erection. (Male and female sexuality, in other words, have a lot more in common than previously thought.)

This whole idea flies in the face of the received wisdom about the interior of the vagina, which—according to a series of famous experiments carried out by the late Dr. Alfred C. Kinsey in the early 1950s—isn't really supposed to have much feeling at all. Dr. Kinsey asked gynecologists to probe the genitals of hundreds of women to identify areas that were sensitive to touch and those that were not. The reason this study found the deep vaginal walls to be "quite insensitive" to touch, the authors argued, was that the decorous doctors probed them only very gently; the G-spot responds best to firm, deep, continuous pressure. (Even so, Dr. Kinsey did mention that "most of those (women) who did make some response (to vaginal touch) had the sensitivity confined to a certain point, in most cases the upper wall of the vagina just inside the vaginal entrance.")

Drs. Ladas, Whipple and Perry went on to describe its location more precisely: "The Grafenberg spot lies directly behind the pubic bone within the front wall of the vagina. It is usually located about halfway between the back of the pubic bone and the front of the cervix, along the course of the urethra (the tube through which urine flows) . . . The size and exact location vary. Imagine a small clock inside the vagina with 12 o'clock pointing toward the navel. The majority of women will find the G-spot located in the area between 11 and 1 o'clock."

Women who wear diaphragms may have trouble finding it, they added, because the device's rim tends to cover the spot.

What Is It?

Other studies that have attempted to locate the elusive spot in large groups of women have come up with findings that are wildly divergent. In one such study a gynecologist explored the entire vaginal wall in a number of women and found that 85 percent of them reported "high erotic sensitivity" on the top wall, producing responses that were "similar in quality . . . but lower in intensity . . . than clitorally evoked erotic sensations." But another study of over 100 women found that only 10 percent had an area of heightened sensitivity on the top of their vagina walls.

If it's there at all, what is it?

Even among researchers convinced that something is there, there's still no universal agreement about what to call it. Some have called it the urethral sponge or simply Skene's paraurethral glands and ducts, referring to a collection of bulbs and pipes that drain the urethra. But many researchers have taken to calling it the female prostate because of evidence that it appears to be similar in form and function to the male prostate (which is also highly responsive to erotic touch).

European researchers, using a blood test to detect the presence of two substances previously thought to be produced only by the male prostate gland (PSA and PAP), say they've found it in two-thirds of 33 women they examined. Further examination revealed that these women had what amounts to a "female prostate . . . these glands strongly resemble the male prostate glands before puberty." In

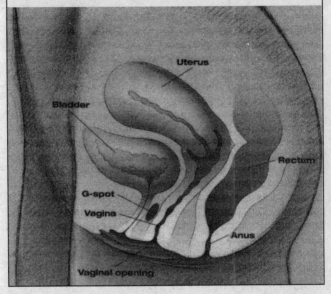

LOCATING THE G-SPOT

Fifty years after its "discovery," the existence of a G-spot continues to be debated. Does this bean-shaped, highly sensitive area actually exist in women? Many say yes, a few inches into the vagina, on the top wall.

Labels in illustration: Uterus, Bladder, Rectum, G-spot, Vagina, Anus, Vaginal opening

women, they say, the glands remain immature because they don't get the blasts of male hormones that cause the male prostate to mature. What the heck do women have them for, then? "No indications can be found for a proper biological function," the researchers report.

How to Find It

Well, so much for other people's science experiments—here's how to conduct your own. Drs. Ladas, Whipple and

Perry say that women often have trouble locating the G-spot on their own. That's where you come in.

The best way for you to search for her G-spot is for her to lie on the bed on her belly, legs apart, with her hips rotated slightly upwards. Then you insert two fingers into her vagina, palm down, and begin exploring the front wall of her vagina (the side closest to the bed). Ask her to guide you by telling you what feels good. She can also lie on her back, in which case you insert two fingers, palm up, and explore the top side of her vagina. Remember to use very firm, strong pressure, not gentle strokes. One clue that you've found it, Dr. Davidson says: She'll often have a fleeting feeling that she needs to urinate. After 2 to 20 seconds of massage, however, the feelings turn to erotic pleasure.

The best way for a woman to find it herself, the authors say, is to sit on the toilet (in case she needs to urinate). With a finger, she should explore the upper front wall of her vagina, at the same time applying firm downward pressure on the outside of her abdomen with her other hand. As it's stimulated, they say, this spot will begin to swell and can be felt as a small lump.

The most interesting way to reach it, of course, is with an erect penis during intercourse. But as Dr. Grafenberg pointed out long ago, in the missionary position, with the woman on her back, a man's penis does not really make contact with her G-spot unless you've got a steeply upcurving penis or her legs are placed up over your shoulders. The best position to reach it, says Dr. Davidson, is in the rear-entry position. She can either be on her hands and knees or you can be lying side-by-side in the "spoons" position. Other women have found that the female-on-top position is best because it allows her to fine-tune the angle of your penis. For more information, see Positions on page 317.

Female Ejaculation

The whole idea of female ejaculation is another one of those "new discoveries" that's not really new at all. Aristotle wrote about it; so did Galen in the second century A.D. In ancient

Taoist traditions female ejaculate is called moon flower medicine.

And in the *Kama Sutra*, a 2,000-year-old love manual, it says: "The semen of women continues to fall from the beginning of the sexual union to the end, in the same way as that of the male."

Among several of the respondents to our *Men's Health* magazine survey, all this wasn't really news either. "Both my wife and I enjoy oral sex very much," a 35-year-old computer systems engineer told us. "I enjoy performing oral sex on my wife so much that sometimes we get right into it with almost no foreplay beforehand. On many occasions she will have multiple orgasms. These orgasms are intense with significant discharge. Sometimes it's like she's 'peeing' on me."

Not all women ejaculate during orgasm, of course. In one study of 233 women, 54 percent reported having experienced this spurt of fluid during sex, but only 14 percent said it happened with most or all of their orgasms. A Masters and Johnson Institute survey of 300 women, on the other hand, found that less than 5 percent said they'd ever ejaculated during sex.

Dr. Davidson believes all women have a G-spot and all are capable of ejaculating—it's just that some women haven't done so simply because they haven't been stimulated enough. "Ejaculation seems to occur more frequently with the second or third orgasm—in other words, after prolonged, intense stimulation," he says.

Skeptics have always maintained that these women are simply peeing during sex. To them, "female ejaculation" is simply stress incontinence, a minor medical problem that should be treated with surgery or Kegel exercises to tighten up pelvic muscles. Others maintain that female ejaculation is real and wonderful, and that the fluids these women release during sex are not urine at all but something else. The ejaculate has been variously described as "colorless, clear or milky," but not yellow. One research team, who actually observed a woman's explosive ejaculation during orgasm, described it as looking like "watered-down fat-free milk." It didn't smell like urine and (unlike urine) it didn't stain the sheets, they said.

But lab analyses of this mysterious stuff have produced differing results. Four studies have found a difference in chemical composition between urine and the "ejaculate" (the most notable difference being the presence of prostatic secretions like PSA or PAP). But two others failed to show it was any different from urine at all. Sometimes it appears to be both: urine mixed with something else.

"The exact origin of the fluid has never been completely documented in a medical setting," Dr. Davidson says. Despite this, you can actually see where it comes out with your own eyes, if she's willing and you have good light. Just below and to each side of the urethral opening (from whence she urinates) at the 10 o'clock and 2 o'clock positions there are two tiny little slits. It's from these "paraurethral ducts" that the mysterious stuff emerges, he says.

But the real bottom line in this whole deal is suggested by the 1,200 women in Dr. Davidson's study. He and his colleagues discovered that there were only "minimal differences in physiological and psychological sexual satisfaction" between the women who ejaculated during sex and those who did not.

In other words, if she knows where her G-spot is and produces a great kablooey of juice during sex, that's wild and wonderful. But if she doesn't, that doesn't mean she's somehow sexually inadequate or any less interesting.

That just means she's wild and wonderful in a different way.

MENOPAUSE
How Lovemaking Changes during the Change

American culture seems almost entirely blind to the beauty of older women—beyond a certain age, women's faces and bodies simply disappear out of TV commercials and magazines. Yet many of these women, perhaps even your wife or lover, remain as alluringly sexual as ever.

Sure, a woman's sexuality often changes during and after menopause (when she has her last period and her reproductive system shuts down, usually around age 50). But menopause should certainly not be the tombstone on the grave of sex—for her or for you.

"One of the most common myths surrounding menopause is that in addition to the loss of reproductive function, the menopause marks the cessation of sexuality as well," observes Sheryl A. Kingsberg, Ph.D., assistant professor in the Department of Reproductive Biology at Case Western Reserve University School of Medicine in Cleveland.

Despite this common notion, "postmenopausal women often retain interest in sexual activity and are fully capable of good sexual functioning," says Dr. Kingsberg.

Another thing most guys don't realize about menopause (and plenty of women, too) is that it doesn't begin the day she has her last period. It's more of a gradual transition, a two- to seven-year period of hormonal turbulence that accompanies the ending of menstruation. In fact, the very earliest stages of this life-change, called perimenopause, may show up when she's in her early to mid-forties. Typical symptoms: insomnia, irritability and stress incontinence (she loses urine when she laughs or sneezes).

The Impact on Sexuality

Studies have shown that about 10 percent of women experience a sort of radiant sexual renaissance after menopause, freshly rediscovering their husbands, paying more attention to their own appearance, suddenly becoming interested in daytime trysts. For them freedom from the fear of pregnancy, the inconvenience of menstruation and (often) the noisy intrusions of children are liberating.

But it's really more common for women to notice a decline in their appetites for sex during and after menopause (about a third of women report this). One study found that more than half the women involved had a decrease in sexual thoughts and fantasies during the years around menopause.

It's hard to predict exactly how your partner's sexuality will change during menopause. But therapists have found that one of the best predictors is her sex life before menopause. If she loved it before, she'll probably love it after. If not, she won't. "For some women menopause can be the long-awaited excuse to abandon sexual activity" because she never liked it anyway, says San Francisco sex therapist Lonnie Barbach, Ph.D., author of *The Pause: Positive Approaches to Menopause*.

The Physical Changes

The physical changes are easier to predict.

Usually the opening to her vagina gradually grows smaller, especially if she's not sexually active. The depth and width of her vagina gradually shrink, and it becomes less elastic, William H. Masters, M.D., and Virginia E. Johnson, of the former Masters and Johnson Institute in St. Louis, discovered. And as her estrogen levels decline, the vaginal lining becomes thinner, drier and less elastic. Masters and Johnson reported that some older women's vaginas eventually become "tissue-paper thin" and "almost give the impression that they can be seen through." Thinner, more delicate tissues mean less cushion against the thrusts of your penis.

At the same time, her vagina's ability to produce lubrication during arousal is reduced. When a younger woman gets hot, her vagina is fully lubricated within 10 to 30 seconds, Masters and Johnson found. But a woman past age 60 may take one to three minutes of stimulation before she's lubricated—even if she really loves what you're doing. As a consequence, if you're too fast or too rough, intercourse can produce a "mild burning sensation during lovemaking and sometimes for hours or even days afterward," says Dr. Barbach. The most common complaint of older women seeking gynecological help, she adds, is pain during intercourse.

The bottom line here is to go gently and slowly. Older women need more foreplay to stimulate their natural lubrication. And they often need some added, store-bought lubrication as well. Lubricants, like K-Y Jelly, are often available without a prescription in drugstores. So are Gyne-Moistrin and Replens, a relatively new type of feminine lubricant that's inserted like a tampon and can work wonders in making sex pleasurable again. (Tell her to avoid cold medicines, too, which dry out her genitals along with her sinuses.)

She may also want to try an estrogen-containing, lubricating cream, like Estrace (available by prescription only), which delivers estrogen directly to the target without spreading it through her whole system. (Nevertheless, these products often do have systemic effects— "I've had women stop having hot flashes within 24 hours after using these creams," says Dr. Barbach.)

Women's skin sensitivity may change after menopause begins, too—a spot that was once highly erotic now just tickles or even hurts. Her breasts often become far more painful both at midcycle and during the last week before menstruation begins. Try suggesting that she take 400 to 600 international units of vitamin E, "which really makes a big difference in relieving breast pain," Dr. Barbach says.

Sex As Medicine

But nearly all these age-related changes in a woman's sexual anatomy can be kept to a minimum by one simple, pleasurable prescription: Have sex regularly.

One of our *Men's Health* magazine survey respondents, a 55-year-old metallurgist, told us that "when my wife was 48 she became concerned that she didn't seem to be going through menopause yet, so she went to the doctor. (I was concerned a little, too.) She came home with a big smile on her face and told me that as long as we continue to have sex regularly, her menopause would be delayed."

Well, not exactly. But by staying sexually active, her sweet spots will stay sweet longer. Among the hundreds of women Masters and Johnson studied, they found three women over age 60—one was 73—whose vaginas began lubricating in response to sexual stimulation as rapidly as girls in their twenties. Their only explanation: These women had had satisfying sex once or twice a week for their entire adult lives.

Hormone Replacement Therapy

Of course, many postmenopausal women also take estrogen in pill form to replace the estrogen their bodies stop producing at menopause. Hormone replacement therapy (HRT) has a host of benefits, including reducing hot flashes, improving a woman's cholesterol profile, reducing bone loss—and keeping vaginal tissues "plump, lubricated and pain-free," Dr. Barbach says.

Though not all women are candidates for HRT (for instance, breast cancer patients are generally advised against it), it can really help keep sex pleasurable later in life. Of course, what difference does it make if a woman's vagina is soft and youthful if she's lost interest in having sex at all?

Which is where testosterone comes in. Testosterone, it now appears, is what boosts sex drive in both men and women, and by spicing up the estrogen with tiny amounts of testosterone, researchers have found they can put a certain glint in the eyes of many women who take it. (Giving women testosterone is not "unnatural": Testosterone is produced in small amounts by a woman's adrenal glands and ovaries, which gradually cease producing it if menopause occurs naturally, and abruptly stops if the ovaries are surgically removed during a hysterectomy.)

"Adding androgens (male hormones, like testosterone) to estrogen therapy may be the answer for women who report loss of sex drive, especially in those who can date a decline in drive to the start of menopause," observes Dr. Kingsberg.

In the early days of experimenting with these estrogen/androgen mixes, there were unwanted side effects, mainly facial hair, lowered voice, weight gain, acne and higher cholesterol levels. (Real sexy.) Now, though, testosterone is added in such tiny doses that side effects are rare, mild and easily reversible, according to John Arpels, M.D., a San Francisco gynecologist and founding member of the North American Menopause Society.

Keep On Talking

But even if you've recruited modern medicine to help keep your sex life alive, it's not always easy. The big thing is to keep on talking to each other.

"It's really important to keep on getting 'weather reports' about what's happening with your partner," says Dr. Barbach. "Sit down and ask her what's going on, how she's feeling. That constant communication has to keep going on."

And respond to what she says. If she's having trouble lubricating during intercourse, keep some lube in the bedside table and use it without her having to ask. If she says her nipples are sensitive, go gently. It's best to schedule sex for the morning, when you both have more energy. And if intercourse is painful or difficult, just try to take the focus off intercourse—plenty of other things (like oral sex, sensual massage and bathing) can be arousing, too.

Oh, and don't forget one other little thing: There are plenty of "menopause babies" walking around out there—so don't forget to use some kind of contraception until a year after her last period.

MENSTRUATION
How It Affects Sex Drive

There's one very modern reason to be worried about love-making during her period—AIDS. There are also a few very old, fairly weird reasons to wonder about it.

But the bottom line is this: If you're certain she's not HIV positive and you don't mind a little additional mess, there's absolutely no reason not to make love while she's having her period.

Plenty of other people do. Of the thousands of men polled for the *Hite Report on Male Sexuality*, 67 percent said they enjoyed making love during her menses. And William H. Masters, M.D., and Virginia E. Johnson, of the former Masters and Johnson Institute in St. Louis, found that out of 331 women they studied, only 33 objected to having sex during menstruation (either for religious reasons or because of all that extra laundry). Almost two hundred, in fact, said they were often pretty randy during their periods, especially toward the end of the menstrual flow. And 43 of the women confessed that having an orgasm during their periods actually triggered a pleasant kind of sexual healing by relieving the cramping and backache that often goes along with menstruation.

Risk of AIDS

In case you flunked high school health, here's how things work. The ovaries of a woman generate an egg every month or so. Once the egg is mature enough, it breaks out of the ovary and works its way through the fallopian tubes, waiting for a sperm to come along and fertilize it. At the same time, the walls of the uterus get lined with thick, blood-rich cells; the concept is that if the egg gets fertilized, it will have a home ready to nourish it. If no fertilization occurs in ten days or so, this bloody uterine lining sheds out through the vagina—a process called menstruation.

For men exposure to a woman's menstrual blood is really just a minor aesthetic problem—unless of course it's infected with the HIV virus. In one European study of 563 heterosexual couples, researchers tried to identify precisely what it was that put people at risk of getting AIDS. "The only sexual practice associated with increased risk of female-to-male transmission," they concluded, "was unprotected vaginal intercourse during menstruation."

That's because, though HIV is present in vaginal secretions, it's present in much higher concentrations in blood. If she is infected, lovemaking brings you into direct contact with infected body fluids—the thing all "safer sex" guidelines beg you to avoid.

It should go without saying in the 1990s, but: If you don't know a woman's HIV status and she's having her period, always wear a condom. If she's HIV positive, having unprotected sex with her during her period is like jumping out a fifth-story window: You might survive, but you have to be nuts to try it.

And don't forget, gentlemen, that lovemaking during menstruation can also be hazardous to her health—if it's you who's infected with something. There are a couple of reasons for this. For one thing the vagina is normally fairly acidic (pH 3.5 to 4), which helps kill invading bacteria. But during her period, blood's higher alkalinity raises the pH of her vagina to 5 or so, making her more susceptible to infection. Also, menstrual blood flushes away some of the mucus that partly plugs the cervix (the doorway into the uterus), making it easier for microorganisms—like gonorrheal or chlamydial infections—to penetrate the deeper regions of her reproductive system.

When she's bleeding, she's vulnerable.

Horniness and Periods

From an evolutionary point of view you would think that both men and women would tend to feel sexiest during times when a woman is most fertile in order to ensure maximum baby making—in other words, that our lovemaking would be tied directly to her menstrual cycles. After all, in the lower mammals (like squirrels and rabbits) and among most nonhuman primates (like apes and monkeys) almost all sexual activity takes place during the time when the female is ovulating (producing eggs). The rest of the time, neither party seems especially interested.

But when it comes to the human female—well, nothing is that simple. The legions of sex researchers who've studied fluctuations in women's interest in sex over the course of their periods haven't found any consistent pattern. Some women say they feel horniest toward the end of their menstrual flows, others at the beginning, in the middle or never at all. One study that looked at a whole slew of other such studies concluded that "there is no consistent evidence . . . that either subjective or physiological levels of sexual response vary systematically across the menstrual cycle."

Since nobody we know of has studied men's sexual interest during her menstrual cycle, we'll hazard a guess: It doesn't change at all.

A more important question is whether or not you can get her pregnant while she's having her period. (In the age of AIDS it's easy to forget that pregnancy used to be the main reason guys feared sex!) The short answer: It is possible, though unlikely, especially if her periods are irregular, according to Philip M. Sarrel, M.D., and Lorna Sarrel, co-directors of the Sex Counseling Program at Yale University. For more information, see Pregnancy on page 146.

> It is an undoubted fact that meat spoils when touched by menstruating women.
>
> —British medical journal, 1878

Weird Taboos and Wild Women

Actually, there's a very old tradition, common to many cultures all over the world, that women are unclean—and sexually off-limits—while they're having their periods. The Old Testament, the Koran and the Torah all forbid sex during menstruation. Among Orthodox Jews if a bride is menstruating on her wedding night, by custom a young girl is sent to accompany the newlyweds to their wedding chamber so they'll keep their hands to themselves. And the Carrier Indians of British Columbia—who really got carried away with the whole thing—used to banish young girls who'd just begun menstruating to the wilderness, where they'd spend three or four years in total seclusion. Tattered adolescent ghosts, they were thought to be a danger to anyone who saw them out there, and even their footsteps were said to taint the path they walked on.

In some ways it's not hard to understand the primitive awe and fear inspired by a woman's monthly bleeding. Blood is associated with both birth and death and, hence, is mysterious. But menstrual blood is doubly mysterious—it flows but does not bring death or sickness; it affects only healthy adult women and it comes and goes for no apparent reason. The fact that a woman "bleeds from that very place of mystery that—for male and female alike—is both the gateway to life and to erotic pleasures has always and in all cultures been regarded as a sign of magical power," observes Rufus C. Camphausen in *The Encyclopedia of Erotic Wisdom.*

If it's filled with magic and power but you don't know what it is or where it comes from—well, no wonder men from 10,000 cultures just decided to stay away, whether there was any real reason to or not.

ORGASM
How to Make It Happen

To most guys a woman's orgasm is a wonder to behold. It can also be baffling beyond belief.

How, exactly, are you supposed to get her to climax in the first place? (The sex literature varies on this point, but studies suggest many women don't reach orgasm during intercourse anywhere from 20 to 80 percent of the time.) And if she does come, did she really come or was that just a realistic simulation? (Two-thirds of the women surveyed in one study said they'd faked an orgasm, most often in casual relationships.) And if it wasn't real . . . well, what does that mean?

Sometimes guys wind up feeling so confused, uncertain and uncomfortable about it all that they just flat out ask her if she made it over the top.

"With my wife sometimes I'll ask (if she came)," was what one man wrote who responded to a sex survey sent out by researcher Shere Hite. "She'll usually laugh and say, 'Can't you tell?' or 'What difference does it make?' "

Which is exactly the sort of answer that's been driving guys around the bend for the past ten thousand years.

No, he usually can't tell.

And yes, it makes a big difference.

A Moment Suspended in Time

Strictly speaking, female orgasm is the third stage of the sexual response cycle as laid out in a series of classic observations by William H. Masters, M.D., and Virginia E. Johnson, of the former Masters and Johnson Institute in St. Louis. During the first phase, called excitation, a woman's vagina begins to lubricate (normally about 10 to 30 seconds after stimulation begins), its interior begins to dilate, her muscles grow increasingly tense and her clitoris and nipples begin to swell with dammed-up blood. Phase two (the plateau) is a continuation of this tension buildup—her heart rate and respiration increase, her skin begins to flush and the outer third of her vagina begins to swell dramatically. Up out of sight her uterus also swells, in some cases actually doubling in size.

All of this comes to a dramatic climax at orgasm, when all that muscular tension and engorged blood are suddenly, ecstatically released. Her orgasm is accompanied by muscular contractions of the uterus and the outer third of the vagina (the so-called orgasmic platform) at 0.8-second intervals. (Men experience muscular contractions during orgasm at precisely the same interval.) In some women the sphincter muscles in the rectum also contract spasmodically in synch with genital contractions.

Strictly speaking, nobody really knows what triggers a woman's orgasm, or even exactly what it is. Researchers from Rutgers University in New Brunswick, New Jersey, note that "there is no universally accepted definition of orgasm," and go on to suggest a half-dozen reasonable-sounding (but quite different) definitions. We won't bore you with the details except to point out that at the very center of sex lies something so powerful we are all drawn to it like moths to the flame—yet in many ways it remains fundamentally mysterious, radiant and inscrutable as a star, after all these years still impervious to the impudent probes and charts and studies of researchers.

What's it feel like? Here's what women have said.

"A moment suspended in time, a hot rush—a sudden

breathtaking dousing of all the nerves in my body in Plea-sure," women have written. "Beautifully excruciating . . . an explosion of unbelievable warmth and relief."

In other words, almost exactly the same way it feels to you. One researcher has actually observed that when you delete the anatomical references, "written descriptions of orgasm by men and women are indistinguishable."

So at least we have something in common.

Her Orgasm As Enigma

One of the biggest differences, of course, is the difficulty some women have in getting there.

In fact, inability to have an orgasm is the second-most common complaint of women visiting sex therapists. Even love is no panacea: A University of Pittsburgh study found that over half the women who said they were happily mar-ried also admitted they had trouble reaching orgasm or becoming aroused.

The really mystifying thing about all this is that, in many ways, "the female has an infinitely greater capacity for sex-ual response than a man ever dreamed of," as Dr. Masters once remarked. It's women, not men, who have an organ (the clitoris) with no other known purpose than to provide sexual pleasure. It's women, not men, who are capable of leaping from one orgasm to the next without pausing for a postorgasmic time-out, or refractory period, in between. It's women, not men, who are often capable of an astounding series of orgasms, one after the other: "The female may have had two or three or even as many as a dozen or more orgasms in a relationship in which her husband had ejacu-lated only once," the late Dr. Alfred C. Kinsey remarked of the 14 percent of women in his sample who were multior-gasmic.

Part of the problem, and much of the glory, lies in the fact that all women are different.

"Men need to learn that women are very different from one another—much more so than men," says Donald Strass-berg, Ph.D., a sex therapist and psychology professor at the

University of Utah in Salt Lake City. "For men pretty much anything works. Apply some friction to his penis and he's happy. Women, on the other hand, become aroused in different places on the body; they respond to different levels of stimulation, different tempos. And they are even variable from one time to the next."

One respondent to our *Men's Health* magazine survey, a 51-year-old manager, told us that "it has been my experience that while a specific stimulus may consistently result in orgasm for a given partner, the specific stimuli can vary for different partners. My current partner reaches orgasm occasionally through penetration but consistently reaches orgasm through cunnilingus. Previous partners who reached orgasm consistently did so through one of the following: penetration only, very rapid stimulation of the clitoris or seemingly unending orgasms through finger stimulation inside the vagina."

And if the methods needed to arouse each woman are different, so is a woman's own interior experience of orgasm. Some sex researchers have taken to using the term orgasmic fingerprinting to suggest the uniqueness of each woman's sexual ecstasy.

In other words, as a male lover you should give up on the idea of becoming an expert on women in general and instead become an expert only on your woman.

There is no sweeter purpose under the sun.

Hooey from Dr. Freud

Is there a difference between a clitoral and a vaginal orgasm? Quite possibly, you don't give two hoots about this question, but it's worth mentioning (briefly) because it's caused men and women a world of grief over the years. In many ways the whole debate arose with Sigmund Freud, who shortly after the turn of the century came up with what came to be known as the clitoral/vaginal transfer theory. He argued that little girls tend to discover their own sexuality through direct stimulation of the clitoris during masturbation, but as they mature beyond their childish years, they learn to transfer the focal point of their sexual responses from the clitoris to the vagina. Silly, childish clitoral orgasms turn into mature, satisfying vaginal orgasms, achieved through penetration during intercourse. If a woman can't achieve this amazing switch, she's a neurotic nut case.

Freud's influence on the culture was so pervasive that this idea was handed out to millions of women (maybe even your mother) in marriage manuals and articles in popular women's magazines by the score. One 1936 book advised: "If this transition (from clitoris to vagina) is not successful, then the woman cannot experience satisfaction in the sexual act. . . . The first and decisive requisite of a normal orgasm is vaginal sensitivity."

There were just a couple of problems with this idea. Number one, the whole notion that a woman's sexual responses could just magically leap from the clitoris to the vagina like that is "a biological impossibility," as Dr. Kinsey was later to note rather coldly. Number two, as he also noted: "There is no evidence that the vagina is ever the sole source of arousal or even the primary source of erotic arousal in any female."

When Masters and Johnson revisited this question in the mid-1960s by actually studying women having orgasms, they concluded: "Are clitoral and vaginal orgasms truly separate anatomical entities? From a biologic point of view, the answer to this question is an unequivocal no."

Although "there may be great variation in duration and intensity of orgasmic experience, varying from individual to individual and within the same woman from time to time," there was no real physiological difference between an orgasm triggered by intercourse, clitoral stimulation or stimulation of some other part of the body (like the breasts).

In all of its splendor and mystery and variety a woman's orgasm is an orgasm is an orgasm. All that really matters is helping her get there.

Helping Her Get There

To hear the feminists tell it, the biggest problem is us: We're selfish, clumsy, impatient and focused primarily on our own pleasure. But to hear the respondents to our *Men's Health* magazine survey tell it, women need to bear their share of the blame: "Men want to satisfy as much as they want to be satisfied sexually—but unfortunately, most women do not assert themselves or verbalize their wants during lovemaking," one guy told us. "Most of my male friends agree that they would like their lovers to tell them how they can please them better. We love directions, if only, 'higher,' 'lower,' to the left,' 'to the right.' "

Still, most of the magazine survey respondents seem to have figured out how to communicate sexually because when we asked, "Have you discovered anything that consistently enables your partner to reach orgasm?" 62 percent said they had. Among their various suggestions:

After you, ma'am. "One surefire method of getting every mate I've ever been with to experience orgasm is to hold off penetration for a considerable time and spend much time just on them," wrote a 36-year-old paramedic. "I find that giving a woman an intense and satisfying orgasm orally before I even consider penetration will do the trick every time."

"If a guy is having erectile problems, he obsesses, he worries, he gets performance anxiety—but very few things can give a man confidence like seeing her come," adds Jude Cotter, Ph.D., a psychologist and sex therapist in private practice in Farmington Hills, Michigan, who insists that ladies should always come first. "If she comes first, that takes away 90 percent of his fears."

> Women complain about sex more often than men. Their gripes fall into two major categories: not enough and too much.
>
> —Ann Landers

Studies demonstrate the benefits of being a sexual gentleman: In one survey of 805 nurses the women who reported the least trouble reaching orgasm were those whose partners delayed their own orgasms until after the woman had experienced hers. Another study, this one of 709 adult women, found that women who usually came after their male partners were less physically and psychologically satisfied by the whole experience than women who came first.

Give her the oral exam. For the humble authors of this book one of the biggest revelations of the *Men's Health* magazine survey was the number of men who said that oral sex is the best way to ring her chimes. Over and over again we heard things such as "oral sex (tongue to genitals) is the only method that consistently enables my wife to reach orgasm" or "if a man knows how to give outstanding oral sex, then a woman will reach orgasm every time."

Studies have shown that oral sex does not always work—but to hear our respondents tell it, it sure comes close. One 50-year-old cattle rancher told us: "As a young man I was taught oral lovemaking as an art, man on woman. My teacher was one of the most beautiful women I have ever known. She taught me that a man must never leave a woman who has not had her own orgasm. To my knowledge, all the women whom I have been graced to have sex with have had orgasms."

A few suggested special tricks, like the 25-year-old student who said that "one of the simplest things I do to help her reach orgasm is to have a glass of hot tea and a glass of ice water next to me while I perform oral sex on her. I take a sip of the tea, go to work, then stop and take a sip of the water and go back. This drives her nuts and she normally has two or three orgasms before I am even inside her."

Give her a hand. The trouble with standard, male-female, in-out intercourse is that it usually does not give much direct stimulation to the clitoris, leading Shere Hite to describe intercourse itself as "something that sounds more like a Rube Goldberg scheme than a reliable route to (female) orgasm." She even went on to suggest that "intercourse was never meant to stimulate women to orgasm."

Well, we don't know about that—but whatever you think of the matter, it's a problem that's not all that difficult to solve. A whole slew of sex studies have shown that women whose lovers give them a little additional, direct clitoral stimulation during lovemaking are more likely to climax consistently. It doesn't matter if it's your hand, her hand, a vibrator or something else that makes direct contact with her clitoris; it often helps. In Hite's sample of 3,000 women, for instance, only 30 percent said they reached orgasm regularly during intercourse—but 44 percent said they reached orgasm regularly if their partners directly stimulated their clitorides during intercourse.

One of our respondents said this rather ingenious method nearly always helped his wife over the top: "After a long period of foreplay I place some lubricant on three fingers of a gloved hand, place one finger directly on the clitoris, insert one finger high up in the vagina and slowly insert one finger high up in the rectum and use all fingers to slowly massage."

Find a Vassar girl. One study of young Czech women found that the two best predictors of whether or not a woman would be able to reach orgasm during sex were education and social standing. Better-educated women with higher professional status were more likely to be orgasmic—a finding confirmed by other studies.

Try asking her who wrote *The Federalist Papers* before you get seriously involved.

Try a new angle. Varying the position you use during intercourse may also help her get there.

A 63-year-old writer said that "with her riding on top of me, this gives her almost complete control as to when and how she'll reach her climax. I have developed the ability to control my orgasm so that when she hits hers, I am within seconds of reaching mine."

"My wife can always 'finish' if she is on top," says a 31-year-old accountant. "She doesn't have to be on top, but it tends to come easier in that position. She says it is easier for her to find her 'spot,' which she describes as an area about three to four inches inside her."

Play show-and-tell. "I've discovered that one thing that almost always works is open communication," said a 28-year-old advertising executive. "Unlike male sexual response, every woman is a bit different. So men can either try endless experimentation (which will probably frustrate both partners) or he can ask her directly, 'What do you like?

How can I make you feel good?' If a man isn't confident enough to ask these questions or the woman isn't confident enough to answer them honestly, then the two of them shouldn't be together in bed anyway."

"Sometimes the best thing to do is just ask her to show you how she turns herself on—there's almost nothing better than watching her masturbate to help you understand where and how she needs to be pleasured," adds sex therapist Judith Seifer, Ph.D., president of the American Association of Sex Educators, Counselors and Therapists.

"I think women should say the same thing to men. After all, what is so scary about this? It's basically just show-and-tell."

Most women know precisely what it takes to make themselves climax; they punch their own buttons when they masturbate. In Dr. Kinsey's sample, for instance, only 4 to 6 percent of the women who masturbated were unable to reach orgasm that way—a far smaller percentage than those who couldn't climax during intercourse.

Interestingly enough, Dr. Kinsey and other, more recent researchers also found that it's not necessarily true that women are innately slower to become aroused and reach orgasm than men are. During masturbation many women can reach orgasm just as fast as males, and some even faster. The big difference, apparently, is that they know exactly how and where to stimulate themselves. So ask them (very politely) to show you how they do it.

If She's Really Having Trouble

Of course, there are some women who seldom have an orgasm no matter what they (or you) try. Others, often referred to as anorgasmic or preorgasmic women, have never yet reached the peak of sexual ecstasy. Many of these women could benefit from sex therapy, Dr. Seifer says, whether individually or in small groups.

Have some blood work done. "Still, before I go jumping in a woman's head and start psychoanalyzing her, I'd want her blood work done," Dr. Seifer adds.

That's because in some cases anorgasmia may be caused by a lesion (injury or abnormal growth) on the anterior pituitary gland. In her six-week workshops she's had excellent success teaching women to become orgasmic—but a few who didn't respond turned out to have pituitary lesions. When the lesions were surgically removed, "all three became orgasmic and fertile," she says. One other telltale sign: Women with these lesions also sometimes have a little drip from the breast (the anterior pituitary produces prolactin, which induces milk production).

Visit a bookstore. On the other hand, she might be able to save the expense and trouble of sex therapy and go to a bookstore instead.

"Most women who are anorgasmic don't need psychotherapy—nine out of ten of them would be greatly helped just by reading Lonnie Barbach's books," Dr. Seifer says. If your lover is still having trouble reaching orgasm, consider giving her one of these excellent books, written (and often recommended) by sex therapists.

For Each Other: Sharing Sexual Intimacy and *For Yourself: The Fulfillment of Female Sexuality*, both by Lonnie Barbach, Ph.D.

Becoming Orgasmic: A Sexual Growth Program for Women by Julia Heiman and Joseph LoPiccolo, Ph.D.

PMS
What It Is—And Isn't

Suddenly, for no obvious reason, she's weepy and irritable and depressed. She doesn't like it when you touch her, especially her breasts. She complains that she feels fatigued and bloated, that she can't seem to lose weight. Then she sends you out in the middle of the night for a chocolate bar and a case of Sugar Wowies.

Premenstrual syndrome, or PMS, is part of the reason lots of guys are completely mystified by women. (Don't waste your time wondering, "Was it something I said?" It wasn't.)

The thing is, PMS is also mystifying to women—and to their doctors, too. It's known that this collection of bizarre symptoms, which in a few women can be extremely distressing, are related to hormonal changes that occur about a week before menstrual flow begins. Various theories have been floated about the exact connection

> There will be sex after death—
> we just won't be able to feel it.
>
> —Lily Tomlin

between those hormonal riptides and all that weeping, but the truth is nobody really knows.

"I have PMS" is one of those expressions that pretty much says it all between women. Actually, though, PMS strikes each woman quite differently: different symptoms (as many as 150 have been documented), different intensities, different lengths, different recurrence rates. While as many as 95 percent of women have premenstrual symptoms at some point during their childbearing years, only 3 to 5 percent ever have symptoms that interfere with daily living—in other words, pose a serious medical condition. PMS generally hits hardest when women are in their thirties.

To soothe milder symptoms, doctors often recommend that women with PMS cut back on salt (to reduce fluid retention and bloating), exercise regularly and reduce their consumption of caffeine (in the form of tea, coffee, soda and chocolate). In one study of 188 Chinese nursing students, researchers found a strong relationship between the amount of caffeine they consumed and the severity of their symptoms (including breast pain and tenderness). Some women have found that vitamin E also helps relieve breast tenderness. Other women have been helped by taking progestin-only "minipills" (a low-dose oral contraceptive) that keep hormones stable throughout the month.

Other than that, though, the best thing is just to be sympathetic, wear a hard hat and wait it out.

PREGNANCY
Why Sex Is Still Safe

Study the question as I will, I can see no law or reason which jus-
tifies the husband in approaching the wife for the purpose of sex-
ual gratification at any time during pregnancy.

—Mrs. Emma F. Angell Drake, M.D.,

"What a Young Wife Ought to Know" (1902)

Well, jeez, lady, we can sure think of a reason!

Luckily, though, there's no longer any need to argue with a doctor with an ostrich-plume hat and 42 buttons on her shoes. The expert advice on having sex during pregnancy has changed dramatically in the past hundred years.

"Normal sexual activity in an otherwise uncomplicated pregnancy does not jeopardize fetal, maternal or neonatal (newborn) health," says Ricardo Loret de Mola, M.D., an instructor in obstetrics and gynecology at the University of Pennsylvania Medical School in Philadelphia, who has conducted an exhaustive review of the medical literature on the subject.

For instance, studies that have compared babies born to women who were sexually active throughout their pregnancies to those who quit at some point during the pregnancy found no significant differences on any measure of infant health. And one Israeli study of nearly 11,000 women found no link between intercourse during pregnancy and premature labor, premature rupture of the membranes, low birth weight or infant mortality.

Nature has gone to great lengths to keep the fetus safe by tucking the uterus deep inside the pelvic girdle and surrounding it with a sort of airbag of amniotic fluid, thus shielding it from the "external trauma" of your amorous intentions, Dr. Loret de Mola explains. That's part of the reason why physical injury to the fetus is only rarely the cause when a pregnancy ends in miscarriage, writes Kenneth Judson Reamy, M.D., professor of obstetrics and gynecology at West Virginia University School of Medicine in Morgantown. In one examination of the records of 250,000 miscarriages, fewer than 0.007 percent were caused by injuries, Dr. Reamy observes.

So there, Emma. Uh . . . ma'am.

A Few Exceptions

Still, there are some women whose doctors generally advise them to abstain from sex during pregnancy, Dr. Loret de Mola says. These include women with abdominal cramps and vaginal bleeding during the first 20 weeks, those with leakage of the amniotic fluid (intercourse might lead to chorioamnionitis, or infection of the fluid), women with a history of premature labor or miscarriages, or any condition that requires bed rest during the pregnancy.

There are also two sexual practices doctors advise pregnant couples to always avoid. One is cunnilingus (oral sex on her vulva). The reason: You may force air into her vagina and an air bubble, or embolism, could pass into her bloodstream, which could be fatal to both her and the baby. In fact, ten deaths of pregnant women associated with cunnilingus have been reported in the medical literature. (You should never blow air into her vagina at any time, "but during pregnancy an embolism is more likely because the veins of her uterus are dilated in order to get more blood to the baby," Dr. Loret de Mola explains.)

And of course, a pregnant woman should never have sex with somebody carrying a sexually transmitted disease, like gonorrhea, syphilis, herpes, hepatitis, group B streptococcus or AIDS. Newborns can contract potentially fatal infections if the mother's birth canal has been contaminated by these pathogens. (See more on these diseases in part eight.)

If your lady is pregnant and you are a new lover (or not her only one), it's best to make a practice of wearing condoms during sex throughout the pregnancy, for the baby's sake.

But if you're in a stable, monogamous relationship and

you're both disease-free, there's really no need to wear condoms, experts say. Bush-league bacteria (with which a healthy vagina is loaded) is not a problem it's just the big-league pathogens that matter.

Sex during Pregnancy

Some people still believe that when she gets pregnant, he's got to tolerate a sexual Sahara for the next nine months or go elsewhere to find some relief. But this is really a throwback to long-gone (duller) days. Back in 1902 Miz Emma advised young wives: "It occasionally happens that the wife during pregnancy is troubled with a passion far beyond what she has ever experienced at any other time. This in every instance is due to some unnatural condition and should be considered a disease, and for it the physician should be consulted."

The truth is that most couples remain sexually active throughout the pregnancy, though their activity and level of interest in sex varies a lot. In fact, the bottom line on all the many studies of sex during pregnancy is how variable they are. William H. Masters, M.D., and Virginia E. Johnson, of the former Masters and Johnson Institute in St. Louis, found that most couples in their study group reported a decrease in sexual activity during the first trimester (when women are inclined to throw up a lot), an unexplained surge of desire, often well above prepregnancy levels, in the second trimester (when women generally feel a lot better) and a drop-off in the third (when just getting around her belly is a trick). But other, more recent studies have found many couples' sexual activities steadily decline throughout the whole pregnancy.

In one study of 260 women the most common reason given for reduced sexual activity was plain old physical discomfort. Many pregnant women complain of pain during intercourse, and these complaints often become more common as the pregnancy progresses, the study found.

Expectant fathers also go through emotional changes that can be as volatile as those their wives are going through.

One study of 59 couples found that "expectant fathers were less emotionally satisfied than their wives through pregnancy." The women felt more peaceful and fulfilled in the pregnancy, more self-accepting sexually and enjoyed sex more than their mates did. One big surprise: Both men and women underestimated how much more attractive the guys would find their wives when their bellies were swollen with child.

Still, some men may discover that pregnancy puts a real damper on their sexual desires. The reasons, observes Dr. Reamy, may range from the reasonable (fear of hurting the baby, lack of attraction to their wives' burgeoning body) to semireasonable (a feeling that sex during pregnancy is immoral) to the genuinely loopy (a fear that "somehow the fetus would be an observer to sexual activity and could hurt the man's penis").

The take-home message in all of this is to just relax, big guy. Pregnancy is bound to cause short-term changes in your sexual life, but whatever they are, other men (and women) have experienced them, too.

Late-Pregnancy Sex

Many couples become particularly worried about having sex toward the end of the third trimester, when she's enormous and the birth is imminent.

"It's widely believed that intercourse, with or without orgasm, can precipitate labor," says Dr. Loret de Mola. Normally, this is no problem—in fact, if the baby is at term, doctors and midwives often suggest lovemaking as a sweet way to trigger the beginning of labor. If the mother has a history of premature birth, though, physicians may advise against lovemaking in the last days of the pregnancy (even though most studies have shown that late-pregnancy coitus does not trigger premature delivery).

One study suggests that it may be best to refrain from using the missionary position during the last few weeks of pregnancy. Medical researchers identified 569 women who had given birth to premature babies or whose waters had broken before they were 36 weeks pregnant. These women were then matched with 569 controls (women of similar age and race) who'd given birth to normal, full-term babies. After interviewing them all about their sexual activities during the pregnancy, the researchers found that making love in the missionary position during the last four weeks was the only thing that was significantly associated with premature rupture of the membranes, or premature birth. It's not exactly clear why, they admit, but "a possible explanation is that the pressure placed on the woman and the resultant trauma caused by movements may make this position unsuitable during the later months of pregnancy."

Just because of the practical difficulties of maneuvering around her belly, many couples prefer rear-entry positions (both of you on your knees), or some variation of the "spoons" position (lying side-by-side, with you behind her). Some couples who like making love face-to-face favor using a chair, with her straddling him and using her feet to adjust the depth. Or she can sit on the edge of a bed, legs spread, feet on a chair, while you enter her between her legs.

Birth and Afterward

After the baby is born, couples are generally told to abstain from sex until the six-week checkup—but lots of people ignore the advice. Studies show that 40 to 60 percent of couples don't wait that long.

"After delivery everything is very raw inside the woman, and the tissues need time to heal," Dr. Loret de Mola explains. "The big danger is that bacteria may attach to sperm cells, swim up into the uterus and cause an infection."

One other drawback to resuming intercourse early is pain from her episiotomy (the small incision made to enlarge her vaginal opening during delivery, later closed with stitches). Episiotomies are supposed to heal within three weeks, but sometimes they may be painful as much as four months later, studies have shown.

Studies of sexual behavior after delivery are as variable as those before it. In one study most couples had resumed intercourse six to eight weeks after delivery—though some started in a couple of weeks and others weren't interested even after three months. Other, larger studies have shown that couples' sexual activities often gradually return to previous levels, but this may take a year or more—something many guys are not quite prepared for.

Women who are breastfeeding tend to have very low estrogen levels, Dr. Loret de Mola says, which means intercourse can be painful because of vaginal dryness. Just use a good lubricant, like K-Y Jelly or Astroglide, he advises. Remember that breastfeeding is not a surefire contraceptive—use some kind of birth control while she's breastfeeding, unless you want all your kids spaced nine months apart. Masters and Johnson also found that, right after orgasm, a woman who is breastfeeding may dribble or spurt milk from her nipples, which can add a little drama to an otherwise uneventful evening.

Shortly after delivery, an estimated 50 to 80 percent of women also suffer through a mild, mysterious depression called the baby blues, and depression has a well-known stifling effect on sexual desire. And then, of course, the fear of another pregnancy often puts a damper on things.

VAGINA
What Pleasures Her and What Doesn't

Male-oriented erotica endlessly conjures up violent images of deep vaginal penetration: Swords, daggers, ramrods, scimitars, all plunging hungrily in to the hilt. It's no wonder that lots of guys think this is what satisfies a woman sexually.

But what many men don't realize is that the deep interior walls of the vagina contain very few nerve endings, so they're relatively numb to the touch. The deepest two-thirds of the vagina "is, in fact, a continuation of the uterus," or womb, according to Kermit E. Krantz, M.D., professor of obstetrics and gynecology at the University of Kansas

School of Medicine in Kansas City. And the uterus, being an internal organ, has about as much tactile responsiveness as your kidney (which is not much).

By contrast, the outer third of the vagina, including the entrance (or introitus), the labia (the folds of skin that surround the vaginal opening) and the clitoris, tend to be wildly responsive. In a series of famous experiments arranged by the late Dr. Alfred C. Kinsey and colleagues, five gynecologists using a device similar to a cotton swab gently touched 16 points in the genitals of about 800 women, including the deep walls of the vagina, the introitus, labia and clitoris. Less than 14 percent of them could even feel it when the probe touched the interior of their vaginas. But when the probe touched the clitoris, labia or anywhere else around the vaginal opening, 97 percent were "distinctly conscious" of the touch, Dr. Kinsey reported.

Even so, more recent researchers have reported that many women do find deep vaginal penetration incredibly pleasurable, triggering a "deep" orgasm that seems different than clitoral ones. The source of these sensations is still not exactly clear—whether it's the deep muscles of the pelvic floor, uterine contractions or the G-spot. Some researchers have even suggested that the cervix (the bulblike opening of the uterus, at the deep end of the vagina) contains nerve endings that respond to deep thrusting, producing a kind of "cervical orgasm."

Of course, don't forget that the vagina is designed to serve two functions: sexual pleasure and reproduction. William H. Masters, M.D., and Virginia E. Johnson, of the former Masters and Johnson Institute in St. Louis, point out that the vagina is tipped inward at a 10-to 15-degree angle partly because it's designed as a receptacle for semen. If it were tilted the other way, the spawn of civilization would spill out. It's also been suggested that men love deep thrusting so much because nature's secret intention is to get semen planted as deep inside the vagina as possible, to improve the odds of pregnancy.

Maybe we're all just helpless pawns of that cosmic longing of sperm for egg.

A Potential Space

Another misconception guys tend to have is the idea that the vagina is a tunnel, a cave or some other kind of hollow space. (The word vagina, also misleading, actually means "sheath.")

But in its normal, unstimulated state, Masters and Johnson have reported, the vagina is "a potential rather than an actual space"—its soft, moist walls of muscle—in some ways similar to the mouth—are collapsed together, like folds of cloth. It's only after she starts to become sexually aroused that the deepest two-thirds of her vagina begin to open up, expanding like a balloon, growing dramatically deeper and wider.

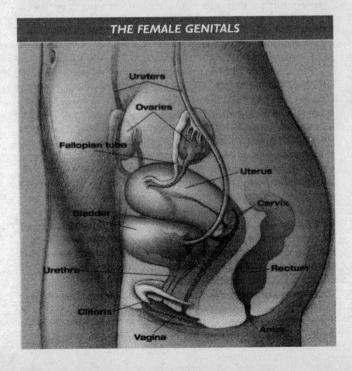

THE FEMALE GENITALS

Ureters
Ovaries
Fallopian tube
Uterus
Bladder
Cervix
Urethra
Rectum
Clitoris
Anus
Vagina

During arousal the cervix also pulls up and back, out of harm's way. (Though if a woman has a retroverted or tipped uterus, the cervix stays where it is, suspended in this ever-widening vaginal cavity—where the man's penis may batter it, sometimes painfully, during intercourse.)

If you enter her too quickly, she may feel uncomfortable at first—but once she's fully aroused, the average woman's vagina has expanded so dramatically it can accommodate virtually any size penis (yes, even yours), Masters and Johnson found. The vagina's capacity for expansion is amazing (after all, it's designed to accommodate a newborn baby's head). In fact, this "ballooning" is sometimes so extreme that it may feel like you're making love to a cavern. Women, especially those who've given birth vaginally, also sometimes complain that it feels like their lover's penis is "lost in the vagina."

Naturally, some men find it more pleasurable to make love to a woman whose vagina is fairly tight. If your penis is not getting the stimulation you need because of the size of her vagina, consider gently suggesting she try Kegel exercises. One guy who posted to a computer bulletin board commented: "Gentlemen, any and all women can have as tight a vagina as they wish. Kegels are a vaginal-muscle tightening exercise that all can do, and they definitely work. My wife (after our son's birth) started doing the exercises, and we have fantastic results. In some positions she can literally 'spit' me out at will. When she comes, the natural contractions that occur during her orgasm are strong and usually send me over the edge within seconds."

On the other hand, of course, just as penises and noses and hands vary from person to person, so do vaginas. In the medieval Indian love manual *Ananga-Ranga*, in fact, women are divided into three classes, according to the depth and extent of their "yonis," or vaginas. The "Deer-woman" has a yoni six fingers deep; the "Mare-woman," nine fingers deep and the "Elephant-woman"—who has large breasts, fierce eyes and "a wicked and utterly shameless disposition"—is twelve fingers deep.

She also never forgets a thing.

Lubrication: An Unreliable Guide

Within 30 seconds after stimulation begins, the vagina begins to lubricate. Little beads of fluid form all over the vaginal walls, making them look almost like a sweat-beaded forehead. The little beads rapidly spread to form a smooth, glistening covering. Many men don't realize that vaginal wetness is not a reliable indicator of whether or not a woman is turned on. Female lubrication is linked to female sex hormone levels, and fluctuations in these hormones—along with many other things—can sometimes make it difficult for a woman to get wet naturally, even if she's sexually aroused. It's also linked to aging: Older women often have trouble producing adequate vaginal lubrication for sex.

At other times, when she's not aroused, her vagina produces secretions that are colorless, odorless and slightly acidic (pH 3.5 to 4.5), according to Rudi Ansbacher, M.D., professor of obstetrics and gynecology at the University of Michigan Medical School in Ann Arbor. These secretions are formed from vaginal "sweating," mucus produced by the cervix and cells shed by the vaginal walls. Their acidity makes the vaginal environment hostile to bacteria that don't belong there—though male semen, with a pH of around 7 (neutral), has a "buffering" effect, which helps to neutralize the vagina's acidity, on a woman's vagina that lasts for hours after intercourse.

A clean, healthy woman's vagina hardly smells at all (sex odors are caused by hormonal secretions outside the vagina), and its sweet secretions do not cause itching, burning, irritation or soiling of her underwear, according to Dr. Ansbacher. If her vaginal secretions have an unpleasant odor or if there's discharge, soreness, irritation or itching, she may have an infection like chlamydia or a yeast infection, which she could in turn pass on to you.

Vaginismus

Another problem that may occasionally develop is vaginismus—an involuntary spasm of the muscles surrounding the vagina. This ring of muscles may clamp down so tightly that penetration (by a penis, tampon or anything else) is virtually impossible, and sex is out of the question. Vaginismus may be caused by a past traumatic experience, fear of or distaste for sex, or some physical injury that makes penetration painful.

It's not really all that uncommon, actually—it's the third most common female sexual dysfunction, after lack of orgasm and painful intercourse, according to Emmanual Fliegelman, D.O., professor of obstetrics/gynecology and director of the Human Sexuality Programs at the Osteopathic Medical Center of Philadelphia.

The good news is that vaginismus treatment has one of the highest success rates (nearly 100 percent) of all sexual problems. Basically, treatment involves counseling and relaxation exercises, followed by gentle insertion of a hard plastic "vaginal dilator," which is gradually increased in size. Husbands, of course, are also affected by this closing of the gates of heaven, and many develop erectile problems as a result. That's why therapists like to involve both partners in the cure.

VIRGINITY
Why Men Care about It

When a man loses his virginity, who's to know? There's no physical evidence, no bloodstained sheets, no pain. It's an event almost as ill-defined as "becoming a man." You're never quite sure it really happened, or when or sometimes even how.

The whole business is so murky that, historically, virginity has been a term applied mainly to women. Because for a woman, losing it is generally a more clear-cut, tangible affair. The first time a penis penetrates her vagina is often memorialized with blood, pain or both. That's from the rupturing of her hymen, a fibrous membrane that may partly or completely cover the opening of her vagina. Still, it's hard to know quite what to expect: Women's hymens are extremely variable, gynecologists have found. In some women it may be nearly nonexistent; in others, quite thin and flexible, like cellophane covering the mouth of a jar, or so thick it bleeds profusely when broken.

In most women the hymen begins gradually disappearing by a natural process shortly after birth, so that "lack of blood on the honeymoon sheets or a pain-free first intercourse does not mean that a woman has had sexual intercourse before," according to June M. Reinisch, Ph.D., former director of the Kinsey Institute for Research in Sex, Gender and Reproduction in Bloomington, Indiana.

Things may go smoothly for you not because she's already met Mr. Right, but because nature has paved the way for you.

The Lord's Right

Down through history, cultures all over the world have placed extraordinary value on a woman's virginity at marriage. Newly married Kurdish tribesmen, for instance, will often triumphantly display a sheet stained with blood to demonstrate that their brides were untouched before they came to the altar, according to Reay Tannahill in her wonderful romp of a book, *Sex in History*. (A male's virginity at the altar is usually a matter of considerably less concern—the double standard goes way, way back.)

Many societies have even figured out the exact, dollars-and-cents market value of a bride's virginity. According to ancient Chaldean and Jewish law, if a virgin strayed from the straight and narrow, the husband, father or fiancé had to be compensated for the woman's "depreciation in value."

Virginity has also been greatly valued by men who were not exactly looking for an unblemished bride. In London during the Victorian era there were actually "virgin" brothels, which had their own doctors who issued certificates of authenticity to customers who asked for untouched women. Naturally, this led to a whole new cottage industry: the production of fake "virgins," who could simulate a wedding night hemorrhage by slipping a bloodsoaked sponge into their vaginas, or simulate a virginal vagina by tightening themselves up with an astringent such as myrrh water or vinegar. In fact, says Tannahill, in some brothels professional "virgins" were tightened up several times a week.

As recently as the 1950s, in fact, some gynecologists in the United States were still performing a minor surgical procedure known as the lover's knot—putting several stitches in the labia of young women who were engaged but deflowered. On her wedding night when the stitches were broken, a newly-minted virgin would feel pain and bleed—and hopefully convince her husband that he was her one and only.

At various times in history the conquest of virgins has been so highly prized that it was actually reserved for kings. *Droit de signeur*, or lord's right—a practice that dates back to Sumerian times and was still in vogue in Europe up until the twelfth century—meant that if you were a king or a feudal landlord, you had the legal right to bed a virgin bride before her own husband did. In other cultures the lord was a lord indeed—not a fleshly man but a god. In ancient Rome before a marriage was consummated, the bride would sometimes lower herself onto the sculptured stone phallus of a fertility god before she went to bed with her new husband.

Even so, if she hands you the old fertility god line, take it with a grain of salt.

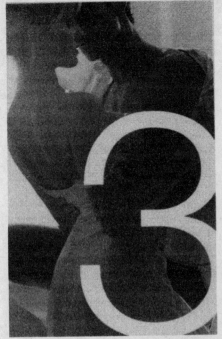

GOOD HEALTH, GOOD SEX

BODY IMAGE
How We Think about How We Look

It's a given: Women are unhappy with the way they look.
Even when we sweetly disagree with them. They're practically entitled to complain—it almost seems part of their
femininity. Or so the old stereotype goes.

Men are supposed to be the opposite. We don't bother
worrying about the way we look. We're practically entitled
to be oblivious. It's part of our big-palooka charm. Bad
assumptions. Fact is, many men are unhappy with the shape
they're in. Literally.

A psychologist at Old Dominion University in Norfolk,
Virginia, Thomas F. Cash, Ph.D., made a huge survey of
people's body images. He got over 30,000 replies, from men
and women both, and found a lot of unhappiness out there.
Two out of five women express what he calls a wholesale
dissatisfaction with their body image. (In other words, when
asked "How do you like the way you look?" the answer was
"I don't.") Surprisingly, one out of three men feel just as bad
about themselves. And roughly another one-third of men
express dissatisfaction with a particular feature—their
height, hairline, weight, waistline, that sort of thing. Only 28
percent of men (and 15 percent of women) were content
with their appearance. Happiness is the exception, not the
rule.

In a way, men's discontent is worse. Women are permitted to share their insecurities with each other, and boy, do
they. ("God, I hate my legs." "Are you kidding? Honey, I'd
kill to have those legs!") Psychologists have a label for that
kind of shared complaining: normative discontent. It brings
women together. Most guys, on the other hand, would not
dare to say to the guy at the next locker, "God, I hate my
legs." Not unless they have a deep-seated need to collect
put-downs. They don't even like complaining to themselves
about it; worrying about such things is what weak men do.

"They're upset that they're upset," says Dr. Cash. "They're thinking, 'I'm a wimp.'"

It wasn't always thus. Think of your father's generation. If memory serves you, weren't they awfully cavalier, as a bunch, about their flabby muscles and big guts? And didn't they look like hell? You've sworn not to let yourself get that bad, haven't you? Our point exactly: Men care more about body image these days. We had to start caring around the time that personal image became more of a key to success.

And it's just a theory, mind you, but greater insecurity about body image might be part and parcel of a time when men are feeling insecure about basic gender issues. With the very definition of masculinity now up for grabs, some men get nervous. Some men. Not you, of course.

What Is Sexy? Not What You Think

The big thing to remember, when you're most worried about your ability to wow 'em anymore, is that both men and women judge themselves more harshly than they are judged by the opposite sex. Most women think men want busty, blue-eyed babes. Most men think women will accept nothing less than Fabio. The truth is, both sexes are more forgiving than that. And beauty is in the eye of the beholder—the range of personal preferences is enormous. Or, as Dr. Cash puts it, "It's reassuring to know there are different strokes for different folks."

Not that there isn't a masculine ideal. Several studies over the years have revealed, with remarkable consistency, the average woman's taste in men. What they find most repulsive is the pear-shaped look: small shoulders atop a rear end that's just begging for a big, black-and-yellow "Wide Load" banner. What they crave is the inverse of that: a tapered "V," with broad shoulders, a trim waistline and trim legs. In other words, a guy who's healthy. A guy who's in shape.

Note that their ideal is *not* a big muscle-bound guy. Most women find the heavy-workout look a tad excessive. Instinctively, they arch one eyebrow in suspicion; like Belle in

Beauty and the Beast, they don't want to play the little gal to some self-involved Gaston.

It's still true, of course, that men pay much more attention to a woman's physical attractiveness when choosing a mate. Although women notice what we look like, our physical appearance is just not their first priority. So men may never be as insecure, collectively, as women—who, after all, must face a beauty contest every day of their lives. Nonetheless, if we are more concerned about body image, it follows that we're probably more vulnerable to feelings of inadequacy. We'll have to start being careful not to get into a rut of forever comparing ourselves to male models, the way some women defeat themselves with comparisons to images of female beauty.

One of our survey respondents, a 26-year-old program director for a nonprofit agency, says he got fed up with erotic videos for that very reason. "I am satisfied with my own body," he says, "and not obsessed with being Mr. Muscle-Bound Super Schlong who can hold his partner in the air with huge arms and screw standing up for an hour."

Buff That Image!

If you're among the majority of men who are unhappy with at least some aspect of their body image, you have two choices. You can change the way you look or change the way you think. You can also do a little of both, of course, but we suggest you begin by tackling whichever is more amenable to change.

If you've ever heard a supermodel criticize her own body, you know that what we see in others is not necessarily what they see when they look in the mirror. For them, Dr. Cash has written a book, appropriately titled *What Do You See When You Look in the Mirror?* Early in the book he states his thesis: "Negative body image has little to do with outward appearance; it's a state of mind." Dr. Cash makes the particularly persuasive point that those who suffer from negative body images don't fully realize what they're saying to themselves: "That's pathetic. That's so goofy. I can't believe you're going out like that!" Now imagine if a spouse or friend said that to you. "You'd say, 'I don't need you in my life,' " says Dr. Cash. But we insult ourselves ceaselessly.

Some things we can change, some things we cannot. And as we all know courtesy of Oprah, body weight is highly resistant to change. Most dieters end up replacing their lost pounds—and then some. Dr. Cash says, "I'm offering another alternative for taking control that is not trying to fix your body or make it fit some idealized standard."

For those of you who are determined to make a change and get back in shape, you'll be reassured to know that even a modest improvement can dramatically restore your feelings of sexiness. In a study done by Ronette L. Kolotkin, Ph.D., at Duke University's Diet and Fitness Center in Durham, 64 men and women participated in a one-month weight-loss program. At month's end, they'd lost an average of 20 to 25 pounds and felt better about several aspects of their lives: health, relationships, sexuality, daily activity, mobility and self-esteem.

> The position is ridiculous, the pleasure momentary and the expense damnable.
>
> —Lord Chesterfield on sex

Dr. Kolotkin says that men who are overweight still feel it has less impact, in general, on their quality of life than do women. But that's shifting. When she began working at the Diet and Fitness Center in 1984, she says only 10 percent of the people coming in for help were men. Now it's more like 50 percent. "The change is remarkable," she says. "Men's consciousness has been raised."

Now Let's Bust That Gut

According to Dr. Cash's survey, half of all men are unhappy about their midtorso areas. In plain English: that damn spare tire, the bane of the middle-age male. As we age, we discover, to our dismay, that some of our other goals conflict with fitness—that great job, for instance, that keeps us deskbound 70 hours a week, the hectic travel schedule that confines our leisure time to hotel bars or a great family life that has kept us from seeing the inside of a gym since the Reagan Administration.

The bottom line is that between the ages of 30 and 55 it's common for guys to gain a pound a year. With undue haste, it goes to our waist.

To slim down that blob, you need to hit the trifecta of good health: diet, aerobics and muscle exercises. For easy ways to take fat—but not taste—out of your diet, see Low-Fat Diet on page 177.

Next, you need a general aerobics workout, starting at 20 to 30 minutes three days a week, and increasing if you can to 30 to 40 minutes four to six days a week. Do whatever is most fun: running, racquetball, bicycling, stair-climbing. . . . You name your game.

Finally, stomach exercises are necessary to help you build the muscles in the abdomen. Good muscle tone here can help hold your belly up and in, making you appear thinner even before all the excess weight comes off. Now, we know what you're thinking. You're thinking, "Oh, no, sit-ups. I hate sit-ups!" Sit-ups are the Model T of stomach exercises. We suggest you try these late-model versions.

Don't go nuts, by the way. We're talking 10 to 15 minutes a day, three times a week.

Knee raise: Lie on the floor on your back, arms at your sides, palms down. Slightly raise your knees, pressing the small of your back against the floor. Now raise your head and shoulder blades off the floor. Slowly draw your knees up to your chest, hold for two seconds, then lower your legs back to the floor. Repeat 10 to 15 times.

Knees-up crunch: Lie on your back with your feet flat on the floor and knees raised and bent at a 90-degree angle. Raise your legs until your thighs are perpendicular to your body. Now cross your arms and lift your head and shoulder blades off the floor. Slowly bring your torso toward your knees in a curling motion. Hold for two seconds, lower your torso back to the floor—but keep your head up to sustain tension on your abdominal muscles. Repeat 10 to 15 times.

The bicycle: With your thighs perpendicular to your body,

as in the knees-up crunch, cup your fingertips behind your ears, twist your torso to the left, bring up your left knee and touch it with your right elbow. Then touch your left elbow to your right knee. Your feet will move as if you were pedaling a mountain bike up the side of the Sears Tower. Repeat 20 times, going slowly so that you don't start rocking from side to side and lose your balance.

Frog crunch: Lie on the floor and put the soles of your sneakers together so your knees angle outward. With your fingertips cupped behind your ears, raise your head and shoulders in a forward-curling motion off the floor. Hold for two seconds and lower. Repeat 10 to 15 times.

Double crunch: Lie on your back, feet flat on the floor, fingertips cupped behind your ears. Lift your right foot and rest the heel on your left knee. Raise your left foot off the floor a couple inches. This is the starting position. Slowly curl your head and torso up while bringing your right knee toward your head. Hold for two seconds and return to the starting position. Repeat ten times, then switch leg positions.

Straight-leg crunch: Lie on your back, legs straight and together. Slowly raise your legs until they point toward the ceiling, keeping your knees slightly bent so you don't strain your hamstrings. With your fingertips cupped behind your ears, slowly raise your head and shoulders off the floor, curling forward. (Only your head and shoulders should lift, not your back.) Then slowly lower yourself back to the floor and repeat 10 to 15 times.

EXERCISE
Drop Your Lard and Get Truly Hard

When we surveyed readers of *Men's Health* magazine, we asked them, "In your own life, have you observed any connection between being fit and healthy and having a better sex life?"

Do they ever.

Talk about exercise and sex: Virtually all of the people

who answered our survey say exercise *is* sex. Because they're in shape, their love-making is hotter, more pleasurable and lasts longer. In describing the benefits, both mental and physical, the same words came up, over and over again: Energy. Desire. Performance. Stamina. Endurance. Confidence. Virility. Self-esteem.

These people have found a more proximate reason to get fit than, say, the threat of a coronary bypass in 40 years.

"Now that I think about it, sexuality is probably the single underlying reason for working out," says one 34-year-old public relations man. "Getting pumped. Getting noticed by shapely women in spandex. It's what keeps me returning to the gym on a regular basis."

For some guys the benefits are so immediate, they get horny while working out! "I sometimes wonder if my weight training regimen exercises my libido more than my physique," writes a 31-year-old accountant. "Sometimes during a workout it's hard to focus on any muscle group except the 'one-eyed muscle.'"

Other survey respondents said their workouts left them feeling unaroused and just plain wiped out. But not for long—a couple hours later it's like puberty all over again. In the words of one office supply store manager, "I want it and I want it badly!"

Our survey confirms what more formal studies have also found to be true: Exercise revs up the libido. In the most recent study of this sort, at the University of California, San Diego, 78 sedentary middle-age men (mean age, 48 years) were put through some serious aerobics an hour a day every other day. After nine months they were making love 30 percent more often—and masturbating 50 percent more often. (Alas, their wives were not included in the study.)

So we know that these delightful effects are not merely "anecdotal," to use the word scientists use when they want to scoff at findings. We know exercise works. But we learned much more than that from our talkative survey respondents, whose insights can be summarized in four general points.

The mental benefits are just as important. "Being in

great physical shape provides a mental edge," says a 29-year-old vice president of a corporate image development firm. That mental edge comes in the form of a keener awareness and greater involvement with the world, for one thing. Men talk of feeling more awake, more alive; "I feel more alert," says a 27-year-old electrical engineer. But it's also "a natural ego booster," as another respondent put it. Exercise, they say, makes them feel more "manly," more in control. Says a 45-year-old real estate consultant: "I feel better about myself."

There's no one right exercise for sex. Any exercise regimen will work. Do whatever pops your cork. "After a great run or bike I experience an increased desire to do the wild thing," says a 33-year-old general manager in the food service business. Whereas a 36-year-old musician found his salvation at the gym. "I began a serious weight-lifting, body-building program a year ago," he says. "Sex is getting better and better."

In truth, there are sexual benefits to be gained by both aerobic exercise *and* muscle building. Those who prefer one over the other naturally tout theirs as superior. "Stamina and breath control are far more important than musculature," a 27-year-old electrical engineer insists. While a 26-year-old naval officer warns, "If you're with a lover who needs a long and wild ride to achieve orgasm, you'd better have those butt muscles and lower back muscles in shape." To which we would add: good abdominal muscles for thrusting power and strong shoulders, especially if you like to linger in the missionary position.

Obviously, a well-rounded fitness program is your best bet. We cannot recommend any one exercise for better sex, other than the Kegel. (Learn all about it in the next chapter.) But we want to emphasize that sexual benefits accrue from vigorous workouts. You may have read that health experts say a routine of merely mild activity, like walking or raking leaves, helps protect against the kinds of chronic diseases that can ravage us in later life. We're not quarreling with that. But we're talking about sex, not diabetes and high blood pressure. In the University of California exercise study mentioned above, a "control" group of 17 middle-age men were put on a program of walking an hour a day four days a week. Their sex lives, if anything, diminished over the nine-month time frame. By the end, they were reporting more erection problems and greater failure to achieve orgasms. The 78 aerobicized guys reported exactly the opposite.

For some, exercise is foreplay. "We shower together when we get home to work out our other muscles," says a 21-year-old business law student. A 32-year-old designer seems to have fallen upon the same routine with his partner. "She demands to be entered under the shower," he says. "It's a 'total body workout.'"

A 37-year-old architect doesn't even wait until they hit the shower to get together. He claims he brings his wife to multiple orgasms right on his exercise bench because it's perfect for deep, hard penetration. "She lies down and holds the two vertical supports for the bar bell," he explains. "I stand over her by straddling the bench and am able to push hard and deep. She is able to push by holding the vertical bench supports."

Another couple says a good, long tennis match makes them shout, "Love!"

If you don't work out alongside your sexual partner, all your heavy breathing leads to self-arousal—the 1990s equivalent of riffling through a girlie mag. "When I come home I feel like I could drive nails with my penis," says a 44-year-old chemicals salesman. Part of what makes exercise the right aphrodisiac for these times is that it's non-sexist—it works for women, too. One 29-year-old self-described "stay-at-home mom" who answered our survey says, "After a hard run and a hot shower, sex is truly awesome!"

What's going on here? You'd think a long, hard, exhausting regimen that leaves people in a puddle of sweat would make them beg to be left alone. But on the micro level, it elevates blood levels of endorphins, adrenaline and testosterone, all of which play a part in the brain chemistry of arousal. On the macro level, it chases away stress, making room for more enjoyable feelings. It makes you more aware of your body—and more aware of other bodies. Asked whether he becomes aroused soon after a great workout, a 48-year-old chiropractor says, "It depends mostly on what the women at the gym are wearing."

Being out of shape sacks your love life. We heard from a lot of guys who had been grossly out of shape and had battled their way back to good health. A 31-year-old programmer who put himself through a major makeover, dropping 150 pounds in 1994, says, "My wife swears I'm stiffer. And the belly is out of my way, making for more creative positioning."

Other men who've achieved major weight loss say it's not just the newfound fitness that makes sex better but it is also the improved body image that goes along with the weight loss. They're more confident of their sexuality. They aren't afraid to be naked any longer.

Could exercise actually reverse the waning sexual responsiveness that haunts the aging male? That's what the University of California study concluded, and that's what this 65-year-old retired government nuclear engineer seems to be saying: "Over the past ten years I've never been healthier and more fit, and my sex life has been the best it ever has."

A 55-year-old high school biology teacher also tells us that sex doesn't have to flicker with age. "Some years ago, a long summer of beer and barbecues left me 30 pounds overweight and in terrible condition," he writes. "During sex I tired very easily and somehow seemed to lose touch with what was going on because of cramps in my legs or back, or because I started to worry that I was sweating too much. And my wife began to complain that I was too heavy. It took me quite a few months to get back in shape and lose most of that 30 pounds, but in terms of sexuality it has been more than worth it."

Let's end with this testimonial from a 39-year-old radiology technologist.

"I had back surgery three times and was plagued by a lack of sex drive and stamina. This cost me the relationship I was in at that time. Two years later, after becoming disgusted with myself (and my increasing waist size), I set out to regain the 31-inch waist I had prior to my back injury. At first I had increased back pain and sciatica. After a month or so the pain decreased. Now, years later, I still have back pain occasionally—but I have my 31-inch waist back, I can do anything I want, I am very active in youth sports management and coaching, my body fat measures 16 percent versus the 40 percent I once carried and I went from a copulation time of five minutes to hours of passionate lovemaking. Exercise, working out with weights, diet and dietary supplements have saved my life mentally, physically and sexually."

If that doesn't inspire you couch potatoes, nothing will.

KEGELS
How to Exercise Your Love Muscle

In our *Men's Health* magazine survey we asked the readers if they have discovered anything that helped them achieve more than one orgasm during a single session of lovemaking—and how they learned to do that. One 32-year-old stockbroker replied, "It's not so much a learned thing as much as it is one's own ability. I've learned to prolong orgasms by stopping a good urination stream in midstream."

All by his lonesome, apparently, this fellow has stumbled across the Kegel exercise.

The exercise is named after Arnold Kegel, M.D., a gynecologist who practiced in suburban Los Angeles during the 1940s and 1950s. Like any gynecologist, he had postpartum patients who lost urine when they coughed or sneezed or laughed. This common condition, which is caused by pelvic muscles that are stretched out or even torn by childbirth, is called urinary stress incontinence. In Dr. Kegel's time the condition was usually treated by surgery (the muscles were cut and retied, in the hope that a lump of resulting scar tissue would provide more clamping power). But Dr. Kegel had a better idea. He taught women to strengthen their pelvic muscles—specifically, a group of muscles called the pubococcygeal muscle group. The formal name is such a mouthful doctors call it the PC muscle for short.

Dr. Kegel taught his patients to exercise their PC muscles via repetitive contractions (the way we exercise any muscle). He knew that stronger PC muscles would hold urine better. But what started out as better bladder control soon revealed itself to be a major development in better sex. Dr. Kegel soon discovered that the women who developed stronger PC muscles not only got over their stress incontinence but were having more and better orgasms. In some cases women were reaching orgasms for the first time.

Both men and women have PC muscles, but in America in the 1950s and 1960s you never heard them talked about, even in impolite conversation. Dr. Kegel's breakthrough was nearly lost to obscurity. It wasn't until the late 1970s, with that era's openness about sexuality and especially female sexuality, that Dr. Kegel's work resurfaced. Finally in 1982 the "Kegel exercise" was introduced to a mass audience with the publication of *The G Spot and Other Recent Discoveries about Human Sexuality*, by Alice K. Ladas, Ph.D., Beverly Whipple, Ph.D., and John D. Perry, Ph.D.

In a nutshell, here are the specific sexual benefits that accrue with Kegel exercises. Women with strong PC muscles say they get sexually aroused more easily, lubricate faster, have more and better orgasms and may achieve orgasm from G-spot stimulation alone. Men who do Kegels find that they have more intense orgasms and sometimes multiple orgasms. It also helps to curb premature ejaculation and it shortens the recovery time between orgasms.

That's been said before, but the respondents to our surveys said it again. "Since performing Kegel exercises," says a 51-year-old accountant, "I enjoy longer and more intense orgasms almost continually without ejaculation during foreplay," even though that can involve oral and manual stimulation from his wife. And a 33-year-old firefighter says, "By working on my PC muscle, my erections at times will enable me to continue until I climax again."

Squeeze, Please

The PC muscle forms a "floor" at the base of the pelvis, helping to keep our internal organs from sagging. "Imagine a hammock," says one of the authors of *The G Spot*, Dr. John D. Perry. "The PC muscle looks like a hammock with three holes in it: one for the urethra, one for the anus and in the case of women one for the vagina." In animals this muscle wags the tail. In the female of our species, it is stretched and

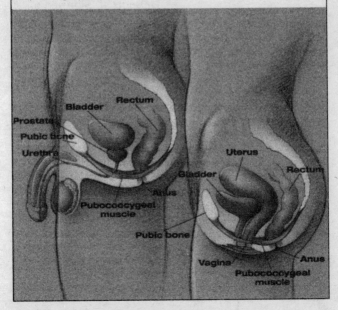

THE KEGEL MUSCLE

In both men and women the urethra and rectum pass right through the pubococcygeal muscle. By constricting it, both sexes can cut off the flow through those tubes. For men Kegels are the key to orgasm control.

weakened by the carrying and delivery of babies—a burden, says Dr. Perry, that was borne by our more powerful abdominals before we began walking upright. Kegel exercises are taught regularly in childbirth classes to help women ease the trauma of delivery and shorten their recoveries.

But knowing its location is not enough. To find it, you have to move it. In other words, the first step in doing Kegels is learning to *isolate* the PC, moving that muscle and no other. Lucky for us, this is one activity where it's still advantageous to be a guy. "It is easier for men to learn Kegels," says Dr. Perry. "It's just so easy to see when you're doing it."

> I learned a little exercise during my visits to a childbirthing class. I call it a pelvic quickie. You tighten your muscle as if you were trying to stop urinating . . . contract and hold for as long as possible, start by holding the contraction for 5 seconds— then repeat about 10 times. See if you can work up to a hold of 15 to 20 seconds with about 6 to 12 per set. Trust me, I have no reason to lie to you, *it works*!
>
> —Survey respondent, age 35, in Ohio

All you do is imitate our 32-year-old stockbroker friend: Stop your urine in midstream. This not only teaches you to find it but gets you going on the exercise itself. Stop and restart your urination five times during every trip you make to the men's room. (Okay, maybe you don't want to do this during halftime at a football stadium.) For some men this first step is easy. Others may need to work on this a while because their PCs are particularly weak.

Once you can do this for several days with ease, you'll be ready for the next phase. You can skip the bathroom trips, which may be unseemly long by now, and you can start doing your Kegels anytime, anywhere. Every time you stop at a red light, for instance. You'll learn to contract the muscle for a count of 3. Then a count of 10. Then, by the end of six weeks you'll be contracting for 20 seconds at a time. Some sex therapists call that the Super Kegel. Maybe you call that excessive.

Fine. The point is, you want to squeeze your PC on a daily, systematic basis. If you get so good you're doing 100, 200, 300 contractions a day, that's okay. Just remember: As with any exercise, you should start out gradually so you don't hurt yourself.

Here's a second way to see your PC power at work. This has been called the towel trick. Drape a handkerchief over your erect penis. Can you raise and lower it at will? Good. Now do it with a washcloth. If you can raise and lower it, try a small towel. If you can still make it move up and down, you've been workin' your Kegels, pal.

Do Kegels sound too good to be true? After all, how could one inconspicuous little muscle do so much good for a man's sex life? We asked Dr. Perry that question, and here's his explanation: "Notice where the PC muscle is. The penis passes right through that hole in the hammock. Now, when the PC muscle is contracted, it pulls the base of the penis up against the prostate. The effect of that is to increase prostate stimulation, which is responsible for the emission phase of orgasm, the phase that gets the juices into your tubes. Then in the expulsion phase of orgasm the PC muscle contracts and you ejaculate." In other words, a stronger PC muscle gives you greater sensation during both phases of orgasm, especially the ejaculation phase, which is produced in part by the PC muscle's rhythmic contractions.

> I want you to do Kegels in the car—not while driving! And I want you to look over at the people in the car next to you ... and wink.
>
> —Dr. Ruth Westheimer

But how would that affect premature ejaculation? "My theory is Kegels help simply by increasing awareness of that muscle," says Dr. Perry. "With premature ejaculation, a major problem is that men aren't aware of how rapidly they're coming to a climax." Men can recognize their point of ejaculatory inevitability, that is, the time after which ejaculation can't be stopped, says E. Douglas Whitehead, M.D., associate clinical professor of urology at Mount Sinai

School of Medicine of the City University of New York and co-director of the Association for Male Sexual Dysfunction, both in New York City. If they learn to do the Kegels just before that point, they can slow down their sexual excitement, which delays ejaculation. Men can learn to do this several times during each love-making session. For more on this, see Lasting Longer on page 281.

Now You Can Help Her

Women can isolate their PC muscles by stopping urination, just like we can. But they cannot see it at work, the way we can wag our joysticks under handkerchiefs and the like. Nor can they move it and feel that movement while masturbating, as we can. So, if your partner is having trouble isolating her PC muscle, it might be in both your interests to help her find it.

If she's willing. Don't start nagging her about this, okay?

You can actually see her muscle working by watching her perineum, the span of skin between her genitals and anus. Ask her to alternately pull up (as if holding in urine) and push out (as if moving her bowels). You should be able to see the surface of her perineum move in and out. If she's unabashed about this rather clinical activity, you can show her with a mirror.

Now you're both going to feel her PC at work. Insert a finger in her vagina. Slowly, half an inch at a time, move your finger toward her cervix while she flexes the muscle at each stop. Underneath the spongy tissue you should be able to feel the muscle, and perhaps determine its thickness. A weak PC is pencil-thin; a strong one can be as much as three fingers thick. When you feel you've located it, try the "two-finger test." Insert two fingers and open them like a pair of scissors. Have your partner tighten her muscle. If she's been doing her Kegels, she'll be able to squeeze your fingers together. If not, she could use the exercise.

If she has difficulty isolating her PC muscle, even with your help, there's still hope. A sex therapist can help her isolate and develop the PC.

One final note: Kegels will gradually enable a woman to tighten her PC during coitus. Some men find that frightening—they imagine a castrating vulva. Other men say it's like discovering the thrill of *l'amour* all over again.

LOW-FAT DIET
How Healthy Food Helps Erections

Most mornings, Joseph Khoury runs a couple of miles, or in the late afternoon he may swim half an hour to blow off stress. He gets more exercise than most guys, but what he's really fanatical about is his low-fat diet. Forget substituting olive oil for butter: "I've tried to cut out oil, period," he says. "I use white wine for cooking. I use those no-stick sprays." He relies on *Cooking Light* magazine for a constant source of new recipes.

Then again, Khoury's job isn't like most guys'. He's associate professor of urology and the medical director of urophysiology at the University of North Carolina at Chapel Hill. He has expertise in the mechanics of maleness. He knows what a high-fat diet does to an erection, sooner or later. "Men who have a high-fat diet have a higher chance of getting clogged arteries, so to speak, and that impedes blood flow to the penis, just as it impedes blood flow to the heart," he says. "With a low-fat diet, your chances of impotence are lower." E. Douglas Whitehead, M.D., associate clinical professor of urology at Mount Sinai School of Medicine of the City University of New York and co-director of the Association for Male Sexual Dysfunction, both in New York City, goes a step farther. He tells his patients over age 50 that just like a heart attack, they can get a "penis attack"—permanent impotence—if too much gunk clogs the arteries of the penis. That, he says, usually makes the point about diet.

The causes of impotence are incompletely understood, and only a few studies have correlated its onset with fat in the arteries. But those few studies are rather convincing. In one of the latest, doctors examined 3,250 middle-age men who'd come in for preventive checkups at the Cooper Clinic in Dallas. The patients whose total blood cholesterol measured 240 (that's high) had an 80 percent increase in the risk of impotence over those men whose cholesterol reading was 180. Further, those men who had lots of the "good" kind of cholesterol (high-density lipoprotein, or HDL) in their blood—a reading over 60—were at one-third the risk of those men who had abnormally little HDL—a reading of 30 or less. "These results suggest that the present diet or physical activity programs for preventing cardiovascular disease . . . may also lower the prevalence of erectile dysfunction," the researchers concluded in the *American Journal of Epidemiology*.

Add to that benefit the maintenance of a better body shape and you have a pretty good sexual argument for refusing that third helping of scalloped potatoes. This isn't the sort of thing Jenny Craig talks about; let's just say it's our dirty little secret.

The big problem with a low-fat diet, of course, is that men tend to crave high-fat foods. In one study women were found to crave sweets over high fat entrées, two to one, while men craved high-fat entrées over sweets, two to one. Women dismiss our hankering for steak 'n' eggs as just a macho thing, but the gender difference in food cravings shows up in lab animals, too. Because we have more muscle mass, we have a biological interest in getting the protein we need to build strong bodies.

Too often, that interest goes overboard. One in three Americans is overweight. You know all about the more general health problems that go along with obesity, but you may not know that those problems affect men disproportionately. "In general, weight is more dangerous for men than for women," says Ronette L. Kolotkin, Ph.D., of Duke University's Diet and Fitness Center in Durham, North Carolina. And although the simple answer is dieting, the vast majority of diets fail because people eventually go off their diets and gain back all the weight they lost. The only real dieting solution is to make permanent changes in the way you live and eat. "I tell both men and women," says Dr. Kolotkin, "figure out what's livable for you for the rest of your life."

There must be 50 ways to leave your blubber, but we'll give you just 20 to get you started. These are minor changes, which is good. But they can add up to major weight loss over time, which is also good.

A key point: It isn't always necessary to reduce the amount of calories you consume each day to lose weight. You merely have to reduce the percentage of your calories that come from fat. Why? It takes very little effort for fat to get digested and absorbed into your body, while proteins and carbohydrates take lots more calories to process. So equal caloric amounts of bacon and cereal, for example, will yield far different amounts of stored energy (that is, fat) in your body.

The following tips are designed not to sacrifice taste, and in most cases you won't notice the fat you're not eating unless you're some sort of gourmand or something. Say, aren't you the guy who keeps a stash of Twinkies in his desk? You're no gourmand.

For Breakfast

1. It's the egg yolks that kill your waistline, not the whites. If you want a three-egg omelet, use one whole egg and two egg whites. You'll be saving yourself ten grams of fat. If the taste difference is too great, start with two whole eggs and one white. Work the same magic with French toast.

2. If you love bacon, switch to Canadian bacon. Two medium slices contain 4 grams of fat, compared to 9.4 grams in three pieces of regular bacon. Maybe it'll help your hockey game.

3. Pop a pancake in your toaster instead of frying it in your pan. Aunt Jemima Low-Fat Pancakes are just 1.5 grams of fat per stack of three, instead of the 6 grams that come in regular pancakes. Then cover 'em in real maple syrup instead of that corn syrup stuff you use now.

4. Lighten your coffee with evaporated skim milk instead of half-and-half. It's creamy because it has less water, not more fat. Savings: 3.5 grams of fat.

For Lunch

5. When ordering a sandwich, keep in mind this hierarchy of lunch-meat health: turkey and chicken, roast beef, ham, processed meats like salami, olive loaf. Okay, you're at the deli counter and you're trying to decide between a roast beef sandwich and an Italian sub with cheese and mixed cold cuts. Answer: "I'll take the roast beef sandwich, please." Fat savings: 30 percent.

6. When selecting ham, "extra lean" or "reduced fat" contains half the fat of regular ham.

7. For a less-greasy grilled cheese sandwich don't fry it in butter. Instead, toast the bread first, then slip in some reduced-fat Cheddar between the slices and microwave on high for 25 seconds. Fat savings: eight grams. Time savings: 10 or 15 minutes, including cleanup.

8. Slather on the mustard the way you used to slather on the mayo. More taste, far less fat.

For Dinner

9. Men barbecue. That's what we do. And as it turns out, that's a much better way to cook, fat-wise, than being your own short-order chef.

10. When it comes to red meat, choose leaner cuts, like "loin" and "round." A top round steak contains 8.4 grams of fat per six-ounce serving, whereas a six-ounce rib eye contains 20 grams. Replace fat with flavor. That's why man invented marinades.

11. Always trim visible fat from meats before cooking. You can easily knock off half the fat right off the bat.

12. Go on a seafood diet. No, not the "I see food, I eat it" diet, yuk-yuk, but a diet with more shellfish. Clams, crabs, shrimp, oysters and scallops got a bad rap as high cholesterol foods a few years ago, but scientists are now saying their *mea culpas*. Shellfish are low in fat, free of saturated fat and loaded with beneficial omega-3 fatty acids. They'll stay that way when broiled, grilled,

steamed, blackened or baked. But serve them in a pool of melted butter and you're backtracking.

13. When sautéeing, be sure the oil in your pan is heated before adding food. Cold oil tends to soak into meats and vegetables.

14. In a fowl mood? White meat contains about one-third less fat than dark meat.

15. When grilling chicken, try this fat-free marinade: three cups apple juice, two cloves pressed garlic, one cup low-salt soy sauce.

16. Nobody's trying to take your weenie roast away from you, but try the new reduced-fat variety. Ball Park Lite brand has 12 grams per hot dog, which is better than the 17 grams packed into most doggies. Turkey franks have 9 grams—but they can be a little trickier to cook. No dietary penalty for gobs of mustard and ketchup.

For Dessert

17. Substitute nonfat frozen yogurt for ice cream and save more than seven grams of fat per single-scoop cone. Make sure it's nonfat; some frozen yogurts have as much fat as ice cream, and what's the point of that?

18. Angel food cake has no fat. Top off a huge slice with fresh fruit and a scoop of nonfat frozen yogurt.

Snack Time

19. Pretzels are better than chips. As in 8 percent of calories from fat, rather than 58 percent. Even pork rinds are lower in fat than potato chips!

20. Beware the bowl of mixed nuts; 80 percent of the calories come from fat. Unshelled nuts are better. They are lower in fat, plus you spend so much time getting them out of their shells, you eat less.

Faster! Lighter!

It takes roughly ten half-hour lovemaking sessions to lose one pound, according to Dr. Whitehead. That's based on using up about 200 calories in a "very active" sexual encounter. "That's a weight-loss program that's hard to say no to," the good doctor notes.

MUSCLES
Strength Is Good, Obsession Isn't

Men are supposed to be strong—and the stronger, the manlier. We have bigger muscles than women because we have all that testosterone floating around in our bloodstreams. They bulk up our gender identity.

Okay, granted this is the post-industrial age, and muscles have undergone more devaluation than the Mexican peso; whether you can tote that barge or lift that bale is no longer a matter of survival. Women don't view rippling deltoids as a sure sign of a good provider. But most women still admire a well-built man. Just as most men admire a well-built woman. All those delicious curves along her shoulders, her thighs, her calves? Muscles.

To the extent that sex is a physical activity, being strong and in shape will allow you to go through its motions with grace and ease, with relaxation and confidence. Mentally and physically, you feel more alive, energetic and sexier. It's not muscles alone, but a combination of strength and aerobic fitness that results in being perfectly ready for love—at least that's what our survey respondents told us. As they also told us, nothing is worse than being grossly out of shape and getting easily fatigued. Great sex doesn't have to be an athletic event, of course, and bulging muscles aren't essential. The average lovemaking session uses only about as much energy as walking up two flights of stairs. But if you're climbing a stairway to heaven, you'll be needing extra stamina.

The more toned your muscles, the more pleasure you'll get from the total-body contraction that occurs during the crescendo to orgasm, and the release afterward. (And you will not be as sore the next day.) When William H. Masters, M.D., and Virginia E. Johnson, of the former Masters and Johnson Institute, were busy watching hundreds of men and women achieve more than 10,000 orgasms in their St. Louis laboratory, they saw, time after time, the act of lovemaking gather into its climax virtually every muscle in the body. This buildup of muscle tension, "obvious from forehead to toes," they promptly tagged with a clinical label: myotonia. In their book, *Human Sexual Response*, it was worth a chapter unto itself. During orgasm, if it's a good bed-creaking orgasm, most people aren't aware that their muscles are contracting spastically, but the next day they might notice that their muscles ache. Well, no wonder, said Masters and Johnson: "In response to effective sexual stimulation individuals may accomplish feats of muscular coordination that would be unattainable in sexually unstimulated states."

Good Muscles for All

These delights are not the sole domain of virile young men who don't know how good they have it. Every man can attain more muscle power. In 1989 scientists at the Noll Physiological Research Center at Pennsylvania State University in University Park conducted a study to determine the effects of weight lifting on the very, very old. Their oldest participant in the study was a 96-year-old dentist who lived in a nearby nursing home. The men in the study increased their muscle strength by more than 200 percent.

When the study was over, the dentist wouldn't leave. "He ended up working out with us once or twice a week for the next four or five years," recalls center director William J. Evans, Ph.D. The man kept pumping until he died—at the age of 101.

Old age withers everything, including our muscles, but Dr. Evans thinks our muscles don't have to decline nearly as rapidly as we let them. Aging men get into a vicious circle—

the less they exercise, the more muscle tissue they lose. The more muscle tissue they lose, the more fat they store from fewer calories. The more fat they store, the more sedentary they get.

And you thought the most important function of muscles was to be able to open the new jar of relish. Hmmm, not quite. What bigger muscles do for you is help to maintain a stable metabolic rate by burning calories faster, even when you're parked in Sofa City. Extra muscle mass means increased metabolic rate, and that means extra calorie burning. In fact, when Dr. Evans's lab put men ages 56 to 80 on a thrice-a-week strength-training program, the men had to eat 15 percent more calories just to maintain their weight. If that training program were a diet pill, it would be hailed as a miracle by every tabloid in the supermarket.

Extra calorie burning means a better body image, more sexual self-confidence—and a younger you. "The loss of muscle is at the root of many age-related problems we've seen," Dr. Evans says, "including risk for chronic diseases such as heart disease and diabetes." You wouldn't get those diseases if your body didn't store so much fat, and you wouldn't store so much fat if you had more muscle, which sucks up calories before they're converted to lard. "Although the metabolic rate does go down with age," he says, "it's not age per se that's the culprit, it's declining muscle mass."

Too Much of a Good Thing

Let's review, then. Muscles keep you looking and feeling your sexiest. They help keep your weight down and your arteries clean. You'll have more power from your engine, more gas in your tank and a bigger smile after the last mile.

But—to stretch this metaphor to its limit—you can lose control.

"There's a downside, too," says Bryant Stamford, Ph.D., the director of the Health Promotion Center at the University of Louisville. "The harder you train, the less time and energy you have for other physically demanding activities, like sex."

You might expect an exercise physiologist to encourage more and more exercise; you may think it just keeps on improving your sex life. Not at all. Not only is there "no huge spillover effect," he says, but beyond a certain point, exercise begins to affect your sex life adversely. "Think of it as a bell-shaped curve. If you're totally out of shape, sex is going to be more of an ordeal than a pleasure." Your sex life will improve with more fitness as you go up the one side of the curve to the top, where you get the best of both worlds. Up there is the optimum: Your weight's in check, you exercise pretty much daily, maybe you do a little weight training—and you can enjoy a lively session between the sheets. As Dr. Stamford puts it, "You're a classically balanced person."

> Someday he'll come along, the man I love. And he'll be big and strong . . .
>
> —Billie Holiday

Go beyond that, however, and you begin to develop what Dr. Stamford calls "a compulsively driven fitness fetish. That kind of person is setting goals for himself. He's feeling the need to conserve his energy. He approaches sex thinking, 'How is that going to impact my workout tomorrow?' He's going to put his workout ahead of his sexual performance—so he's going to have a headache."

Men who want more and more and more muscle don't know when to stop. It's almost like our version of anorexia. Beyond a certain point these guys lose friends and family, and their appeal to the opposite sex. They have no time or energy for anything or anyone who doesn't help them add more muscle mass. They worry about themselves. Nothing else matters.

Anyone in danger of getting drawn into the musclehead subculture should read *Muscle: Confessions of an Unlikely Bodybuilder* by Sam Fussell. It's good reading as well for those of us who've felt insecure all these years for not looking like Charles Atlas or Arnold Schwarzenegger. How reassuring to learn that body-builders are even more insecure than we are! But more startling, when you rip back the curtain, is this revelation: The masculine ideal is awfully unhealthy.

At the age of 26, Fussell was a tall, skinny, slouched-over son of two English professors who had graduated from Oxford. He was working in New York City, terrified of its streets and the crazies who populated them, and he decided that working out would give him some armor. Two years and 50 pounds later he was moving to Southern California, the mecca of the bodybuilding scene. There he joined a gym and lived the life: squats, deadlifts and bench presses, a diet of baby food and protein powder and distilled water and supplements by the bucket. Finally, he was ready to enter a local competition. Two days before it, he appraised himself in the gym's mirror.

> In modern paintings of India and Japan, as well as in the splendid ivory works that decorated the golden throne of the King of Tanjora of the fifteenth century, I have seen the most curious and daring erotic positions, making me believe that all people of the earth have strained their fantasy in the invention of new kinds of voluptuousness.
>
> —Italian anthropologist Paolo Mantegazza in *Sexual Relations of Mankind*, 1932

"The mirror did not lie. I had effected a most extraordinary mutation. The man staring back at me was, unquestionably, a bodybuilder. With the reduction of my waistline and the tightening of my abdominal muscles, my chest looked twice its normal size. Veins covered my thighs and chest like cobwebs. Thanks to my diet, my skin was thinner than airmail paper. And with my varnish, I was browner than a buried pharaoh. 'I've done it,' I thought to myself. 'I've actually done it.'

"Then why did I feel so awful? Thanks to the rigors of my training, my hands were more ragged, callused and cut than any longshoreman's. Thanks to the drugs and my diet, I couldn't run 20 yards without gasping for air. My ass cheeks ached from innumerable steroid injections, my stomach whined for sustenance, my whole body throbbed from gym activities and enforced weight loss. Thanks to the competition tan, my skin was breaking out everywhere. Vinnie and Nimrod explained that all this was perfectly normal."

"What, do you think this has anything to do with health?" Nimrod asked, shaking in mirth at the idea.

He entered that competition and another. Then, four years after first walking into a New York City YMCA, he left bodybuilding. Within four months, he would look like he'd never lifted a weight in his life. Poof. All those muscles, just a bad dream.

STEROIDS
More Sex Drive, but Not More Pleasure

Back in 1913 a doctor in Chicago implanted a human testicle into a man who had lost both of his. Four days later the man demanded to leave the hospital to satisfy his regained sexual desire.

That was the crude beginning of modern hormone therapy. For thousands of years mankind had suspected that something in our testicles spurs our carnal appetites onward and upward. Yet it wasn't until 1935 that scientists in three different laboratories across Europe managed to isolate that substance, give it the name testosterone and synthesize it in the laboratory. These artificial versions are now known as anabolic steroids.

Today we know that steroids increase sexual appetite, just as testosterone increases it. In one study, researchers recruited three groups of 15 amateur bodybuilders from Pittsburgh-area gyms—current steroid users, past users and "natural" bodybuilders, men who never touch the stuff. The 15 current steroid users had nearly twice as many orgasms as "natural" bodybuilders during a four-week period, and almost three times the orgasms as ex-users. Their average was 28 times—once a day.

Both the current and former steroid users in the study

firmly believed that steroids do increase sexual functioning. But the big question is, were they having any more fun? "It doesn't in any way seem to increase pleasure," says Howard B. Moss, M.D., professor of psychiatry at the University of Pittsburgh Medical Center who directed the study. "It's much more the animal desire to copulate."

Ironically, the steroid users reported far more sexual dysfunctions, such as troubles in getting and maintaining erections and achieving climax. Steroids make the mind more willing—but sometimes the body is weak. Even on these big guys.

And big they are. Steroids, a.k.a. juice, can add 20 to 30 pounds a month of pure muscle to the frame of a man who works out with weights. Which is why the synthesized steroids were quickly taken up half a century ago by athletes with practical benefits in mind. Bodybuilders in Southern California began experimenting with steroids in the late 1940s and early 1950s. By the 1960s they were part of professional football. From there they descended into college athletics, and then to the high school level. Despite the fact that steroids are illegal (in 1991 nonmedical steroid distribution became a federal offense), it's estimated that a million Americans are injecting their rear ends with black market steroids.

Half are male adolescents. Anywhere from 5 to 11 percent of high school students admit to steroid use on anonymous surveys. Most teen users say they started steroids before age 16. Some play on sports teams, but not all do; in any case, the predominant reason to take steroids is to improve appearance—to make themselves more attractive to teenage girls, and more intimidating to other boys. And so they each spend hundreds, if not thousands, of dollars per year to get these drugs. The drugs may be stolen from the local pharmacy or start out as veterinary medicine half a world away. Much of it is bogus—from 30 to 50 percent of it. Kids call 'em blanks. That doesn't discourage anyone. The international black market for steroids is a one-billion-dollar industry.

Rages and Repercussions

The risks of unsupervised steroid use are far from understood. Clearly these drugs can cause severe side effects in
adults, to say nothing of their impact on a kid who's only
halfway through puberty. The quick laundry list of their side
effects includes acne, baldness, an increase in body hair, rectal bleeding, dizziness, gallstones, liver and kidney malfunction, smaller testicles, plummeting levels of high-density
lipoprotein cholesterol (the good kind) and swelling of the
breasts from the body's desperate attempt to counteract the
steroid overload by pumping out more estrogen. Doctors
call it gynecomastia. Bodybuilders call it bitch tits.

Do teenage boys need any *more* acne and sex drive? But
they're not easily dissuaded. First of all, there's a credibility
problem: Authority figures have a history of weaseling on
this topic. For years the medical community denied steroids
had any effect on athletic ability; it then turned to hyping the
dangers. All the while, famous athletes were taking steroids.
The drugs gained in use not just among bodybuilders but
also among endurance athletes who used them to train
longer and harder, with less recuperation time.

Charles Yesalis, Sc.D., professor of health and human
development at Pennsylvania State University in University
Park and a leading expert on the topic, argues that the dangers of steroids have been overblown. He says most professional athletes use safe doses of steroids—about 100
milligrams a week. That, he says, is less than the dose of 200
to 300 milligrams per week that the World Health Organization deemed safe to administer to men around the world during the late 1980s when it tested steroids as a "male pill." At
the levels taken by professional athletes, Dr. Yesalis says,
"there are no remarkable side effects." Furthermore, he
believes steroid use in athletics will become more acceptable as its uses expand: the treatment of "male menopause"
in older men, relief of suffering in AIDS patients and possibly as a contraceptive.

As of now, the only completely uncontroversial reason to
dose men with testosterone is the treatment of hypogo-

nadism, when the testicles, because of age or inherited disorder, aren't pumping out enough male hormone on their
own. The doses for that, and the doses taken by many amateur athletes, differ by a hundredfold. Amateur athletes often
resort to "stacking," the taking of two or more steroids at a
time. Says Dr. Yesalis, "It's not uncommon to see people
taking a gram a week."

These doses are alarming even to someone like Arnold
Schwarzenegger, who admits to using steroids himself back
in his Mr. Universe days. But in an interview for a 1992 *U.S.
News and World Report* cover story on steroids, he said he
always got them from a physician. And the doses were
lower: "The dosage that was taken then versus what is taken
now is not even 10 percent."

In addition to the physical distortions created by steroids,
there is psychological damage, too. Some guys develop a
warped body image. They gain 100 pounds of new muscle,
but it's not enough. They want more. It's been called reverse
anorexia. And indeed, it is the standard of male beauty gone
haywire. But far more common—and more dangerous—is
the increase in hostility and aggression known as 'roid
rages. Dr. Moss says all the headlines of reported assaults by
professional athletes makes him wonder about the possible
connection: "A part of me wants to attribute that to steroid
use," he says.

Steroids may yet find an official acceptance among professional athletes—they've already found a place. But
nobody wants to see kids taking steroids, much less wildly
excessive doses. Will more scolding do any good? In Dr.
Yesalis's view steroid use among adolescents will get worse
before it gets better. "It's driven by societal values—which
are, win at all costs," he says. "We're telling kids at a
younger and younger age, it's inappropriate to play sports
for fun. You play to win." Given that game plan, he calls
steroid use "a very rational behavior." Maybe we should stop
blaming the kids.

VITAMINS AND MINERALS
From A to Z, They Don't Improve Sex

More exercise is generally good for you and your sex life. The same cannot be said of vitamins and minerals.

As far as anybody knows, there is no vitamin or mineral that acts as a magic sex pill. If you're an average guy who's already getting enough of the basic nutrients in the foods you eat, then taking more of them in pill form will not make you a better lover. You will merely be passing a richer urine. As for the reputation of some vitamins and minerals as natural aphrodisiacs . . . forget it.

That reputation seems to cling to zinc and vitamin E, mostly because of studies that show what happens when you take away these nutrients. But there is a big difference between a deficiency, when the body is simply starved of these nutrients, and a superabundancy, when the body is getting more of these nutrients than it can possibly absorb on a daily basis. In short: More isn't always better.

Zero from Zinc

Take zinc. Nutritionists know that a diet devoid of zinc can retard growth and delay sexual maturity. In the 1960s researchers studied groups of young men in Egypt and Iran who were eating something in their diets that prevented them from properly absorbing the trace amounts of zinc that were also in their foods. "They looked like they were 10 years old, when actually they were 20 years old," says Philip Reeves, Ph.D., a United States Department of Agriculture (USDA) chemist. "When they got zinc supplements, they actually began to change from boys into men."

But would super amounts of zinc have turned them into supermen?

Nah.

What happens when you suddenly take zinc out of a normal diet? Only the USDA would want an answer to that question, and answer it they did. USDA biologist Curtiss Hunt and others gathered 11 male volunteers and put them on strict diets with varying amounts of zinc. Zinc, they reasoned, is thought to play an important role in several aspects of male reproduction, so what happened when the male body's intake was lowered to 1.4 milligrams per day—about a tenth of what the body seems to require? The result was a lower level of testosterone in the blood, and the amount of total semen ejaculated dropped by a third. But the number of sperm in the semen stayed the same. "The sperm count, per se, did not change," notes Hunt.

"It's probably very difficult to have a zinc deficiency," says Drogo K. Montague, M.D., director of the Center for Sexual Function at the Cleveland Clinic Foundation. Are you the exception? It's possible. Everyone's body chemistry is slightly different, and individual diets vary greatly. But if you aren't getting enough zinc, a disappointing ejaculate may be the least of your troubles. Zinc plays key roles in growth, skin health and even digestion.

> The Ten Questions of Good Sex
>
> "What do you like?"
>
> "Does that feel good?"
>
> "Show me what you like."
>
> "Do you like that?"
>
> "Harder?"
>
> "Softer?"
>
> "What don't you like and why?"
>
> "What's your favorite position and why?"
>
> "Slower?"
>
> "Faster?"
>
> —28-year-old musician's manager

The recommended dietary allowance for men is 15 milligrams a day. Foods rich in zinc include lean beef, lamb, crab-meat, oysters, turkey, cereals, beans and shiitake mushrooms. Too much—defined as over 100 milligrams a day— can be as detrimental as not enough. Excess zinc intake could increase your risks of copper deficiency, anemia, suppressed immune function and the worsening of Alzheimer's disease. It would be extremely hard to get too much zinc from diet alone. There are really just a few ways: Eat 12 or more oysters daily, or two pounds of roast beef daily.

An E for Effort

As for vitamin E, its reputation as a love potion may date back to the original study in 1922 that identified the substance as an essential nutrient. Female rats without the stuff couldn't carry a pregnancy to term. When wheat germ oil was added to their diets, bingo, baby rats.

The substance was given the scientific name tocopherol, which in Greek means "to bring forth birth." "But that has nothing to do with male potency or virility," says Jeffrey Blumberg, Ph.D., of the Human Nutrition Research Center at Tufts University in Medford, Massachusetts.

That said, supplements of vitamin E may prove beneficial—but for a very different set of complaints. There is evidence that taking 100 to 600 international units a day may lower the risk of heart disease and boost the body's immune system. But a big, conclusive, long-term clinical trial has yet to be done. Also, large doses of vitamin E are toxic. The recommended dietary allowance is only ten milligrams for men—and perhaps a fourth of us aren't getting anywhere near that from our diets. Vitamin E may yet prove itself to be a potent antioxidant, battling toxins at the cellular level. But an aid to sexual potency? Not likely.

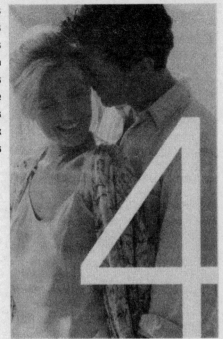

GETTING READY FOR LOVE

APHRODISIACS
Sometimes Magic Works. But Are You a Magician?

Take a tip from all those fancy hotels. Leave a piece of fine chocolate on your lover's pillow.

That first kiss afterward will be especially delicious. Then you can say, "Did you know that chocolate contains an amino acid that stimulates the brain to make phenylethylamine, a chemical released when we fall in love?" If she responds with, "That has to be the geekiest thing you've ever said," maybe you should soften your approach. Try something more romantic, like: "You know, Casanova always drank chocolate before entering the boudoir." Tell her that chocolate has been regarded as an aphrodisiac ever since the Aztecs handed a box to Cortés.

The sudden appearance of chocolate can even become your own little bedtime ritual. Whenever either of you wants to invite the other for a walk in the garden of earthly delights, you can reveal your intent, wordlessly. It will be your own private sex signal. Perhaps there will be nights when both of you find chocolate on your pillows. Those nights we live for.

But all that aphrodisiac stuff, is there really anything to it? Well, maybe there isn't, and maybe there is. Stop being such a little inspector about it. It's all in the suggestion. You see, when researchers have tried to prove the claims about aphrodisiacs, they often get a big placebo effect. For example: In one Canadian trial of the drug yohimbine, 42 percent of a group of impotent men responded to treatment—but so did 28 percent of the "control" group, who were slipped a simple sugar pill. Santa Monica family practitioner Cynthia Mervis Watson, M.D., writes in her book, *Love Potions: The Doctor's Guide to Aphrodisia*, "It is entirely possible that as long as your brain *thinks* that any given substance or ritual will work, it will trigger the appropriate chemical responses and your body will experience all the physical signs of arousal."

An old Cole Porter love song said it: "Do, do that voodoo!"

Coming Soon to Your Local Pharmacy

If you insist, we'll tell you about some real, actual, bona fide, scientifically tested aphrodisiacs. They are drugs with names such as L-dopa, apomorphine, trazodone, bupropion and fenfluramine. Unfortunately, you wouldn't take these drugs unless you were suffering from clinical depression, bulimia or Parkinson's disease. Patients who have been put on these drugs have experienced a quite unintended zing in the libido department. But when they were subsequently administered to healthy groups, the drugs produced only mixed results, and their various side effects ranged from uncontrollable yawning to irregular heartbeats.

Nonetheless, the medical research community's experiences with these drugs have led to a greater understanding of arousal and the brain chemistry behind it. In the last few decades we've seen some drugs dampen sexual arousal—notably, drugs commonly prescribed for high blood pressure, depression and high cholesterol. Other drugs—those mentioned above, plus a couple others—awaken the libido. Most of them do it by mimicking a brain chemical called dopamine, one of the neurotransmitters that brain cells use to communicate with each other. Raymond C. Rosen, Ph.D., professor at the Robert Wood Johnson Medical School in Piscataway, New Jersey, and a leading researcher in the field, has coined a term for these medications: prosexual drugs.

The perfect aphrodisiac, says Dr. Rosen, would heighten sexual desire, pleasure and performance. That magic substance "is still eluding us," he says. But drugs that match part of that job description are in the pipeline. Specifically, drugs to treat erection problems are in clinical trials—oral medications, not the currently available drugs that you must, alas, inject into your penis before each use. "There's great interest and enthusiasm" about these drugs among researchers, he says. Also coming soon: a drug treatment for premature ejaculation. "We're understanding more and more about the neuropharmacology," Dr. Rosen says. "The future of prosexual drugs looks very good."

Well, that's nice for guys with performance problems. But what about desire? What about pleasure? What about people who can summon neither? The major pharmaceutical companies seem not to be so interested in that. "A few efforts to increase libido have not worked out," Dr. Rosen says. "We don't have a good libido drug that's free of side effects at this point." A few years ago researchers had high hopes for the drug quinelorane. It went as far as clinical trials; once nausea appeared as a side effect, its maker, Eli Lilly, suddenly stopped the research.

So. We're back to using . . . what? Spanish fly?

Eating Wild Yams?

Once upon a time, when the authors were callow youths, we couldn't spell aphrodisiac but we'd heard about Spanish fly. It was supposed to make a woman beg you for sex. As pimply 14-year-olds we figured that was the only way we would ever enjoy a liaison with the opposite sex. The whole notion of aphrodisiacs appealed to the era's playboy philosophy, magnified by early adolesence—the ultimate way to trick a young woman into having sex. Big fun.

Dr. Watson, in *Love Potions*, debunks our dweeby dreams of Spanish fly. She says it isn't an aphrodisiac at all. The extract from a Spanish "blister beetle" (real name: cantharides), it does cause extreme irritation of the urogenital tract, among other horrid symptoms, although an indiscriminate roll in the hay is not the sort of relief that will leap to the poor sufferer's mind.

Forget Spanish fly. There are thousands of traditional aphrodisiacs, devised by every major culture, and most of them are listed in Dr. Watson's book. She argues that many traditional aphrodisiacs contain the vitamins, amino acids and enzymes that nourish our brain chemistry, creating the chemistry for love—"which is why they really do work," or so she claims. You should know that the Food and Drug Administration claims they really *don't* work.

The plant world is where the pharmaceutical industry finds its compounds, so if you have any interest in herbs you can eliminate the middle man. Among the venerable herbs of love: damiana (a shrub that grows in the desert of Mexico and Texas), saw palmetto berries (the saw palmetto is the palm tree that grows in the American Southeast), wild yams (native to Mexico), licorice root, kola nuts, ginkgo, sarsaparilla, red clover and bee pollen.

> If you cannot inspire a woman with love of you, fill her to the brim with love of herself—all that runs over will be yours.
>
> —Charles Caleb Colton, British poet

The strength of Dr. Watson's book is that she gets down to recipes. A recipe for damiana, for instance, involves soaking an ounce of the dried herb's leaves in a pint of vodka for five days, straining and then soaking them in three-fourths of a pint of water for another five days, heating the water, adding some honey and recombining with the vodka. Dr. Watson says she has "personally observed its amatory effects."

For love potion ingredients try the Health Center for Better Living, 6189 Taylor Road, Naples, FL 33942; 1-800-544-4225. Health Center for Better Living sells blends containing most of the aforementioned aphrodisiacs. Just look for the labels "Love Formula," "Male Power" and "Man's Rejuvenator" in the catalog. If you've always intended to become a junior herbalist, you're all set.

As for the rest of you . . . looking for something a little more conventional? There's always alcohol, America's favorite aphrodisiac. Only one problem: Alcohol is technically a depressant. It does remove inhibitions—hence the bit of bathroom-wall wisdom, "Candy is dandy, but liquor is quicker." But in anything more than moderation it can render you temporarily impotent. Numerous studies show that, at best, it reduces arousal and the intensity of orgasms in both men and women. Likewise its modern counterparts, the "recreational drugs" such as amphetamines, barbiturates, cocaine and marijuana. Perhaps you already know that, based on unfortunate personal experience.

Based on fortunate experiences, here's what does work: A great meal. A crackling fire. Candlelight. Soft music. Fragrances. Lingerie. Sweet nothings whispered in the ear. In short, all the preliminalia discussed in the rest of this section.

Have a piece of fine chocolate, and keep reading.

ATTRACTIVENESS
It Isn't Cheesecake or Beefcake

Remember the Diet Coke TV commercial with the hunky young construction worker? He leans back against a girder and downs a soda while all the women in the office building next door stand at the windows, ogling and sighing.

Cute. Very cute. Don't fall for it.

Sure, it was a fun reversal of the usual sex role behavior. It was a great ad. But it's not a great sexual strategy. Imagine, for a moment, that guy actually asking one of those ogling career women out on a date. Whoa, wait a minute, pal! Imagine him highlighting his beefcake, implying that's the chief reason she should go out with him.

Pfffft.

The actor in that commercial, Lucky Vanous, went on to make a successful exercise video. Good for him, and if it gets you pumping, good for you. Look your best! Absolutely! If you can look more like Lucky Vanous, we can practically guarantee three results.

You will get noticed.

You will get a higher salary.

You will not automatically get more sex.

In a study entitled "Tactics for Promoting Sexual Encounters," 50 students at the University of Michigan in Ann Arbor were given a long list of hypothetical tactics for getting a member of the opposite sex into bed with them, and were asked to judge which were the most effective. The guys all said that women would be most effective when using the direct approach. Like: Asking the guy if he wanted to have sex or guiding his hand to her genitals or simply undressing in front of him.

The women, on the other hand, rated these actions as the seven most effective ways to seduce a date.

1. He told her he really loved her.
2. He implied that he was really committed to her.
3. He took her to a private or secluded area.
4. He told her he really cared about her deeply.
5. He offered to give her a massage.
6. He treated her with respect.
7. He made her a gourmet meal with wine and candlelight.

As you can see, "men were perceived as most effective when they performed behaviors *not* directly about sex but about expressing love or commitment," the authors wrote in the *Journal of Sex Research*. The vast majority of women, although they find sex pleasurable, simply do not seek out sex as an end in itself—the way you probably do. They're not interested, generally, in something that doesn't have long-term prospects. Therefore, men need to imply love, commitment and generosity. And the sexually successful man has always implied these things. Whether he means it or not, well, that's an old, old story.

One of the study's authors, David M. Buss, a psychology professor at the University of Michigan in Ann Arbor and author of *The Evolution of Desire*, is an evolutionary psychologist. He's most famous for his huge study of mating preferences among 10,047 individuals from 37 cultures on six continents and five islands. He found that sexual attractiveness, despite some cultural differences, is basically the same all over. Men have been shaped by evolution to equate sexual attractiveness in women with youth and beauty. Men's brains are hardwired to desire a sweet, young thing, because that union produces a maximum number of offspring. Whereas women the world over show a greater desire for mates with good financial prospects and/or the qualities that could lead to future wealth—status, ambition, industriousness. Thus the tubby, balding

tycoon is a virtual babe magnet. Apart from the world of
television commercials, cute, young construction workers
are not.

How to Attract

"What is sexy?" asked another television commercial a few
years back. This one, for Jovan Musk, answered its own
question with jump-cut images of lovely bodies striking various poses. The usual television fare. Nothing was said
about evolutionary forces nudging men into viewing women
as sex objects, and women into viewing men as success
objects. Fancy that.

But it's a darned good question. It's been asked since
Adam, and the answer has yet to be boiled down to a 25-
word reply. If anything, the answer is getting longer. A
thoughtful response includes biology, upbringing, beliefs,
family life and cultural values as the various forces that all
have a hand in what we find sexually attractive about
another person.

Although Buss has found cross-cultural truths about men,
women and mating choices, there's still plenty of room for
diversity. In parts of Greece, men put their handkerchiefs
under their armpits at festival time, and then present these
odoriferous gifts to the woman of their dreams as an invitation to dance. (Just try that the next time you go out to a
nightclub.) And if you lived in northeast Uganda, you'd be
attracted to a gal with a hole in her lip. Even within the same
culture, standards of beauty shift with time. Marilyn Mon-
roe, for example, would be too pudgy to get any modeling
work were she alive and young today.

Then there's the whole question of what happens in each
little household of every particular culture. Sexologist John
Money invented the intriguing word "lovemap" to describe
your own, very personal collection of erotic ideals. He
believes people form lovemaps between the ages of five and
eight in response to what we find appealing or unappealing
in our parents, siblings, friends, relatives and strangers. At
the time, we're not aware they're being formed. But later on

in life, as we reach sexual maturity, these become our quirks—our very own list of turn-offs and turn-ons.

> The old man, especially if he is in society, in the privacy of his thoughts, though he may protest the opposite, never stops believing that, through some singular exception of the universal rule, he can in some unknown and inexplicable way still make an impression on women.
>
> —Giacomo Leopardi, Italian poet

All these forces are powerful. Therapists say we can't do much about what we find attractive in others. It's easier to change what others find attractive about us. As every stand-up comedian knows, many laughs can be gotten over the fact that women invest more time, money and energy in their appearance. Supposedly, they have to—that's how they're rated by society, blah blah blah. But, hey, no one is stopping men from investing more time, money and energy on their appearance. Indeed, a little vanity is perfectly acceptable in the modern man. You, too, can perform a "male makeover" on yourself. The question is, why don't more men do this? Hmmm. This sounds like a multiple choice question. The choices:

a. It doesn't pay off with other men, not the way a woman's makeover pays off with other women.

b. It may not pay off with women, either, who are ever on the alert for the first sign of an Overblown Male Ego.

c. It's easier to put the same amount of time and energy into improving our wealth and status, and the end result is the same.

d. We're really, really bad at it.

Maybe this is a stupid thing to say, but we suspect that for most guys, sexual attractiveness is a bit of a mirage. If we can't attract women directly with sex, then why should we be able to directly attain sexual attractiveness? For men sexy is as sexy does. Like happiness, it's obtained only in the pursuit of something else.

BEDROOMS
How to Make Them Hot Spots Again

The final question we asked in our *Men's Health* magazine survey was, "What's the most bizarre place you've ever made love?" More than a few wise guys answered, "our bedroom."

They were joking, but not really. After a relationship gets beyond the infatuation stage, a bedroom is the last place on the list of exciting locations. Bor-ing. No wonder so many people relocate their sex lives to the living room, the garage or the laundry room. As relationships mature, the bedroom gets de-coupled from its former role as passion pit and instead becomes a place to zonk out, watch TV or work. Those of you who drag your Power Books to bed, you know who you are.

And when you do turn to love, its sameness conspires against you. The same old routines of getting ready for love—getting up to lock the door, peek out the curtains, set the alarm—turn sex into the night's final routine.

You can either give up bedroom sex completely—in which case we wish you luck in not getting caught—or you can do something about this problem. In a nutshell think of what you've done to de-eroticize your bedroom, and then think of ways to re-eroticize it.

Your first task is to get rid of a lot of extraneous stuff. "A bedroom should be a retreat, a place where you can push away all distractions," says Shirley Zussman, Ed.D., a certified sex therapist and co-director of the Association for Male Sexual Dysfunction in New York City. That means moving the television, the computer and the treadmill to other rooms. Dr. Zussman calls them seductive rivals, and they're very powerful rivals, at that. At the very least they fill the room with an anti-erotic mood (especially the local TV news). At their worst they provide ways to avoid intimate contact. Dr. Zussman says flatly, "The bedroom should be devoid of other activities.

There. Now you're ready to start putting things in the bedroom. The right things.

Soft lights. For many couples the ideal bedroom lighting represents a compromise. Men tend to want the lights on, being creatures of visual stimulation and all. They get excited by the sight of their partners. Whereas some women feel that their sensations are heightened by turning off the lights. That way, there's less distraction, they can focus on sex and they can enjoy a freedom from distress over appearances, especially if they have a negative body image.

> One can learn technique, but never feeling, and feeling is the main factor, for the art of giving pleasure is the art of love and devotion; without love the most perfect technique is worthless and becomes merely a soulless artifice.
>
> —A. Costler, M.D., in *Encyclopedia of Sexual Knowledge*, 1937

Solutions: candlelight. It's easy on the skin, making it look warmer, smoother, younger and purer. Or a black light. "A black light near the bed helps because it gives us both a pleasant-looking tan without having to destroy our skins in the sun," says a 42-year-old Kansas man. Or quite possibly the answer to your prayers is a 99-cent dimmer switch. You always said you were good with your hands. . . .

Soft sheets. We hate to be the ones to say something, but maybe you need to ditch that scratchy set of polyester sheets you bought at a discount mall ten years ago. You're spending a third of your life between the sheets, can't you treat yourself to something nice? Satin? And while you're out shopping, how about new pillows? New positions require new pillows.

Once you start arguing about which sheets to buy, it could escalate into a battle over the whole room's decor. Good. "Many bedrooms are extremely feminine," says Dr. Zussman. "They're very frilly. I don't think the man feels as if he quite belongs in there. To the extent that a couple can share the decorating, that's a very good idea. Because then, when the man walks into that room, he instantly feels good."

Soft music. The famous first line of Shakespeare's *Twelfth Night* is, "If music be the food of love, play on." A radio is the only piece of electronic equipment that belongs in the bedroom. Just leave it off the talk radio stations. Search the airwaves: You probably want to tune in to the very stations that you wouldn't listen to during the rest of the day. Try an oldies station—it may take you back to the backseat of your father's Oldsmobile. "Melodies associated in memory with love's happiness in the past have a compulsive power," wrote the Dutch physician Theodoor Van De Velde in *Ideal Marriage: Its Physiology and Technique*, the ubiquitous marriage manual of the pre-World War II years. Of course, he went on to cite his deeply sexual response to Johann Strauss's "Wiener Wald," as "interpreted by an adequate orchestra with rhythm and élan." So to each his own.

A soft touch. All kinds of books and videos teach you how to give a massage. Try it. Don't make a big thing of it; don't even call it a massage if the idea seems too corny. The real purpose is a few minutes of touching. Slow, deeply relaxing, you-feel-terrific touching. Some couples recommend scented oil or baby powder—they can amplify the sensations.

The "Bic Cure"

Your bedroom is now ready. Are you? Given your complicated lives and frenetic pace, many of you have no time or energy for dalliances at the end of the day. Life is just one rush job after another, and unfortunately, love's not one of them. As you know all too well, things that keep falling to the bottom of your ASAP list tend not to happen.

You need to make a date.

Many sex therapists tell their clients to go all the way back to what worked in the first heady days of their relationships: scheduling time for sex. (It's come to this? Yes.) This is even being called the Bic Cure, because therapists know that the only way some clients will really stick to their agreements is to write down the day and time in their planners—in ink. Sex is not mandatory; the two of you can sit in bed with a pint of ice cream. But it does create an opportunity for sex. The only opportunity some people get.

Patricia Love, Ed.D., a marriage and family therapist in Austin, Texas, advises the Bic Cure in her book, *Hot Monogamy.* "By reserving a time to make love and then deliberately creating a positive attitude, you can greatly increase your ability to give and receive pleasure," she writes. "Once these mental habits are firmly established, you begin to transform your bedroom into a sanctuary—a place of comfort, safety and sensuality."

CHILDREN
Romance Is a Good Lesson for Them

"Two young kids is the best birth control method," said one of our survey respondents. In his house, and many houses, love is a matter of getting past the Big Wheels.

Judging from our other survey respondents, it seems most people have trouble reconciling a great family life with a great sex life. Children annihilate your leisure time ("We have no time for ourselves.") and energy ("The kids sap our strength.") and whatever spontaneity was left in your romance ("They're night owls.").

If you were to flip through the women's magazines on a regular basis (and we're not suggesting you do), you'd see articles from time to time on what *really* happens after the baby's born. These articles are filled with new mothers' voices saying they've just totally lost interest in sex, and for a gamut of physical and emotional reasons. Coitus can be painful for several months after the birth, hormonal changes are brought on by breastfeeding, baby has replaced hubby as her center of attention . . . all that, and more. The consensus is: You can just forget about sex for a year, guys. If it's any consolation, these articles usually end with a gentle reminder that mothers should really, really try to (sigh) start having sex again if they want their marriages to last.

To the extent that a couple shares this problem, it can be

something that unites you, instead of driving you apart. And believe it, kids will do their best to drive you apart.

Anybody who says they got right back into the *schwing* of things—bully for them. Most of us don't. That's life, and you'd have to be a pretty dim bulb to expect otherwise.

Children Are for Life

But some couples find that their children make mincemeat of their sex lives for years and years. We suspect this is a bigger problem than in past generations. Working moms and dads get so few hours with their kids that they stay up late with the kids, and go to bed with them, instead of marching them off to their own bedrooms by 7:30 P.M.

In other words, today's mom and dad don't get a spare nanosecond to themselves. Part of that is from too much to do and too little time to do it; part of it is the parental guilt-o-meter going nuts about spending so much time out of the house. To the extent that Dr. Spock's parenting style is still with us today, parents make themselves available, at any hour, to their kids' every whim so nobody feels unloved. And to the extent that the American household is small, confined and extremely casual, not much room is left for privacy.

CHILDREN AND SEX

In our written *Men's Health* survey we asked: "How have your children affected your sex life?" More than one answer was allowed. The responses:

Altered when and where we have sex	88%
Too tired to have sex	34%
Sex is less romantic	30%
Not altered sex life	9%
Enhanced our sex life	3%

Thus, Judith Seifer gets plenty of clients who complain they have no sex lives anymore. Seifer, an R.N. and a Ph.D., is a certified sex therapist in West Virginia and the president of the American Association of Sex Educators, Counselors and Therapists. She's reared three kids with her husband, Bill, an osteopathic physician, so she has lots of I've-been-there sympathy.

But she also can be very clear about the necessity to make changes. When one couple said they had no lock on their bedroom door because they didn't want the children to feel shut out, she told them: Stop at the hardware store on the way home. If they say they simply don't have any time for sex, she'll tell them: Set the alarm 30 minutes earlier in the morning. If they can afford it, she'll advise getting out of town one or two nights a month—that's what she and Bill do. If they can't, she'll tell them to look their kids straight in the eye and say, "For the next hour it's time for your dad and me to spend some time together, just the two of us."

There may be some consolation in knowing your life would probably be this way right now, even if you decided not to have children. "Whenever you have a busy life, good sex isn't just going to happen," says Dr. Seifer. You'd still have to make a date to keep the home fires burning. The big difference now is your planning has to include a babysitting budget. Every marriage finds its own solutions—you don't need us to say, "Tell your parents you'll plant their new azaleas this weekend if they take the kids next weekend." Chances are, you can figure out stuff like that for yourself.

Who's Denying Whom?

But, just to placate us for a moment, ask yourself this: Are some of your favorite solutions still a fantasy? Maybe you really don't act on those solutions? And why is that? Because, when you get right down to it, you're hugely conflicted about standing up for yourself? Are you uncomfortable being a sexual creature around your kids? Do you make love but pretend you don't?

Ten years from now, we guarantee you, your kid will be

sitting in a dorm room at college and saying, "Gawd, I can't ever imagine my parents, like, doing it."

Seriously, are you sending mixed messages about sex? If so, your kids will grow up with a little voice inside *them* that says that sex is something to be ashamed of. They certainly won't think they can come to you with questions about sex and later on with their problems that involve sex. All their lives you've been busy pretending it doesn't exist. Your conflicts will become their conflicts. It wouldn't be inconsistent if they became sexually active but didn't own up to their sexuality by seeking out birth control until much later.

So you owe it to yourself *and your children* to preserve and defend your romance. Dr. Seifer has a phrase for this: Sex-positive parenting. It's two principles are, and we quote:

1. Parents have to acknowledge their kids as sexual beings from the cradle on.

2. Kids have to get comfortable with their parents being sexual creatures.

"This is a win-win lesson for a family to learn," she says. "It's a gift to teach children that, as much as you love them, other things take priority at times. It's teaching children what they need to know as adults. As parents we're modeling for our children all the time—we can't lose sight of that. By showing our kids that we know how to take care of ourselves, we're modeling functional adult behavior." Moreover, you're providing an antidote to the skewed images of sex they pick up from peers, video games and *Baywatch*. Says Dr. Seifer, "It's our responsibility to model what's good about sex and affection."

It's also our responsibility to teach our children about privacy. "We want our kids to learn all about 'boundaries' these days, but that begins with enforcing household boundaries. Chances are, if the parents aren't getting any privacy, it's because they don't respect their kids' privacy either." How about it? Do you knock on the door when your kids are in the bathroom or bedroom? Or do you barge right in? By teaching the fundamentals of privacy, you're also teaching kids how to say, politely, "I have a life, too." "A closed door doesn't mean you're not welcome," says Dr.

Seifer. "It means you knock and wait for an invitation to enter."

What to Say When You Get Caught

"Our game is not getting caught by the kids," says a 33-year-old advertising executive. "It's fun to sneak into the utility room on a Saturday morning while they watch cartoons—or tarry in the alley while we take out the trash after dark. Whatever."

It's refreshing to hear this couple approach matters with a light heart. And while some couples live in fear that their kids

---

REGARDING DADS AND DAUGHTERS

"In this culture, we don't give men permission to give their daughters what they need," says Judith Seifer, Ph.D., a certified sex therapist in West Virginia and president of the American Association of Sex Educators, Counselors and Therapists. "And what they need is a wonderful, nonseducible adult male on whom they can try out their social skills, their vamping skills and all kinds of adult behaviors. They need a dad who will acknowledge their emerging sexuality by saying things like, 'What a remarkable woman you're growing into.'"

Given today's gender wars and the fact that thousands of fathers have been falsely accused of incest because of supposedly "recovered" memories, you might be saying to yourself right about now, "Judy—are you insane?" Dr. Seifer definitely thinks you should say these things in front of your wife, so nothing's misconstrued. But by the same token, you should not be frightened away from giving your daughter the affirmation she needs.

There are precious few ways in this culture to acknowledge our children's coming-of-age, says Dr. Seifer. And we're poorer for it: "Men have lost the opportunity to celebrate what's supposed to be one of the sweetest times of a woman's life."

might actually catch them in the act, others live . . . dangerously. A 28-year-old karate instructor says the most bizarre place he ever made love was on the living room couch—while their kids watched TV in the next room. "The 4-year-old asked if Mommy would get off me because he wanted to sit on my lap. I said, 'No way, this is Mom's seat!' "

Potential conflicts with kids are amplified in second marriages where the usual peak of, ahem, romantic activity takes place while small children from the previous marriages are already running around. Dorothy Strauss, Ph.D., a sex therapist in Brooklyn, has worked on this issue with clients. Her advice: "Anticipate the problem and deal with it in advance."

But what if a child comes charging into your bedroom while you are in *flagrante delicto?* What do you say if they see something?

What you would do next depends on the age of the child. If it's a preschooler, Dr. Strauss advises attaching as much normalcy as you can to whatever the child saw. Remove the actions, if possible, from any sexual aspects, because at that age they really don't get it. Put it in terms of hugging or wrestling. But if the child is, say, ten or older, then Dr. Strauss's advice is, "Allow the child to ask whatever the child wants to ask. Call the child back into the room. Say, 'Why did you run out?' Now, you know the answer, but it gets them talking. Try to contain your own unease and say, 'Let's talk.' "

Some parents get jittery about this topic. They have vague fears that such a scene might scar their child for life. Hardly. In fact, the idea that you'd be permanently damaging your kids if they ever caught you making love verges on the puritanical. In our *Men's Health* magazine survey we asked what attitudes people want to pass along to their kids. Many respondents said they don't want to pass along the guilt or shame they feel, the sense that sex is "dirty." But isn't that exactly what you teach if you're so afraid to be caught? And if you were caught, wouldn't a flipped-out reaction on your part be much more damaging than anything the child might see?

"Please be openly, physically close," says Dr. Strauss. Otherwise, you'll have a loveless marriage—and your kids will grow up to be the sort of obnoxious teenagers who think they invented sex.

The Disappearance of Desire

The months when a new infant is brought home from the hospital are overwhelming, but then life gradually begins to find new patterns, and the opportunities for making love again come with setting limits—teaching about privacy, establishing bedtimes. But there's opportunity, and there's libido. A more intractable problem is the disappearance of sexual desire. You may have heard husbands complain that "things change" with their wives after a pregnancy or two. We heard it, too.

A 40-year-old civil engineer wrote: "Although we used to have a great sex life, after the birth of our third child four years ago, it completely disappeared. I could write pages on the agony I've gone through, the excuses I've received, the behavior changes I've tried and the books I've read to get a grip on this situation. Whether it ever really existed or just got lost is the only question. It is my opinion that women just use sex to get you to marry them or have kids or buy them a house or whatever, and as soon as they have what they want, they forget completely about it. But you are expected to keep up with your end of the bargain and keep working, keep making the mortgage payments. There is a book titled *Celibate Wives*; please think about a book called *Celibate Husbands*."

Can this marriage be saved? It is true that many women feel a drop-off in sexual desire in midlife. A gender gap begins to show up in the reported frequency of intercourse, and by the time they reach their late fifties, more than four in ten women say they are no longer having sex with a partner. Only one in ten men at that age say the same thing. So three in ten men at that age are either lying or cheating. Neither is a good choice to make. We hope our friend here is getting help by now.

FRAGRANCES
The Alluring Sense of Scents

You've given her roses before. But not this way.

A 55-year-old university professor offers the most romantic tip we received from our *Men's Health* magazine survey respondents: "I like to take fresh petals from a long-stemmed red rose and scatter them over the body of my lover just prior to engaging in intercourse," he writes. "Kissing and licking around the rose petals on her stomach, breasts, nipples and thighs add a new dimension to this experience. Finally, intercourse with rose petals between the lovers provides a very sensuous addition to sex—the petals cling to both bodies because of the sweat generated and leave interesting patterns when sex is over."

When you're done marveling at the possibilities of this idea, take just a second to note what the professor has left out. He praises the visual and tactile aspects of this very romantic act—but says nothing about smell.

Yet what's the first thing you do with a rose? You sniff and say, "Aahh."

Nothing much is ever said about smell and sex. And yet they are inextricably linked. Certainly, odors have the power to arouse you sexually—mankind has known that for thousands of years, and not for nothing has perfume been called sex in a bottle. The fact that women spend billions of dollars each year basically to enhance their sex appeal through sweet smells should not be lost on you.

But this is bigger than Chanel. Your sense of smell affects who you fall in love with and whether you stay in love. It has the power to improve everything from your mood to your penile blood flow. Lose your sense of smell, and you actually lose sexual function.

The Train to the Brain

"Every person smells slightly different; we all have a personal 'odor print' as distinctive as our voice, our hands, our intellect," writes Helen Fisher, Ph.D., an anthropologist at the American Museum of Natural History in New York City, in her book, *Anatomy of Love*. "As newborn infants we can recognize our mother by her smell, and as we grow up, we come to detect over ten thousand different odors. So if nature be our guide, we are probably susceptible to odor lures."

Does that mean a special someone can lead us around by our noses? In a word: yes. "When you meet someone new whom you find attractive, you'll probably like the 'smell' of him, and this helps predispose you to romance," writes Dr. Fisher. "Then, once infatuation flowers, the scent of your sweetheart becomes an aphrodisiac, a continuing stimulant to the love affair."

There's an anatomical reason why that would be so. When an aroma wafts your way, it gets picked up by some of the thousand-or-so odor receptors that are lumped together in a small patch of tissue in your nasal cavity, right behind the bridge of your nose. Via an elegantly versatile nerve network that scientists have teased apart in just the last few years, we know that these receptors feed their findings to your olfactory bulbs, which process the raw data and send it on to various portions of your brain. One of those places is the limbic system, a primitive region developed early in our evolutionary past that controls emotions and sex drive. Among the five senses, smell is unique, because it has a nonstop flight to this region. (The limbic system is also the seat of long-term memory, which is why you can remember odors years later, while sights and sounds fade after a few days or weeks.)

> I put my arms around him yes and drew him down to me so he could feel my breasts all perfume yes and his heart was going like mad and yes I said yes I will Yes.
>
> —James Joyce, Irish writer

"Anatomically, smell and the emotions overlap in the brain," says Susan S. Schiffman, Ph.D., professor of medical psychology at Duke University Medical Center in

Durham, North Carolina. "So if you smell something nice, it's going to make you feel better."

Dr. Schiffman's research interest is nonhormonal ways to improve patients' moods. In pursuit of this interest, she's discovered that food odors can boost the immune systems of the elderly. But more to our point here, she studied the effect of perfumes on 56 women in midlife (ages 45 to 60). She found that nice smells did indeed make them feel better. Then she tested 60 men between the ages of 40 and 55. For 12 days these men doused themselves with either a cologne or placebo, and rated their moods twice daily in diaries. Result: Colognes improved men's moods, too. Not wildly— overall, the moods were boosted by a point or two on one-to-ten scales that attempted to measure such factors as tension, anxiety, dejection, anger, fatigue and confusion. If these all-male fragrances didn't give middle-age men the power to seduce young models, at least the scents gave them a lift.

You should know that Dr. Schiffman's research was funded by the fragrance industry. (Men now spend $1.5 billion on colognes every year.) But that does not make it mere propaganda. If colognes can make you feel calmer, more confident and therefore sexier, well, that's money well-spent. You can make that decision for yourself.

> In bed her heavy resilient hair— a living censer, like a sachet— released its animal perfume, and from discarded underclothes still fervent with her sacred body's form, there rose a scent of fur.
>
> —Baudelaire, French poet

But what about the opposite sex? Does our odor print have any measurable effect? Although Dr. Schiffman hasn't researched that avenue yet, she does offer an interesting anecdotal observation. She counsels couples, and she says many differences can be overcome—except odor. If one person dislikes the other's smell, they've got trouble: "There's no amount of counseling you can do to make that go away." In one longtime marriage the husband disliked the wife's smell, so Dr. Schiffman counseled the wife to wear fragrance. (She refused, saying perfumes were unnatural.) Fragrances do not so much mask your odor print as meld with it. "What you come out with is a new odor," she says. She believes fragrances are useful in smoothing your interactions, both at work and at play. "It probably makes initial encounters more neutral," she says.

Popped Flies and Pumpkin Pies

One of the leading researchers in this field is Alan R. Hirsch, M.D., a neurologist and psychiatrist who runs the Smell and Taste Treatment and Research Foundation in Chicago. On the treatment side, he works with people who've lost their sense of smell. More than four million Americans suffer from noses that no longer know; the impairment can be brought on by head injury, age (half the elderly have lost their ability to smell) and diseases, like Parkinson's, Alzheimer's and hypothyroidism. Whatever the cause, its consequences involve more than just a bothersome inability to stop and smell the roses. For instance, says Dr. Hirsch, "Approximately 90 percent of patients with head trauma describe a loss of sexual function after losing their sense of smell."

On the research side of his foundation, he has conducted over 100 studies in the last decade. Among his discoveries:

Odors may be useful in treating impotence. Dr. Hirsch tested a group of medical students and found that the smell of cinnamon buns increased blood flow to the penis. He then did a larger study of 31 guys ages 18 to 64 and found that a combination of lavender and pumpkin pie increased penile blood flow 40 percent. Also effective: the scent of doughnuts and black licorice (32 percent) and doughnuts and pumpkin pie (20 percent). Why this is so is still anyone's guess.

> I will be arriving in Paris tomorrow evening. Don't wash.
>
> —Napoleon to Josephine

Odors can help you lose weight. In a massive, six-month study of 3,193 overweight people he instructed them to sniff an inhaler containing banana, mint and green apple scents whenever they got hungry. Those who felt bad about being overweight—but did not feel bad about themselves overall—were able to lose nearly five pounds a month.

Odors can help you learn faster. Men and women were able to complete a series of tests 17 percent faster when wearing a floral-scented mask. The effect was even more pronounced on children. One more good reason to keep flowers around the house.

Odors can make you spend money faster. One of the latest trends in retailing is the subliminal odor strategy—pumping just enough scent into the air so that we don't notice it, but our moods improve and we open our wallets. Dr. Hirsch tried this at a Las Vegas casino one weekend and got people to spend 45 percent more on the slots.

The loss of smell is linked with other maladies. Migraine sufferers suffer disproportionately from an impaired sense of smell. And 35 percent of patients with smell problems are clinically depressed. Odors can affect people with anxiety disorders; the smell of green apple and cucumber, for example, eases the panic of claustrophobia.

The Smell and Taste Treatment and Research Foundation currently has 85 research projects in progress. Among them is a study of odors and male-male interaction. In other words: If you wear a cologne, does that have any effect on the other guys at the office? "It's not as simple as we thought," Dr. Hirsch says of the results to date. It seems that different scents work differently, depending on your age, the ages of the men around you and who's in a position of authority.

The bad news is, we'll have to wait until the late 1990s for some answers. The good news is that maybe there is such a thing as the sweet smell of success.

LINGERIE
Is It the Ultimate Erotic Aid?

Really, we had no idea. In our *Men's Health* mail survey
when we asked, "Have you discovered any sexual aids (toys,
games, lingerie, fantasies) that enhance your sex life?" we
were not prepared for the landslide vote in favor of lingerie.
Without a doubt, it is the U.S. male's favorite erotic aid.

What comes to mind when thinking about lingerie is that
flimsy, filmy torso item, the teddy. But men's interests range
far beyond that. From our survey, we'd judge that the lingerie drawers of America are also filled with briefs, plenty
of thigh-high stockings and garter belts. (No pantyhose,
please—one respondent says it only gets in the way.)

Our survey respondents may be crazier about lingerie
than the average man on the street, but their interest is in no
way a fetish. These guys are not aroused by the garments
themselves. And they all say the stuff doesn't stay on for
long. One 38-year-old investor put it simply: "Lingerie," he
says, "makes me want to attack her."

Because if fires up a man's imagination, there's no sense
in limiting its usefulness to a momentary parade in the
boudoir. "It's not so much what she wears to bed," says a 36-
year-old former defensive back in the National Football
League, "but what she wears under her clothes while she is
out with you. Knowing that she is wearing a pair of thigh-
highs and no underwear under your favorite dress makes the
anxiety of getting back to the bedroom unbearable."

The only problem is, not all women share the enthusiasm.
Some respondents bemoan the fact that their girlfriends and
spouses just aren't interested; other respondents stress the
importance of achieving exactly that—getting them interested. Here's sage advice from one 26-year-old respondent:
"I always go to Victoria's Secret and have girlfriends model
for me so I can get a free peep show as well as get them into
what they feel best in. I have found that if they are comfortable with it, they will try even harder to please you."

There's really no alternative. If it's no fun for her, it won't

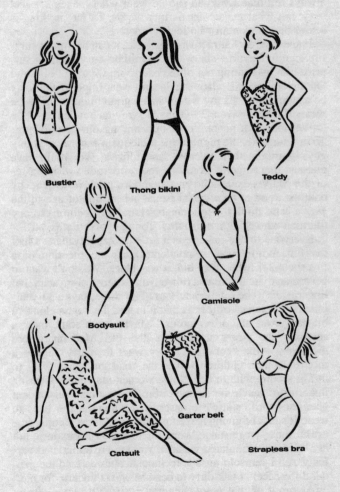

Bustier

Thong bikini

Teddy

Bodysuit

Camisole

Catsuit

Garter belt

Strapless bra

be any fun for him. "Lingerie on a woman works magic for me," says a 28-year-old advertising executive. "But I've always felt that a woman should wear what makes *her* feel sexy, not what makes her partner happy. To me, nothing is sexier than a woman who feels attractive."

If she does feel attractive in lingerie, it can become a sure-fire signal. Anytime she wants to initiate a tryst, she'll surprise him by coming out of the bathroom wearing . . . Wow! On the other hand, when she doesn't wear lingerie, that may be a signal, too. "If my wife wants a good night's sleep, she wears flannel," says a 26-year-old x-ray technician.

We noticed a generational bias among our respondents. To our surprise, the biggest, most eloquent fans were young guys—guys in their twenties and thirties. We would have guessed that lingerie would be too retrograde for the tastes of the MTV generation. The men who pooh-poohed it, by contrast, tend to be either the ones who came of age in the 1960s, who think it's too unnatural and artificial or grumpy old men who think it's naughty. Too naughty, that is.

Everyone thinks lingerie is a *little* bit naughty. That's half the fun. While most respondents made no mention of a favorite color, when they did, it was black. We don't want to get too analytical here and ruin anyone's sense of mystery, but lingerie lets us be safely racy. Part of its allure, says a 34-year-old chief financial officer, is that it makes the woman look "a bit dangerous and adventurous." Maybe, with some men, a spouse who wears it resolves the old Madonna/whore dichotomy—the "good girl" they want to marry and be a mother to their children versus the "bad girl" they want to thrash around with in bed. Some women may enjoy wearing lingerie for much the same reason. One woman respondent used the word "slutty" to describe the lingerie she likes to wear. It's part of giving herself permission to freely enjoy sex.

But make no mistake: Women's lingerie pleases him, not her. Men are stimulated visually, women are stimulated verbally. A 35-year-old missile technician summarized the gender difference: "I talk dirty to her, she wears lingerie for me."

As proof of that point, lingerie is virtually a nonitem in lesbian relationships. In one study researchers in Texas compared a group of 34 heterosexual women with a group of 34 lesbians. All women were in their twenties or thirties and living with someone. The greatest difference between the two groups: 33 out of the 34 heterosexual women reported incorporating "exotic clothes" into their sexual activities. Only 2 of the 34 homosexual women reported likewise.

If you're buying lingerie for a woman, the best advice comes from the fellow we quoted above who takes his sweetheart to Victoria's Secret. That way, they try it, they like it, you like it. Ba-da-bing, ba-da-boom. Your efforts will probably be appreciated more than if you buy through catalogs. Of course, it never hurts to look. Victoria's Secret's catalog (1-800-888-8200) is still chugging along, operated by the same huge mega-billion-dollar company, The Limited, that owns the retail chain of over 500 stores nationwide. Don't be fooled by the British accents when you call for a catalog, and the British spellings in the catalog. These people are strictly Columbus, Ohio.

The Limited's nearest competitor is Frederick's of Hollywood. Frederick's is the granddaddy of this business; it was started as a mail-order company in the 1940s by the late Frederick Mellinger. Today, the company consists of more than 200 stores nationwide, plus its venerable catalog (1-800-323-9525).

Many of our survey respondents said they liked it best when their partners wore lingerie in combination with high heels and lots of makeup. Think about that for a second. Isn't that what some women put on every day to go to work? No wonder so many guys daydream of having sex while on the job.

OPENING LINES
Open Your Eyes before Your Mouth

Men are of two opinions about opening lines. Either they think they have a great opener and it works like magic in getting any woman to talk to them—or they can't screw up the courage to meet a woman because they just don't know what to say. (As one tongue-tied survey respondent said, "I'd rather eat rusty nails than run the risk of being rejected.")

What a bunch of blockheads we are.

This focus on opening lines is crazy. What most men don't realize is that by the time they walk up to a woman and open their mouths, she's already sized him up and said yes or no. "The decision has already been made," says Monica Moore, Ph.D.

Dr. Moore should know. A professor of psychology at Webster University in St. Louis, she has been studying the courtship dance since 1978.

Specifically, she has pioneered the study of nonverbal cues given off by women at dances, bars and other places where singles mingle. Her findings should be of great interest to all men, everywhere. All men, that is, who would like to meet someone tonight, instead of getting rejected over and over again. Her advice is: "Men can do better if they will pay attention to the women who are signaling them." And stop hitting on the redhead who won't look their way.

Signals? Women send out signals? Luckily for you, Dr. Moore has spelled them out for you. Her research has discovered 52 "flirting gestures," most of which would probably make you say, "That means she's interested in me?" We won't overwhelm you with all 52 of them. Here are the top ten to watch for.

Eyebrow flash: An exaggerated raising of the eyebrows of both eyes for a couple seconds, followed by a rapid lowering to the normal position. Often combined with a smile and eye contact.

Lip lick: Very common. Some women use only a single-lip lick, wetting the upper or lower lip, while others run the tongue around the entire lip area.

Short, darting glance: Usually occurs in bouts, with an average of three glances per bout.

Hair flip: She pushes her fingers through her hair. Some women make only one hand movement, others stroke their hair.

Coy smile: A sort of half-smile, showing little if any tooth, combined with a downward gaze or eye contact that is very brief.

Whisper: She leans over and speaks into a friend's ear. Just like junior high school.

Primp: Clothing is patted or smoothed, even though there is absolutely no need to do so.

Skirt hike: Up goes the hem to expose just a little more leg.

Object caress: She fondles her keys, slides her palm up and down her glass or toys with stuff on the table.

Solitary dance: While seated, she moves her body in time to the music. Ask her to dance, you fool!

Dr. Moore says a lot of men have a real tough time understanding these signals. Not all men—in fact, she says she once met a young fellow who would go out to bars with his fraternity brothers and in exchange for beers, read all the signals in the room and tell his buddies which women to approach. But in general, she says, "men are poorer decoders than women of nonverbal cues." Some men, in order to improve their shortcomings, need merely to be told about this phenomenon and start paying attention. Others need lots of practice.

Armed with this knowledge of flirting gestures, you're all set to charge out the door. But before you go, Dr. Moore wants you to know one more thing. Picking up someone is a *process*, not an *event*. Huh? In other words, the first phase of courting is initiated by the woman sending nonverbal signals. In the second phase it's the man's turn to respond, by walking up to her and introducing himself. At this point she may change her mind because now she gets a good look at him up close and doesn't like what she sees, or he says something tasteless or scary and she doesn't like what she hears. But, assuming this meeting goes well, the process continues all night, dancing, talking, stopping to chat with others. The man or the woman may at any time rethink this tête-à-tête and back off. That's the rule of the game, and you can't get huffy about it if she says goodbye. In this situation, both of you enjoy the prerogative of changing your minds and, in effect, saying "no" after having said "yes."

The Importance of Being Earnest

Opening lines do matter—but only in the sense that if you've picked up signals, an opportunity can be yours to lose. And with some lines, you will lose. But once again, you are in luck. Another professor has devoted himself to finding out which opening lines work best. Michael R. Cunningham, Ph.D., a psychologist at the University of Louisville, has spent years forcing hapless graduate students to approach strangers of the opposite sex in order to determine the varying success of opening lines. (Success, in these instances, is if a conversation ensues. Failure is when she leaves tread marks up your face.)

In research done in suburban Chicago bars during the 1980s, Dr. Cunningham tried opening gambits that fit one of three different strategies: direct, innocuous or cute/flippant. Direct won, hands down. The line "I feel a little embarrassed about this, but I'd like to meet you" scored highest with an 82 percent success rate. The innocuous approach was runner-up; the line "What do you think of the band?" scored 70 percent. It bested a plain old "Hi," which scored 55 percent.

Trailing badly was the cute/flippant approach. The line "Bet I can out-drink you" edged out "You remind me of someone I used to date," 20 percent to 18 percent. As it turns out, women don't think it is cute or clever when strange men say this stuff to them. They suspect it's a sign of insecurity, irresponsibility or dominance. They exit promptly.

In his latest research Dr. Cunningham's hapless grad students must have revolted, because now he's merely handing out questionnaires to female undergraduates. You can't blame the grad students; some of the new lines sound like they were taken straight from the pages of *How to Pick Up Chicks*. Like, "I'd like to wake up in your arms." Ugh!

Dr. Cunningham also tried a new twist—varying the attractiveness of the guy delivering the line. It produced an interesting result: "When a really good-looking guy deliv-

TEN WORST PICKUP LINES

10. "Care to dance with a gun-toting loner?"
 9. "You're ugly but you intrigue me."
 8. "Can I lick your fingers?"
 7. "Bond. James Bond."
 6. "I collect dead things and keep them in jars in my closet."
 5. "Is that a false nose?"
 4. "Did you know these pants are reversible?"
 3. "You look like a hooker I knew in Fresno."
 2. "Hey! Your eyes are the same color as my leisure suit!"
 1. "Does this look infected to you?"

ered a line that was bragging," says Dr. Cunningham, "he was less successful than a not-good-looking guy delivering the same line." That was true of three opening lines in particular: "Can I buy you a drink?," "I just bought a new car. Would you like to go for a ride?" and "Would you like to listen to some new CDs?"

Good-looking guys did best of all by delivering the line "What would you like me to serve you for breakfast?" Smile when you say that, mister: It also got the highest marks for humor of the ten lines tested. The absolute worst line for handsome devils: "I'd like to watch the sun set and rise with you."

Nerds did best with a straightforward "Can I buy you a drink?" They did worst with the line "That's a nice sweater. Could I talk you out of it?" The ladies thought that opening line could be semihumorous when delivered by a handsome guy. Uttered by an unattractive guy, it's really unfunny.

So you see, if you're going to try anything more than the direct approach, you have to take a hard look in the mirror first. "Good-looking guys did best with humor that would make them look less pompous and more modest," Dr. Cunningham says. "Somebody who's too good-looking could be dangerous." Or, at the very least, too slick and overbearing.

The woman's fear would be that he's only looking for a one-night stand. That's what most women want least of all.

P.S.: The line "I'd like to wake up in your arms" finished near the bottom of the pack. It scored best—fifth place out of ten lines—when delivered by unattractive guys. Most women still wouldn't want to go out with the guy, but they gave him a fair-to-middling rating for having a sense of humor. Apparently, today's coeds have an ear for irony.

PILLOW TALK
The Best Use of the Mouth

A 30-year-old retail store planner is ecstatic about the results. He calls it "the best sexual aid I have found."

What's this guy's secret? It's, uh, well, "verbal stimulation." That's what a paramedic calls it.

You know. Talking.

> Men may love women, but they are in a rage with them, too. I believe it is a triumph of the human psyche that out of this contradiction, a new form of emotion emerges, one so human it is unknown to animals even one step lower in the evolutionary scale: passion.
>
> —Nancy Friday in *Men in Love*

To be a man of few words may be wise and admirable and earn you respect and praise everywhere you go—except the bedroom. Consider yourself warned.

Back before World War II the British had a wonderful phrase for the kind of intimate conversation between two people whose heads are propped up by the same pillow: pillow talk. It was quickly borrowed by Americans. Unfortunately, it was also borrowed for the title of a forgettable 1959 comedy starring Doris Day and Rock Hudson; they share a party line, but he's a playboy who hogs it to chat with his many girlfriends.

Today, the phrase is as out of date as a party line. Maybe because no one has time for pillow talk anymore—it suggests a slower pace, an era when people weren't asleep before their heads hit the pillow.

Some lovers are trying to bring it back. If not the phrase, at least the notion. One program director for a nonprofit organization writes, "The thing that enhances our sex life the most is talking. I ask my wife if she likes what I am doing, what she would like me to do, if I should do it faster or slower. She does the same for me. It allows for honesty, safe exploration, nurturing, kindness and increased awareness of what is being shared. We not only use talking to teach each other but to support and compliment one another during lovemaking. A strategically said compliment does wonders for both. It's not quite talking dirty, but the effect is the same. It makes my experience more real by using words to describe the pleasure I'm feeling."

If he sounds so earnest, hey, that's him and you're you. You don't have to be superheavy to be intimate. You can be playful and silly. Play is a natural entrée to loveplay. Here's one man's secret: "I talk like a munchkin," says a 54-year-old sales rep. "Drives 'em crazy."

When all is said and done, women are different from men. And one of the big differences between the sexes is their expectations of sex. Women want a moment that's heart-to-heart, as well as skin-to-skin.

Getting Sex and Getting Love

Two millenia ago the *Kama Sutra*, an Indian love manual, cautioned, "Though a man loves a girl ever so much, he never succeeds in winning her without a great deal of talking."

The more things change, the more they stay the same. In 1988 psychologist Elaine Hatfield surveyed women who were dating and women who were married, asking each group what they wished for more of in their sexual relationships. At the top of both groups' lists was "talk more lovingly."

Women seem to reach a point in their lives where they'd just as soon say, "Forget the sex, just give me a little intimacy." In 1985 advice columnist Ann Landers, in her syndicated column, asked women whether they'd rather just hold their partners close and forget about doing it. Of the 90,000 women who replied, 72 percent preferred affection to sex. (Humorist Art Buchwald thereupon claimed that during his bachelor days he dated all of the 62,000 women who preferred cuddling.) Another study of 100 married couples came up with the same results: The women said they initiated sex for "love, intimacy and holding"; the men initiated in hopes of "sexual release."

That's not quite the same as the adage "women give sex to get love, men give love to get sex." The sexes aren't as starkly divergent in their needs as all that. But it's close. Most women simply need more of a connection between sex and love—and, like it or not, they equate love with talking. When they don't get what they need, resentment builds. Pretty soon you get the stereotypical standoff: She's got a million words to describe the nuances of her every feeling, he has none. She feels like the "intimacy expert" on their little team, forever doing the expressing for both of them. He gets accused of being "emotionally stingy." He's not emotionally stingy. He just needs Cyrano de Bergerac down under the balcony, feeding him lines.

Men want intimacy, too. But many men have other ways of showing their love. To some extent, men have let women define love, and women naturally define it in verbal, rather than instrumental, terms. Coming home after a hard day, sharing innermost feelings about it, asking about your day—that's love. Cooking dinner or refilling the windshield wiper fluid in her car while she's telling you all that—that's not love.

Anyway, both sexes crave the joys of intimacy. It's good for both sexes; it has been shown to be a key to physical and psychological well-being. Those who have it are happier, healthier, more productive and live longer than those who don't. In fact, we thought of calling this section Intimacy, because that's what pillow talk is really about.

But we figured you'd just roll your eyes and turn the page. Especially if you talk like a munchkin.

TURN-ONS, TURN-OFFS
Killer Number One: A Big Ego

And now, presenting the ultimate list of things about men that turn women on. Drum roll, please.

1. A guy who loves kids.
2. A guy who doesn't love kids.
3. A guy who loves his mom.
4. A guy who doesn't love his mom.
5. A man of many words.
6. A man of few words.
7. An affectionate guy.
8. A guy who leaves you alone once in a while.
9. A guy with great lips.
10. A guy with a deep voice.
11. A guy with big muscles.
12. A guy with gold-rimmed glasses.
13. A guy who wears a bandanna.
14. A guy who wears jeans.
15. A guy with style.
16. A good dancer.
17. A good cook.
18. A guy who's aggressive.
19. A guy who's shy.
   and finally . . .
20. A guy who's left-handed.

There. Hope you learned a lot. It should be very authoritative—after all, these items come from a list of turn-ons supplied by readers of *Mademoiselle* magazine. We're sorry that "a guy with a great butt" didn't show up on this list. We know—it has shown up on other lists, or at least it has attained the mythical status of showing up on lists like this.

But there must be something on this list that described you. Isn't that the point? There's a Lucy for every Ricky, an Ethel for every Fred. In the words of the poor *Mademoiselle* writer who had to make sense of it all: "Different blokes for different folks."

Every woman carries around a general idea of what she likes in a guy. She also has a general idea of what she likes in the way of *l'amour*. Her tires go flat when she finds the former without the latter; all hell eventually breaks loose when she finds the latter in a guy who doesn't turn out to be the former.

The whole premise of sex therapy is that problems with the latter can be fixed. Your job is to discover what turns on your partner. Every couple goes through a process of attaining a "sexual equilibrium." That includes not only what you like to do and have done to you, and how often, but your attitudes regarding each other's sexual selves. As long as you both have good attitudes, then all that's left is the process of discovering what floats her boat. Some gals like to keep their sneakers on. Some like it up against the wall. Some like the thrill of doing it in a public place. Some like a friendly game of "handyman" or "doctor." Some like it hot. Cold. Fast. Slow. Hard. Tender. Here. There. Top. Bottom. Lights on. Lights off. Tied, blindfolded or covered in barbecue sauce.

Turn-ons are, by their very nature, personalized. You wouldn't get her a robe with someone else's initials on it, would you?

This subject does not allow much in the way of generalizations. Except this one: "Women love you to pay attention to them," says Barbara Keesling. Ph.D., author of *How to Make Love All Night*. Paying attention to her is not just a turn-on, it is *the* turn-on. Call it what you will—approval, stroking, affection, positive regard. It allows your partner to relax, to open up, to cleanse herself of anxiety so that she can get lost in physical pleasure. And the same goes for you.

And if you get her turned on, then you get turned on.

Oh, you *can* get turned on without her. The curse of

manhood is that we so often do. But being sexually selfish is not the manly thing. "If you only think of yourself, you're a punk, not a man," says a 30-year-old electronic technician.

What Sinks Her Ship

Thinking only of yourself is exactly what turns women off the most. Men run into trouble when that fierce animal drive gets the better of us. We're in bed, both partners are ready for something to happen—but then we start pawing. "Men turn women off when they're preemptory about touching only the erogenous zones," says Theresa Crenshaw, M.D., a San Diego specialist in sexual medicine. "It's almost beyond being rushed. It's being disengaged. It's going through the motions without going through the emotions. She isn't being carried along, and she feels left out." Yes, a woman ought to say something at this point. Like, whoa, fella. But those who do may not necessarily get a response. The guy's not listening. Major turn-off. "A woman can tell whether a guy is there or not," says Dr. Crenshaw. "He can fake an orgasm better than he can fake an emotional response."

Another big turn-off is men who get aggression and sex all jumbled up inside. Dr. Crenshaw blames that darn testosterone of ours. When some men get horny, "that may first manifest itself as growliness," she says. One minute he's being abrupt or picking a fight with her, the next minute he wants her to have sex. He tries to patch things up by reaching out with his hands, not with his words. All she can think is "Are you crazy?"

A third turn-off is ignorance. Some fumbling can be excused in the young; it might even be attractive in its own way. But we all reach a point where we greet ineptitude with one unanimous response: Grow up. A 33-year-old social worker who answered our survey wrote, "Here's hoping Mr. Right doesn't grope, but fondles in a deliberate manner, not haphazardly."

Finally, let's take a moment to sound like your eighth

grade health teacher, and talk about plain old hygiene. Sex therapists say a common complaint of women is that their mates have gotten sloppy about their grooming habits. While you're going, "Whoo!" she's saying, "Phew!" It's a quick fix—but if you don't fix it, she'll fix you.

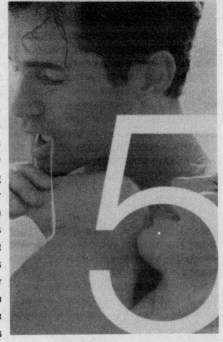

BETTER SEX TECHNIQUES

AFTERPLAY
The Importance of Good Follow-Through

They make love like wild goats, and then what do men do? They immediately fall asleep. Either that or they get up to make a phone call, catch the tail end of Letterman or (in the days before it became a health crime) have a smoke.

And in these innocent acts lie trouble.

She wants to smooch and snuggle and lay there entwined in your arms until you both fall asleep, and if you don't feel like doing that, she feels spurned and lonely, abandoned on the wet spot in the bed. She hates it when you get up and go wash yourself, or check the stock pages or start talking about work. Because for many women, these moments of spent, drowsy, intimate afterplay are all-important. In some ways, women say, they're even better than orgasm itself.

"Going to sleep right away is okay sometimes, but usually I need a little loving after sex," one woman told Oakland, California, sex therapist Bernie Zilbergeld, Ph.D., author of *The New Male Sexuality*. "I want to savor the experience. It makes me feel very close and peaceful in a way that sex itself doesn't."

Well, we're here to tell you there's a reason you fall asleep after sex and she doesn't, and it's not because you're an unfeeling brute. You do it at least partly because there's a difference in your sexual response cycles.

Resolution Phase Resentment

William H. Masters, M.D., and Virginia E. Johnson, of the former Masters and Johnson Institute in St. Louis, spent a lot of time staring at people making love. They described the now-famous, four-part "sexual response cycle"—first, mounting excitement; then a plateau of sustained arousal; then (blammo!) orgasm; and finally, a gradual "resolution phase" return to your prearoused state.

And here's where men and women differ. If you look at a chart of the male sexual response cycle immediately after ejaculation, the guy's body goes into a steep sexual nosedive. You lose your erection amazingly fast, usually within a minute, and then your body clicks over into what's called the refractory period (a time-out before you can get another erection). Your body in general and your penis in particular often feel so hypersensitive they're ticklish. The huge amounts of blood that were diverted to your penis and pelvic area during arousal (so-called deep vasocongestion, the hallmark of sexual arousal) now rush away. Your muscles, which tightened up so ferociously during sex, relax.

Note for the Sexual Trivia Department: In case you've never noticed this, the detumescence, or shrinkage, of an erect penis after ejaculation actually occurs in two stages. It almost immediately shrinks to perhaps 50 percent larger than its unaroused, flaccid state. But after that its rate of shrinkage dramatically slows. And if you and your partner have been involved in sex play over an extended period of time before orgasm, it will linger in this second, partially erect state for much longer than usual, Masters and Johnson found.

A woman's resolution phase, by contrast, is quite different. On a chart it looks more like a long, gentle descent than

---

THE ISSUE IN A NUTSHELL

A 22-year-old legal assistant who responded to our *Men's Health* magazine survey captured the dilemma of afterplay perfectly: "Women must realize that when a man has an orgasm, his energy is zapped ... I don't know why, but I feel so tired after sex, and I get the feeling that most men do. I'm tired of the jokes about how men just roll over and go to sleep after sex. We can't help it. It's physical! It's physical! It's not something that we've planned against women since the beginning of time."

a nosedive. The swelling and florid coloration of a woman's genitals during sexual excitement returns to normal much more slowly than a man's—it often takes five or ten minutes, rather than a minute. Women tend not to get sleepy after orgasm, and their genitals don't become hypersensitive like men's do, Masters and Johnson found. And they have no refractory period either—with sufficient stimulation many women are capable of having another orgasm with no time-out at all.

Coming Together

It's as if, for women, the gentle dalliance of foreplay and afterplay are often the best parts of sex, whereas for guys everything is just warm-ups or cooldowns for the Main

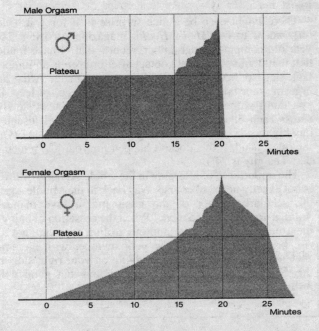

Event. Writer Erica Jong once summed up this whole state of affairs with depressing simplicity: "Men and women, women and men—it will never work."

But of course it has to work.

And finding some common ground that suits the needs of both you and her is usually not all that hard. If possible, try making love in the morning or when you're more rested so you don't immediately fall asleep afterward. Try to pay more attention to the way your actions will affect her; be sensitive to her need for touching and caresses afterward. Try laying there with your penis inside her as long as you can, even though its glory days are—for the moment—over. (Masters and Johnson found that men who maintain body contact with their partners after ejaculation retained their erections longer.) Remember that, like any good novel or movie, the way it all ends is perhaps the most important part.

There might even be a nice surprise in it for you. One respondent to our *Men's Health* magazine survey, a 24-year-old computer programmer, reports that "I have found that maintaining physical contact after orgasm is an important step to becoming a multiorgasmic male. After an orgasm, your body tends to want to relax or go to sleep. If you don't withdraw after your orgasm but instead slowly caress each other, the need to relax or sleep will usually quickly recede behind a new surge of growing arousal." (On the other hand, if this doesn't happen for you, just remember: The guy is 24.)

The importance of afterplay in the whole scenario of love is not exactly news, of course. Way back in the Middle Ages the scholarly author of the great Indian love manual *Ananga-Ranga* advised men: "When the cessation of enjoyment puts an end to your amorous frolics, take care not to rise brusquely, but withdraw your member with circumspection. Stay with the woman, lying on your right side in this bed of pleasure. In this way nothing but good will result."

ANAL SEX
One Step Beyond

Sex surveys invariably show the same thing: While most people seem to find the idea of anal sex about as appealing as inhaling bus exhaust, a significant minority are intrigued by its exotic naughtiness. A few people regularly sample it as a spicy side dish at the feast of love.

One highly respected (and generally quite conservative) 1994 sex survey, conducted by social scientists at the University of Chicago, found that "about a quarter of American men and women have had anal sex in their lifetimes and nearly 10 percent had it in the last year." Other surveys have produced numbers that were considerably higher, like a *Redbook* magazine survey of 100,000 women that found that 43 percent of female respondents (most of them married) had tried anal sex; 19 percent said they did it from time to time; only 2 percent said they did so regularly.

For many heterosexual guys, of course, the big taboo about anal sex is that it is so strongly associated with male homosexual behavior. But a lesser-known fact is that plenty of gay males don't practice anal intercourse—and plenty of heterosexual couples do.

One massive survey of all the studies on the subject concluded that "anal sex among heterosexual Americans is a fairly well-kept secret, possibly involving 16 million people or more."

How Come?

Why do some guys enjoy using the back door when the front door seems so much more convenient? Well, the very fact that it's such a taboo is one of its biggest attractions.

"Feelings of shame and transgression can be highly erotic," observe Anne Semans and Cathy Winks in their book *The Good Vibrations Guide to Sex: How to Have Safe, Fun Sex in the Nineties.* "If the anal taboo is enhancing your pleasure, let us be the first to assure you that anal play is naughty, kinky and downright nasty."

Also, as a practical matter, the anorectal region is laden with nerve endings, just like the vagina or the penis, so it has a vast and usually untapped potential for pleasure. It's "naturally" sexual, so don't be surprised (or ashamed) if you find it to be erotically responsive. Pressure and fullness in the rectum feels good to some women, just like fullness in the vagina. And deep penetration can stimulate the elusive G-spot, located on the top front wall of the vagina, a place that's sometimes difficult to reach otherwise.

There are some other pragmatic reasons for the appeal of anal sex (especially anal intercourse). Throughout history it has served as a sort of contraceptive. People who dislike lovemaking during a woman's period sometimes use anal intercourse as a way of avoiding menstrual blood. And sometimes an unmarried woman who wants to come to the altar as a "virgin," hymen unbroken, will succeed in doing that, but only by the seat of her pants.

The Big Risk

Of course, in the 1990s anal intercourse carries with it one enormous, potentially lethal drawback. It is a very effective method of transmitting the HIV virus that causes AIDS.

"Receptive anal intercourse (being on the receiving end) is the sexual practice carrying by far the highest risk for HIV infection both among homosexual men and heterosexual women," observes Bruce Voeller, Ph.D., of the California-based Mariposa Institute. Medical researchers believe this is primarily because, unlike the vagina, the rectum is not naturally lubricated and penetration causes tiny abrasions in its delicate lining, which opens a direct pathway into the bloodstream. Studies of the pathways of HIV infection have shown that mouth-to-mouth contact, mouth-to-genital contact (including swallowing semen) and mouth-to-anal contact are not nearly as risky as anal intercourse.

So the bottom line is pretty clear: If you don't know your

partner's HIV status, you should avoid anal intercourse entirely, whether as giver or receiver.

On the other hand, if you're absolutely certain your partner is HIV negative, anal intercourse poses no risk of AIDS transmission. This is a point that is surprisingly unclear in the minds of many people. In 1989 the Kinsey Institute for Research in Sex, Gender and Reproduction in Bloomington, Indiana, distributed a Sex Knowledge Test containing this true-or-false question: A person can get AIDS by having anal intercourse even if neither partner is infected with the AIDS virus. Fifty percent of respondents said, incorrectly, that this was true.

You can't get AIDS through anal intercourse if neither of you is already infected. Nevertheless, as a general precaution you should always wear a condom and use plenty of water-based lubricant if you do try it—and only do it with somebody you know is HIV-free.

The How-To Part

If you want to expand your repertoire of erotic delights to include anal sex, the first two things to remember are: You both have to agree to it, and the person on the receiving end should be the one in control. That's because unless she's completely relaxed and you go slowly and gently, it can really hurt.

The anus itself is ringed by two sphincter muscles, like two doughnuts laying on top of one other, Semans and Winks explain. The outer one is the one you voluntarily relax during defecation. The inner one is involuntary, and it will clamp shut if something attempts to enter it too fast. (Hence all the screaming in those prison rape scenes.) But if you're relaxed, the anus is amazingly expandable.

One of the biggest objections to anal sex is its seeming uncleanliness. But the anus is a short barrel an inch or so long, which connects to the rectum, another barrel that's five to nine inches long; together, they only act as a passageway, not a storage area, for feces (which are stored deeper inside, in the colon). Taking a nice bath or shower together before sex, or perhaps using an enema, should ensure that the anus is clean. (Never switch, however, from the anus to her vagina without stopping to wash; you can transport infection-causing bacteria into the vagina this way.)

So, take some time to gently open and thoroughly lubricate her secret doorway, using plenty of water-based lubricant. Once she's relaxed and the anus can comfortably accommodate two fingers, gently insert the tip of your penis and hold it there. Allow her to breathe deeply and relax. Then, when she's ready, let her bear down on you. Hold still until she gets used to it. Then thrust, but not so rapidly or deeply as you would in the vagina.

Anything besides a penis that penetrates an anus should be smooth, seamless and free of rough edges, Semans and Winks advise. And always be sure you're using something that can't get lost up there, otherwise you'll wind up in a medical journal. And, of course, no gerbils.

BETTER-SEX VIDEOS
How to Tell the Good from the Bad

There are certain unmistakable advantages to learning about sexual techniques by viewing a videotape rather than reading a book. For one thing, it's easier to show the exact location and appearance of your typical clitoris than it is to describe it in words. It's also a whole lot more entertaining to watch Julie do the demo than to listen to some disembodied author running at the mouth about it.

Unfortunately, in the burgeoning market for how-to sex videos for couples there's still not much quality control. Some turn out to be low-budget attempts by porn producers to go legit. The joke is that they are nothing more than porn, but with a person in a lab coat first introducing the action.

But others, usually produced and/or narrated by genuine authorities (usually psychiatrists or sex therapists), can have a legitimate role in helping people enhance their sex lives or overcome specific problems, including sex-related relationship problems.

The most useful thing is to watch one of these videos with your partner. But since many of our survey respondents told us that women are frequently offended by sexy videos, this may take a little doing. Even so, we'd be willing to bet it'll be easier to get your wife to watch one narrated by a doctor than one called *Insatiable Cheerleaders at the ASPCA*.

Here are some of the better ones we've found.

Better Sex Video Series. You've probably seen the ads for these heavily promoted tapes in places like *USA Today*, because the producers have aimed them squarely at a mainstream, Main Street audience of heterosexual couples. (They claim to have cornered 80 percent of the U.S. market for sex education tapes.) Each of the three core tapes (volumes one to three, *Better Sex Basics, Advanced Sexual Techniques* and *Sex Games and Toys*) is narrated by a pair of rather somber sexologists, who provide voice-overs during the (very explicit) demonstrations. The tapes are useful, tasteful and even arousing. The four additional tapes, though, nominally about exploring sexual fantasies, are really more like lame soft porn.

To order: 1-800-888-1900.

Intimacy and Sexual Ecstasy. Narrated in an easygoing way by marriage counselor Jonathan Robinson and sex educator Suzanne Rapley, this single 55-minute tape does a good job of covering all the bases, from ways for couples to improve communication to learning Kegel exercises. Interspersed with video clips of a couple making love.

To order: (805) 562-8787.

Loving Better Series. This five-tape series, narrated and produced by Long Island psychiatrist Sheldon Kule, M.D., is like a biology-class version of the sex-ed tape. The advantage is that it's thorough, covering everything from the physiology of male and female sexual responses to do-it-yourself exercises to improve couple communication or understand your partner's (and your own) body. It's also spiced up with live demonstrations of foreplay, oral sex and self-pleasuring. The disadvantage: Like Biology 101, it occasionally gets dull.

To order: (516) 781-5353. Volume one, *The Basics*; volume two, *Discovery*; volume three, *Loving and Caring*; volume four, *Enhancements*; volume five, *Sexual Problems*.

Great Sex Series. This three-tape series features Toronto psychiatrist Frank Sommers, M.D., who claims to offer "a sex-therapy experience in the privacy of your home." The tapes show Dr. Sommers talking in his office, intercut with explicit scenes of lovemaking. His emphasis is on overcoming psychological barriers to good sex. One slightly discomforting oddity: Many of the couples shown on screen are not actors but real people in "permanent loving relationships." (In other words, not very photogenic.)

Volume one, *Taking Time to Feel*; volume two, *Mutuality*; volume three, *Sexual Pleasures*.

Focus International. If you'd rather just make one phone call, you can order this free, tasteful, low-key catalog, which sells many of the tapes listed above. Mark Schoen, Ph.D., president of Focus International, says his company has been providing sexual information since 1974—to enhance adults' sex lives. Tapes are shipped in plain packaging and the company pledges not to sell your name to anybody else. Two videotapes of special interest: *Erection*, about causes and treatment for erectile problems, and *You Can Last Longer: Solutions for Ejaculatory Control*, a demonstration of the stop-start and squeeze techniques.

To order: 1-800-843-0305. You can also request a free "professional supplement," meant for therapists and doctors.

BONDAGE AND DISCIPLINE
The Truth about Dominance

Okay, sure, there are people in Greenwich Village and West Hollywood who, at this very moment, are wearing leather and chains and getting ready to do all kinds of things that you'd rather not know about.

But there are also ordinary married couples who've expanded the bounds of their sexuality a little to include games that are sometimes referred to as bondage and discipline (B/D), dominance and submission (D/S), sadomasochism (S/M) or just plain eroticized power play. Basically, these are fantasy sex games in which one partner has complete power and control over the other, sometimes including physical bondage, for the duration of the game.

Frankly, we were surprised at how many of our *Men's Health* magazine survey respondents mentioned that they'd occasionally tried B/D games as a way of adding spice to their sex lives. As one respondent (we'll call him O) explained it: "None of us really want to be beaten or raped, just like none of us want to jump from a 50-story building. But like the bungee jumper, the participants in D/S play with the illusion to give a special kick to their lovemaking."

Sex surveys suggest that 5 to 10 percent of Americans (most often males) have tried these games at least occasionally, though they usually involve no real pain or violence, according to June Reinisch, Ph.D., former director of the Kinsey Institute for Research in Sex, Gender and Reproduction in Bloomington, Indiana. And of the over 3,000 fantasies men sent in to writer Nancy Friday for her book *Men in Love*, the biggest number were B/D fantasies.

Bound to Please

One 20-year-old student told us he and his lover had recently begun "experimenting with light bondage." At first, he said, "she was uncomfortable with this as she always seemed to associate it with rape (you would only tie someone up in order to force them to do something). Finally, I was able to convince her that it can be done in a very sensuous and intimate way. The first time, I very loosely tied her wrists to the bedposts. This allowed me to do whatever I wanted, however I wanted.

"The second time we tried it, I tied her a little more tightly with her arms and legs spread out, and she did the same thing to me a few days later. It gave the opportunity to be a little kinky and aggressive. The big turn-on for me was her being sexually aggressive and having to be forward in everything that she was doing. I felt very desired and wanted . . . she is now very open to the idea of being tied and we are keen on trying it again."

The way the game is usually played, according to O, is that one partner decides to be the dominant one (or top) and the other plays the submissive role (or bottom). After agreeing on some basic guidelines (how far are we going to go with this?), you begin playing out a fantasy scene that may last anywhere from a few minutes to a few days. Try pirate captain and captured maiden, for instance. Or Cleopatra and galley slave.

"It is the power component that differentiates this form of lovemaking," says O. "The bottom has to please the top in whatever way they wish, but they do not have to make any decisions; they can leave responsibility behind and become lost in the experience. The top takes all of the responsibility for making the experience good for both of the partners. This is an important point: D/S is not about hurting and using another individual. It is about producing the most intense sexual experience you can for the bottom, while enjoying yourself and retaining control of the situation.

"It is a big turn-on for me to know that a woman trusts me enough to put herself in a helpless position on her knees before me, that she trusts me that much," he goes on to say. "It is also the most intense sex I have found, from a physical standpoint. . . . When you finally climax, you can burn out most of the neurons in your brain!"

The Appeal of Submission

In some ways the whole notion of tying your lover to the bedposts as a way of arousing her seems just plain weird. And the association between dominance and rape is troubling to many women (and men). But maybe it's not all that weird—frankly examining your own sexual fantasies may give you some clue about its appeal, write Anne Semans and Cathy Winks in their book *The Good Vibrations Guide to Sex: How to Have Safe, Fun Sex in the Nineties.* After all, they say, two of the most common themes in sex fantasy are being "taken" by a dominating woman, robber, kidnapper, alien or whatever or else "being in complete erotic control of a stable full of love slaves." In other words, controlling or being controlled.

In her book on the subject, *Erotic Power*, sociologist Gini Graham Scott, Ph.D., says that many men who are very dominant in ordinary life (like the high-powered corporate attorney) "may find submission an erotic release or counterbalance to their everyday behavior." For other men, playing the submissive role is a gateway to the suppressed world of feelings. One guy told her: "When I'm treated rough physically by a woman, I feel overcome by a flow of loving, tender, submissive energy. Surrendering to that energy . . . is one of the most joyous experiences of my life."

For others, playing the submissive role is a turn-on because it's a way of relinquishing responsibility for sexual acts: "She made me do it!" Or as Semans and Winks put it: "Abdicating control and putting your partner in the driver's seat is a highly effective way to make an end run around your own sexual shame and self-denial."

By contrast, playing the dominant role also has its own special appeal: "The dominant can explore feelings frowned upon in our society—selfishness, cruelty and lust for power—and act these out in the context of pleasing a partner."

The How-To Part

Be careful. Don't do anything that will cut off circulation, air or constrict a joint. Don't use slipknots (they'll tighten up when pulled) and avoid thin, slippery material such as stockings that also tend to tighten up under pressure. It's best to use square knots, tied very loosely—even thread will work, since the idea is simply to make someone feel bound. Keep a pair of blunt-tipped scissors nearby just in case. And never leave somebody who's bound alone.

Stay sober. Don't try these games while drinking or taking drugs because it could impair a top's judgment and encourage a bottom to exceed his or her physical limits.

Go shopping. All kinds of mind-boggling toys are available from fuzzy handcuffs to paddles. Check out the Good Vibrations catalog, which also offers a book called *Learning the Ropes: A Basic Guide to Safe and Fun S/M Lovemaking.*

Have an escape word. You should always agree on an escape word (like "uncle") that ends the game immediately when uttered. Sometimes couples use "yellow" and "red" to mean slow down or stop. It's good to have a nonverbal signal, like a snap of the fingers, that also ends the game instantly.

CUNNILINGUS
The Rites and Wrongs of Oral Sex

Satisfying a woman sexually is one of life's sweetest and most enigmatic tasks, and one nearly every man would love to master.

So when we polled *Men's Health* magazine readers about their sexual stories and techniques, we made sure to include this question: Have you discovered anything that consistently enables your partner to reach orgasm? We've included those remarkable replies to this question at various other places in this book. But frankly, the thing that amazed us most was how often oral sex was mentioned. The following replies were typical.

"Oral sex has brought about orgasm with every woman I

THE ALPHABET GAME

One of the respondents to our *Men's Health* magazine survey, a 39-year-old bond salesman, shared this titillating tip: "All women I've used the 'alphabet game' on reach intense orgasms—it works every time. Just make capital letters with your tongue very slowly on her clitoris. You might make it to M!"

have ever had a long-term sexual relationship with," a 37-year-old operations analyst told us. "It is said that some women cannot achieve orgasm via oral sex, but I haven't run into such a woman in my sex life."

"Though she is timid at first, my performing oral sex on her never fails to enable her to reach an orgasm," said a 35-year-old medical supply salesman about his wife.

A network engineer told us: "I find that, usually, oral sex works wonders and consistently produces intense orgasms when time is taken to properly stimulate both the vaginal and clitoral areas, paying special attention to the G-spot."

And a 45-year-old biologist said that "my wife achieves orgasm consistently (this means for the almost 17 years that we have been together) only when I lick her clitoris. This is quite an elaborate ritual."

What Women Say

If you needed any more convincing about the pleasure and utility of cunnilingus (a nasty-sounding word that actually means lick the vulva), consider what the women say. In Shere Hite's national survey of female sexuality, for instance, about 42 percent of women reported they were able to reach orgasm through oral sex (that's slightly more than the number of men who reached orgasm through fellatio, according to a separate Hite report). Even if they couldn't, it was still described by many women as "one of the most favorite and exciting activities; women mentioned over and over again how much they loved it," Hite reported.

In another study, 98 Army wives in happy, stable first marriages kept a sex diary in which they noted the frequency of sexual activity, level of satisfaction and experiences. Of all the sexual activities they mentioned, cunnilingus ranked as the most satisfying. Eighty-two percent said having their husbands pleasure them orally was very satisfying; the next-highest activity, intercourse, was rated very satisfying by only 68 percent. The women reported that during intercourse they reached orgasm about 25 percent of the time. But they reached orgasm 81 percent of the time during oral sex.

Understanding Mouth Music

Cunnilingus is sometimes called mouth music, a nice turn of phrase because it suggests all the different melodies that can be played with the mouth, lips and tongue on the labia, clitoris and vaginal opening. Lots of animals, it turns out, are also great music lovers.

"Most mammals, when sexually aroused, crowd together and nuzzle and explore with their noses . . . they make lip-to-lip contacts and use their mouths to manipulate every part of the companion's body, including the genitalia," the late Dr. Alfred C. Kinsey reported back in the 1950s. "They may nip, bite, scratch, groom, pull at the fur of the other animal . . . such activity may continue for a matter of minutes or hours, or even in some cases for days before there is an attempt at (intercourse)."

> Whatever else can be said about sex, it cannot be called a dignified performance.
>
> —Helen Lawrenson, American writer

Since the mouth and the genitals are the two regions of the body that are most abundantly supplied with erotically sensitive nerve endings, it's almost inevitable that they would come into direct contact during lovemaking. Also, a woman may find your lips and tongue more arousing than your fingers, because they're gentler and can produce a much greater variety of sensations.

More subtly, some women find cunnilingus pleasurable because "going down on her," like a respectful bow or the act of foot washing, seems an act of honoring. You put yourself below her in a position of seeming inferiority in order to give her a special gift of pleasure. Lots of women still like that.

A Few New Melodies

If you're wondering exactly how to go about playing this particular tune, consider the following advice.

- The wonderful term *cassolete* (French for perfume box) is sometimes used to refer to the smell of a woman—her hair and skin, her clothing, her sexuality, her whole self. Even so, a fair number of guys refrain from oral sex because they don't care for a woman's body odors, especially her sexual odors.

If this bothers you, it's easy enough to work a shower or a bath into your prelovemaking rituals. Or you can try scented, edible lubricants (they come in exotic flavors such as butterscotch and Irish coffee), which tend to reduce inhibitions and are often favored by folks new to oral sex. Others swear by melted chocolate or whipped cream.

· Some women don't like oral sex performed on them. It could be that it just doesn't feel good, or that there is a psychological or spiritual resistance or even that they are embarrassed or ashamed of their genitals. If your partner starts tugging your hair to keep you from descending, get the message.

· Because the clitoris is so sensitive, it's often best to go gently, first working your way around it. Be creative. Try approaching the clitoris from the upper (hooded) side, which tends to be less sensitive.

"Over many years of practice I've found the best way for me to perform oral sex on a woman is to lay on my stomach with her knees pulled up near her stomach," adds one respondent. "This gives me better positioning . . . inserting my tongue slowly into her vagina and sliding it up to the hood covering the clitoris—repeatedly—will get an orgasm started."

A 26-year-old naval officer advises, "If you use the tongue the way she likes it (usually short, quick strokes) and use one or two fingers to stimulate the G-spot, most women go absolutely wild. You need to make sure she knows she can give you input (harder, softer, faster, slower, etc.) and you need to be careful you don't over-stimulate—most women need you to back off a bit just before they reach orgasm. Then again, the best orgasm tool I've found is being totally relaxed together. If you can laugh during the lovemaking, you're probably on the right track."

- One caution: You should never blow air into her vagina because it could cause an embolism (an air bubble that enters her bloodstream), which could be fatal. A pregnant woman is particularly susceptible to these embolisms because the veins of her uterus are dilated in order to get more blood to the baby, according to Ricardo Loret de Mola, M.D., an instructor in obstetrics and gynecology at the University of Pennsylvania Medical School in Philadelphia. In fact, he says, ten deaths of pregnant women associated with cunnilingus have been reported in the medical literature.

- Sex experts sometimes recommend using sex toys at the same time you're using your tongue. Try this, for instance: Apply a vibrator to the edge of your tongue as a way of transmitting wet vibrations directly into her genitalia. Also, don't forget that sound transmits vibrations, so if you hum or purr during your oral exam, it can be interesting for her.

- Despite all the foregoing, sex surveys continue to report that a small number of men find cunnilingus and other kinds of oral sex repugnant or even "unnatural." Partly because of a sort of institutionalized distaste for it, oral sex between consenting, heterosexual, married adults is still a crime in nine states.

    Well, if you're one of those guys who just doesn't feel quite comfortable with cunnilingus, you might consider this slightly different mental image of the landscape: In ancient Chinese art a woman's genitals are often depicted as a peony flower. And if you take a whiff of a peony, your face is engulfed in a vast, fragrant mass of pink petals.

- "One complaint I've received from a number of women who like oral sex is that they often feel lonely during it," observes Oakland, California, sex therapist Bernie Zilbergeld, Ph.D., in his book *The New Male Sexuality*. "Although the genital stimulation is terrific, there's nobody to kiss, hold or hug." While you're down there, don't forget that you're making love to a whole person, not just a peony.

A Brief Message from HIV

Unfortunately, one other thing that needs mentioning in any discussion of cunnilingus is the risk of AIDS. Since vaginal secretions of women who are HIV positive have been found to contain (small) amounts of HIV, it's possible to get infected by having oral sex with her, according to *Contraceptive Technology*, a celebrated technical manual of contraception and sexually transmitted diseases. It's even more dangerous to have oral sex with a woman when she's having her period (when you'd make direct contact with blood) or when she has a vaginal infection with discharge. So don't do it.

As a general safe-sex precaution it's best to use a dental dam during cunnilingus. Dental dams are thin sheets of latex designed for use by dentists, which can be laid over the whole vaginal opening during sex. (They're often sold in drugstores and displayed near the condoms.) Unfortunately, lots of guys complain that most dental dams transmit sensation about as well as the Sears Roebuck catalog—which is why you might want to try one that's been specially designed for oral sex instead of a root canal. One made for that purpose is the Lollyes dam (Lollyes is an acronym for latex on lips . . . yes), made by an Australian company called Kia-Ora. You can order them through the Blowfish catalog. For more information on ordering this catalog. see page 339.

CYBERSEX
The Virtue and Vice of Virtual Fun

It's a dull Wednesday night in the year 2020, and your main squeeze is out of town. Noooo problem. You slip downstairs into your basement pleasure palace, squeeze into your full-body cybersensual sex suit, pull on the goggles and gloves, crank up the computer and "suddenly, you are in a strange new world where miraculously you can run your hands through virtual hair, touch virtual silk, unzip virtual clothing and caress virtual flesh," according to a scenario envisioned by Kathy Keeton, vice-chairman of General Media International (publishers of *Penthouse* magazine).

Or, better yet, ring up your sweetie on the phone and through wowie-zowie technology that's come to be known as teledildonics—simulated sex at a distance—you could actually (seemingly) meet her in the flesh for a little roll in the hay, even though she's in Sausalito and you're in Chicago.

In perhaps as little as 30 years from now, writes Howard Rheingold in his book *Virtual Reality*, the mating of computers, telecommunications and the ancient human urge to merge will allow people to "reach out and touch someone . . . in ways humans have never before experienced."

What's Available Now?

Primitive versions of the technology that may someday make "virtual sex" a reality are already available. Generally, voyagers into virtual reality don gloves and weird-looking helmets equipped with two tiny TV screens, one for each eye, and two tiny speakers, one for each ear. The goggles have a tracking device that monitors the movements of your head, so that as it moves, new parts of the 3-D picture come into view, as if it (or she, as the case may be) were really there. The gloves enable you to "actually" touch her.

But the majority of what passes for cybersex in the mid-1990s isn't as glitzy as all that. It usually means one of two things: Sexy images or games loaded onto computer discs or CD-ROMs; or adult electronic bulletin boards, where you can have an erotic keyboard encounter with a stranger or download steamy pictures.

And, sure, the image of some pale nerd down in his basement rec room, all alone, caressing "virtual flesh" is pretty sad. On the other hand, cybersex has certain unmistakable advantages. For one thing, in the age of AIDS it's the ultimate in safe sex. If you're contentedly monogamous, you can enhance your sex life through on-line or CD-ROM fantasy play without risking death, disease or divorce. You don't have to visit some sleazy redlight district or depressing singles bar. It doesn't even matter what you look like, where you live or even what sex you are—you can hook up with somebody anyhow. And you can do it all, as they say, in the privacy of your own home.

CD-ROMs and Floppies

Cybersex software on floppy discs and CD-ROMs grew out of the corny sex games of the early 1980s, like the unforgettable "Leather Goddesses of Phobos" (which was all text) and later, the ever-popular "Leisure Suit Larry in the Land of the Lounge Lizards," an interactive picture story in which a dorky dude in a white leisure suit bumbles around from Las Vegas to the South Seas looking for, er, love.

Most of the best stuff now is on CD-ROM, often designed for the Macintosh platform (because of the great graphics and ease of use), say writers Phillip Robinson and Nancy Tamosaitis in their book *The Joys of Cybersex*. Even so, they warn, there's still plenty of overhyped junk out there—magazine photos crudely

> Be good. And if you can't be good, be careful. And if you can't be careful, name it after me.
>
> —Anonymous

scanned onto floppy disks, or skinflicks that have been dumped onto CD-ROM, with bad audio and jumpy Quick-Time action.

To play a CD-ROM, you'll need a computer and a CD-ROM player. A DOS (disk operating system) machine may also need a Microsoft Windows operating system. Where do you find all these types of CD-ROMs? Generally, the software is still not available in stores or through major mail-order outlets—you usually have to search the backs of computer magazines to find them.

It's also possible to download mildly racy "cyber-pinups" through commercial on-line services, like America Online or Prodigy. They're stored as GIF, JPEG or some other type of graphics file; you'll need another program—like a GIFconverter or JPEGviewer—in order to "read" them, but these can easily be downloaded as well.

On-Line Bulletin Boards

"Five years ago, the personal ads were hot—they were the most common way for adults to meet one another for sex. But today it's the electronic bulletin boards," says William Kelly, a sex therapist who works as a consultant to the phone sex industry.

On a board, or BBS, you can engage a stranger in "hot chat" meant to evoke masturbatory rapture. Or you can take things a step farther because many bulletin boards also arrange informal, in-person get-togethers where "Iron-man" can actually meet "Leopardbelly" in the flesh. You can also download erotic pictures that are much more explicit than those you'll find on the on-line services. Some of this may enter the realm of the illegal, particularly when it involves children (and, really, how do you know the person you're faking sex with isn't a 14-year-old with a good vocabulary?). These types of cases are increasingly in the news.

That cyberspace would rapidly develop traffic jams in erotica was perhaps inevitable: France's national computer network, Minitel, with terminals placed in nearly every home at government expense, "has largely turned into a dating service, much to the Socialist administration's chagrin," according to *Barron's*, the weekly financial newspaper.

To subscribe to one of the adult bulletin boards—which have great names, like Adults 'R Us, Heat in the Night or Duke's Doghouse—you have to have a computer, a modem and communications software. Once you log on, you have to register (often giving a credit card number); in a day or so, you'll get a call back to verify that you're an adult.

One respondent to our *Men's Health* magazine survey, a 25-year-old administrator, tells the story of having carried on a two-month "relationship" with a woman he met in cyberspace, including the equivalent of electronic heavy breathing for a couple of hours every night. ("It was great but extremely hard to type with one hand!" he says.) Though they eventually stopped meeting in cyberspace, he says "this is the way people should be required to meet. I felt like I got to know her really well without any preconceived notions that would have been based upon her appearance, hair style, color of her skin, etc. We had a lot of fun together!"

Fishing on the Net

If you already have access to the vast and wonderful electronic chaos called the Internet, you may already know about the usenet newsgroups. Basically, these are bull sessions conducted around the clock, all over the world, by means of interlinked computers. There are tens of thousands of newsgroups, on every subject imaginable—Tim Burton movies, pre-Raphaelite art and (of course) sex. Some of the more interesting ones:

Alt.sex—This is one of the most popular newsgroups on the Net, featuring long discussions of everything from "Do women have rape fantasies?" and "the best songs to make love to" (Pachelbel's Canon in D Minor, anything by Black Sabbath) to seemingly endless debates on the actual entymological origin of a certain Anglo-Saxon word beginning with "f."

Alt.binaries.pictures.erotica—Like other newsgroups using the word "binary" in their names, this one contains codes that can be translated into pictures. Newsgroups like this created a ruckus at Carnegie Mellon University in Pittsburgh when a researcher doing an analysis of erotica available on-line was able to put together a collection of 917,000 pictures and verify that they'd been retrieved by computer users a total of 6.4 million times.

Alt.romance—Discussions of dating, relationships and, of course, "What do women want?"

Alt.religion.sexuality—Mostly theological/sexological arguments.

Hiv.aids.issues and *sci.med.aids*—Both discuss the issues surrounding, and treatments for, AIDS.

FANTASIES
The Pleasures and Perils of Making Them Real

Very likely, most of your sex life is a complete fantasy.

That's not an insult, just a mathematical fact. Think about it: How much time do you spend thinking about sex each week—including the last ten minutes, you sly dog—as compared to the amount of time you actually spend doing something about it? If you're like the rest of us, the fantasy/reality ratio is something like a hundred to one. Human sexuality, especially male sexuality, is very largely a game of pretend.

Sex researchers are forever rediscovering this about men: In one study, when 16-and 17-year-old boys were asked if a sexual thought had crossed their minds in the last five minutes, 51 percent said yes. So did 20 percent of guys ages 40 to 55. Another study found that guys ages 12 to 19 estimated they thought about sex every five minutes; guys in their forties said they had an erotic thought about every half-hour.

Women, of course, are morally superior to men and do not obsess about bumping and grinding like we do. Researchers from the University of Chicago, in the 1994 *Sex in America* survey, found that 54 percent of men say they think about sex "every day" or "several times a day." But less than half as many women (19 percent) said they thought about sex that often. Fourteen percent of the women said they thought about sex "less than once a month" or "never."

During intercourse itself, though, the gender differences tend to diminish: About 85 percent of both men and women have sexual fantasies during sexual intercourse at least some of the time, and 21 percent have them frequently, according to research by Harold Leitenberg, Ph.D., psychology professor at the University of Vermont in Burlington. The study also showed that people who fantasize during sex feel a greater level of sexual satisfaction and have fewer sexual problems in their relationships—even if the person they're fantasizing about is not the same person they're sharing the bed with.

How Women's Fantasies Differ

When women fantasize about sex, it's generally in the form of something akin to a mental daytime soap opera. Compared to men's fantasies, women's erotic daydreams tend to be hazier and more romantic, more personal, often focusing specifically on someone they actually know. They emphasize touching, feeling and emotions, unfold more slowly and tend to include more caressing and nongenital touching. Men's fantasies, by contrast, tend to be dominated by visual images, especially genital images, are more likely to involve multiple, often anonymous partners, are more active and aggressive and move more quickly to explicitly sexual acts.

In other words, the problems we have relating to one another in real life are clearly mirrored in our imaginations.

Nevertheless, though guys fantasize about sex in extremely graphic ways and do so more or less constantly, it's interesting to remember that it's women,

> The male in many instances may not be having coitus with the immediate sexual partner but with all the other girls with whom he has ever had coitus, and with the entire genus Female with which he would like to have coitus.
>
> —Dr. Alfred C. Kinsey in *Sexual Behavior of the Human Female*

not men, who are capable of taking fantasy over the top, actually reaching orgasm simply by thinking about sex. About 1 percent of the several thousand women in Shere Hite's survey were capable of this astounding feat; in the late Dr. Alfred C. Kinsey's sample of 8,000 women, about 2 percent were "orgasm fantasists." More recently, a team of researchers at Rutgers University in New Brunswick, New Jersey, found ten such women and wired them up to various monitors in a lab. First they were asked to masturbate to orgasm (all ten could do it); then to fantasize to orgasm (seven succeeded). Most interesting of all, the researchers found that both kinds of orgasms produced very similar physiological changes: a boost in heart rate, systolic blood pressure and pupil diameter and a significant elevation in the women's sensitivity to pain.

In other words, though triggered purely by erotic fantasy, these orgasms were just as real as any other kind.

Forbidden Flowers

For us cerebral modern creatures sexual fantasizing can be an astoundingly vivid and pleasurable experience, with a variety of practical uses. It heightens your arousal during intercourse or masturbation. It helps you block out work, stress and other distractions during sex. It allows you to "rehearse" new sexual adventures. And what's more, it's free.

In other words, unreeling steamy movies in your mind is an essential part of robust, normal sexuality. Conventional wisdom suggests that people who daydream about sex a lot tend to be lonely, loveless dweebs. But the University of Chicago *Sex in America* researchers found quite the opposite: "The men and women who use fantasy and who use autoerotic materials (like sexy magazines) are those who seem to seek out the most sex with a partner and who find the greatest number of other sexual experiences appealing," they reported.

Researchers have also found that people who lack interest in sex have a curiously sterile, unsexual mental life. These people may consciously squelch such thoughts because they feel guilty or embarrassed about them, or they may simply not have them at all. As part of their cure, many sex therapists help these self-censored folks unleash the erotic potential of their minds by teaching them how to fantasize.

One other great advantage of fantasy, of course, is that it allows you to act out all sorts of things you could not (or wouldn't really want to) actually try in the flesh. For instance, one study found that same-sex erotic encounters were among the most common fantasies among heterosexual men—but that doesn't necessarily mean these guys are "latent homosexuals" (as people used to say). They could simply have been using a delicious taboo as a way of enhancing their pleasure.

Nancy Friday, author of *My Secret Garden* and other books about sexual fantasies, writes that "in my books on women's sexual fantasies the single greatest theme that emerged was that of 'weak' women being sexually dominated, 'forced' by male strength to do this deliciously awful thing." In the same way, these women are not actually harboring some secret desire to be raped. Researchers have pointed out that these dominance fantasies may simply be a way for women to absolve themselves of responsibility for initiating or enjoying sex, or to overcome their feelings of guilt about enjoying sex.

It's a mental trick they use to enhance their sexual pleasure.

And that's the whole point.

Acting It Out

Sharing a secret fantasy with your lover or actually acting one out turned out to be a favorite sexual game among the respondents to our *Men's Health* magazine survey. But sharing a fantasy can sometimes go wrong, warns Friday. "I think that for every person who has written to me about the joys of performing their sex dreams in reality, there have been three or four who knew in advance that it wouldn't work or who tried it and were disappointed."

Still, there's a right way to bring up the subject with your lover. Try picking just one relatively tame fantasy to start, and ask her to share one of hers. If that's as far as it gets, fine. You've still gotten an interesting, indirect clue about what really turns her on. And learning to talk more candidly with each other can be arousing all by itself.

One survey respondent, a 20-year-old student, gave this advice about coaxing a shy and reluctant lover into deeper water, including light bondage and acted-out fantasies: "The key to all of these things that I have done with my girlfriend is respect and understanding. For some reason or other she was uncomfortable or hesitant in some way with all of them.

Feeling comfortable enough to discuss not only secret desires and fantasies but also your fears and discomfort about them has enabled us to try many things that we didn't originally feel comfortable with. By not demanding anything of her and by talking about them with her, I have gotten pleasure beyond my wildest dreams."

A few other suggestions include:

- "An active fantasy life is the key to keeping sex fun and interesting," a 27-year-old law student told us. "It also eliminates all desire to cheat on your partner. Most often we make love without it, but sometimes (approximately twice a month) we do a little role playing. Some favorites: pirate captain/galley wench, pizza boy/bored housewife who lost her purse, Conan/Red Sonja, Prince Charming/wicked queen, Roman centurion/Roman goddess. The improvised dialogue is usually hilarious—but laughter is an aphrodisiac, no?"

- "Fantasies are very good," another respondent said. "I had a long relationship that was also long distance. Phone sex became very necessary. When we were together, it just sort of continued. She would send these letters in which she would describe some sort of scenario, and then I would come home to find it set up. (The Reagans were a favorite fantasy in the mid-1980s.)"

  (We sent him an e-mail message to inquire about this Ron and Nancy thing, but he didn't reply. You figure it out.)

- "I try to make up a new fantasy and trade a new one each month with my lover (when I can get her to 'fess up to one). Then I ambush her with it at an unexpected time. Favorite games: the cat burglar, the detective's interrogation, the flirtatious stranger."

- Sex therapist Lonnie Barbach, Ph.D., in her book *For Each Other*, tells of a woman who was turned on by fantasies of uncontrollable lust—so she and her husband would wear old T-shirts and rip them off each other during sex.

- For more ideas try a nice little book by Rolf Milonas

called *Fantasex: A Book of Erotic Games for the Adult Couple*. Examples: "It's another three years in solitary unless he submits to the warden's attentions; she takes the warden's role." Or "following the doctor's posthypnotic suggestion, the beast in her is freed and she forgets all she believed was proper." Available through the Good Vibrations catalog. For more information on ordering catalogs, see page 339.

FELLATIO
The Song of the Flute

It's not like it's exactly a new concept.

Cleopatra, the Egyptian queen who ruled in the first century B.C., was said to have been so adept at the practice that she was known as the great swallower.

The Indian sage Vatsyayana, in his 2,000-year-old love manual, *Kama Sutra*, called it mouth congress and lovingly described eight different kinds with such names as "sucking a mango fruit" and "swallowing it up."

The ancient Chinese, in their ancient Chinese way, simply called it playing the flute.

But whatever you call it, most guys still love it. In the 1994 *Sex in America* survey conducted by University of Chicago researchers, 83 percent of men ages 18 to 44 said they found the idea of being on the receiving end of oral sex to be "very" or "somewhat" appealing. Fellatio, in fact, was their third-favorite sexual sport, outranked only by intercourse and (believe it or not) watching their partners undress.

If She Doesn't Want To

But here's the rub. In general, women—especially older women—don't seem to have as lusty an appetite for oral sex (whether giving or receiving it) as men do. In this same study only 57 percent of women said they found the idea of giving fellatio to be "very" or "somewhat" appealing; among women over age 45, well over half did not like giving oral sex—or receiving it either—at all. In fact, the whole question of fellatio and/or oral sex differed from other more-or-less standard sexual practices like vaginal intercourse in that "oral sex definitely elicited mixed reactions, from strongly enthusiastic to extremely unenthusiastic," the researchers found.

So, obviously, if you have this real thing for fellatio and she doesn't, you potentially have a problem.

"This can become a huge issue in relationships—and the fact that she is not interested gives her control of the whole situation," says William Hartman, M.D., co-director of the Center for Marital and Sexual Studies in Long Beach, California. A gentle discussion of views later on might reveal deeper reasons for the disdain. Be respectful and supportive; listen, don't beg or coerce. If she still says no way, it's probably best to just drop it and be happy with what you have. "If you really care for her, you should enjoy what she's willing to give, sexually, and not push for something she doesn't want to give."

One thing that might help change her mind, Dr. Hartman suggests, is your own willingness to favor her with oral sex, since oral sex is often part of an unspoken bargain: If you give it to her, and she loves it, it's only fair that she return the favor. Of course, don't keep score. Changing an attitude like this one takes time and patience, and sometimes never happens. If you are giving oral sex only to get oral sex, you both have a problem, and it should be talked out.

What Women Learn at College

Still, if you're having trouble finding a woman who has a genuine appetite for fellatio, you might start out by trying to get invited to sorority parties. Because, amazingly enough, the *Sex in America* researchers discovered that "twice as many

> Sometimes a cigar is just a cigar.
>
> —Sigmund Freud

women who went to college have given or received oral sex as compared to those who didn't finish high school. . . . This practice, it turns out, has gained its greatest popularity among young, better-educated Whites."

Part of the reason that oral sex is so much more widely practiced among well-educated, white women younger than age 50, the researchers surmised, is that oral sex really came into vogue on college campuses during the 1960s. Those coed dorms were hotbeds of revolution.

Not Quite Making It

An amazing number of respondents to our *Men's Health* magazine survey told us that favoring their (female) lovers with oral sex was one of the few things that could consistently trigger an earth-moving orgasm. And at least one female respondent to the survey, a 19-year-old student, said the same thing about fellatio: "Oral sex is a surefire way to enable my partner to reach climax quickly."

Often, though, this is not the case—because despite its delights, lots of guys cannot actually climax this way. In Shere Hite's celebrated, not-very-scientific survey, the *Hite Report on Male Sexuality*, 85 percent of her male respondents said they thought fellatio was a terrific concept, but only 40 percent said they could always or usually reach orgasm by mouth.

So if that's been your experience, don't worry about it—you have company.

Also, don't forget one other thing about fellatio: It's one of the most efficient ways of transmitting the AIDS virus, since blood and semen are the two bodily fluids with the highest concentrations of HIV. If you're HIV positive, or don't know your status, either refrain from asking anybody for fellatio or be sure to use a condom when you do.

Tips and Techniques

The folks at Good Vibrations, a San Francisco-based mail-order shop for sexual accessories, say one of their best-selling videotapes is a half-hour educational video called *How to Perform Fellatio*. A series of actresses do their duty, and narrate, using (slightly glassy-eyed) male actors.

Here are some things to remember.

- In the heat of the action, a woman may take your John Robert so deeply that she begins to gag. Don't forget that retching is a reflex action when something goes way down her throat; if she gags, it's not because she finds you disgusting but because she just can't help herself. Back off, and be gentle.

- The whole question of ejaculating in the mouth sometimes becomes a huge relationship issue. Maybe she likes it, maybe she doesn't. But one nice solution is to agree beforehand on some little signal that will let her know when you're about to come. At that point, she could remove you from her mouth and use her hands, or do whatever else she likes. But at least she has a choice.

- Try playing with temperature. Ask her to hold a small ice cube in her mouth. Or have her drink hot fluids before fellatio.

- Try using weird lubricants. Some kinds will generate heat (they usually contain glycerine or cinnamon, peppermint or clove oils). When you apply them to the skin and blow, a kind of shimmering warmth spreads over you. Other kinds of lubricants contain benzocaine or other mild anesthetics that numb out the skin and trigger a wild sensation when feeling floods back as they wear off. Just remember: Lots of this stuff is oil-based, so it will destroy a condom and can be irritating to the vagina.

FETISHES
When the Object of Your Desire Is a Shoe

A fetish is an inanimate object thought to have magical power—say, a conch shell the local shaman claims has healing power. A sexual fetish is an inanimate object thought to have sexual power. To the fetishist, it becomes the center of erotic interest and satisfaction; it may trigger sexual excitement, or it may even come to displace the real-life person who is normally the object of desire. A foot fetishist, for instance, may be able to ejaculate only by fondling a woman's feet, with no genital contact at all.

The fetish object can be a body part (feet, hair), the look or feel of certain material (latex, leather, silk, fur), a smell (a guy with a shoe fetish might be aroused by the smell of leather and sweat as well as their appearance) or almost anything else. And here's something else about the whole deal that hits kind of close to home: Mental health professionals have found that fetishism is almost exclusively a male practice.

A Hard-Driving, Lustful Desire

How on earth does a person become erotically attached to a foot?

Well, there are lots of theories, but nobody really knows for sure, which just goes to show you how little we understand about human sexuality. Fetishism is one of a group of behaviors that used to be called perversions but are now more politely known as paraphilias (*para* meaning "beyond" or "outside the usual" and *philia* meaning "love"). These include cross-dressing, exhibitionism, voyeurism, pedophilia and others. As a group, these sexual oddities are surprisingly common among males—"2 to 5 percent of males develop a paraphiliac arousal pattern, usually in childhood or adolescence," observes Barry McCarthy, Ph.D., psychology professor at American University in Washington, D.C. More than half these "sexually compulsive" men have a history of childhood abuse (physical, sexual or emotional), Dr. McCarthy says. But that doesn't really explain it all.

Some researchers have suggested that men are more prone to become fetishists because they're more easily aroused by sights and smells than women are; it's easier for them to get so fixated on a sight-trigger that it actually becomes detached from a living person. Others have theorized that because these men are so terrified or revolted by their own feelings of "sinful," "wicked" lust, they learn to transfer their sexual feelings to objects—in effect, to hold their own sexuality at a distance, like a dirty handkerchief. The fetish becomes sinful, arousing and a substitute for a lover. In a crazy way, the object is "blamed" for the arousal, yet necessary for it, according to theories developed by John Money, Ph.D., professor of medical psychology and pediatrics at Johns Hopkins University in Baltimore, one of the foremost experts on paraphilias.

However it's created in the mind, a fetish can become an unbelievably powerful sexual trigger. "The hard-driving, lustful desire evoked by the paraphilia is hard to duplicate," says Dr. McCarthy. "The analogy is to a five-speed car: The [fetishist] male can skip all five gears and switch to his supercharged sixth gear—a powerful, driven, lustful, totally predictable, compulsive sexuality." It's a kind of sexual rush that often makes ordinary partner sex seem dull by comparison. Actually, though, those incredible, lonely orgasms are a sexual dead end—they lead away from a satisfying union with another real person and all the joys and terrors of "real sex," and toward a sad, secret, robotlike sexual world of one's own creation.

In other words, nowhere.

Where Do You Draw the Line?

Still, don't forget, not everybody who responds sexually to a fetish object is lonely or twisted. There are many levels of fetishism. For instance, if you get aroused when your lover wears black, lacy lingerie, in some sense the lingerie is a fetish—an inanimate object that becomes a sexual trigger. It's what you might call a mild trigger, almost a mere mood-enhancer. So what's the problem? Well, there isn't really a problem. It's only a "true" fetish if you can't get aroused unless she is wearing lacy lingerie. The fetish has to be necessary to arousal, not just preferred, to be classed as a paraphilia, according to June Reinisch, Ph.D., former director of the Kinsey Institute for Research in Sex, Gender and Reproduction in Bloomington, Indiana.

In a nice turn of phrase, Alex Comfort, M.D., D.Sc., author of *The Joy of Sex*, calls hard-core fetishism a compulsive ritualism. It has to do with rigid, unvarying behavior, whereas "real sex" has to do with spontaneity, flexibility, variety. You can tell you're getting into trouble if whatever it is

> When sex is good, it's the most beautiful thing in the world. When sex is bad, it's still pretty good.
>
> —Irish saying

that you have to have causes anxiety and interferes with sexual joy. "Refusing to try anything but the missionary position is as much a fetish as only being potent when wearing a diving helmet," Dr. Comfort says.

The good news is that the American public is relatively forgiving of fetishism. In the *Janus Report on Sexual Behavior*, researchers who surveyed 2,700 American men and women found that 22 percent of men and 18 percent of women said they thought fetishes were "very normal" or "all right." Which means they were far more approving of fetishes than, say, cross-dressing. (A few of the women even said they felt more secure with their male fetishist lovers—because they knew the guy would have a hard time finding somebody else who'd feel comfortable with his sexual proclivities.)

But if you feel you may have developed an unwholesome attachment to a fetish object and wish to break free, therapy can be helpful. Twelve-step "sex addiction" programs, which often involve getting support from a group, have been helpful for a fair number of men.

FOREPLAY
Why It Matters So Much

"Why do so many women fake orgasm?"
    "Because so many men fake foreplay."

It's a bad joke, but it pretty much sums up the problem. Studies show three-fourths of men are finished with sex within a few minutes of the time they started. But women often need 15 minutes or more to become sufficiently aroused for orgasm. And therein lies a world of rage, grief and airborne pots and pans.

In a survey of 98 Army wives in stable first marriages, the women were asked two questions. The first question was, "What aspect of partner-related sexual activities do you find to be the most sexually satisfying?" Far and away the most common answer—mentioned by 58 percent of the young wives—was foreplay. (Foreplay, if you don't know, is all the caressing, kissing and stimulating that goes on prior to inter-course.) By contrast, only 16 percent mentioned orgasm.

The second question was, "What aspects of partner-related sexual activities would you like your partner to pay more attention to in your relationship?" Even more of the women (65 percent) again said foreplay. Only 4 percent said orgasm.

Now, we don't know if these young women were married to grunts and noncoms of the old slam-bam-thank-you-ma'am school of sexual fulfillment. But we do know that both the women and their husbands were probably only minutes away from something really wonderful. Because when Paul Gebhard, one of the collaborators on the late Dr. Alfred C. Kinsey's groundbreaking sex studies in the 1940s, went back and re-examined the Kinsey group's data, he found that among women whose lovers spent 21 minutes or longer on foreplay, only 7.7 percent of them failed to reach orgasm consistently.

And when she gets there, too, both of you are bound to be happier.

Foreplay While Fully Dressed

It's sometimes said that, when it comes to sexual arousal, men are like lightbulbs and women are like irons. A light-bulb gets "turned on" with the flick of a switch, almost instantly, and when you turn it off, it instantly goes dark. But when you turn on an iron, it heats up very gradually, and once turned off, it only slowly cools.

But by taking the time for foreplay and lingering over her awakening body while you deliberately delay your own ejaculation, you "handicap" yourself a little—slowing yourself down while speeding her up. Ideally, you'll meet somewhere in the middle. And that's the point.

This is, of course, a simplistic analogy. Dr. Kinsey's studies also showed that during masturbation many women are capable of bringing themselves to orgasm within a couple of minutes, just like males do. It could very well be that women's innate sexual responses are just as rapid as men's, he concluded; it's only during intercourse, widely known to be a clumsy way for women to achieve orgasm, that they're slower. Even so, in lovemaking with a partner a multitude of studies have shown that women simply take more time to get where males get in about 30 seconds flat.

People usually use the word "foreplay" to mean all the sweet skin-to-skin seductions of sex before intercourse— kissing, hugging, licking, touching. But sex therapists say it really means anything that comes before sex—including many things that take place long before you remove your clothes.

"Foreplay doesn't have to start in bed—in fact, sometimes it can start the day before, with anticipation, looking forward to it, even a kind of teasing," says Shirley Zussman, Ed.D., a certified sex therapist and co-director of the Association for Male Sexual Dysfunction in New York City.

To enhance the anticipation, try developing some little "sexual signal" that lets your partner know you're thinking about having sex later, suggests Jude Cotter, Ph.D., a psychologist and sex therapist in private practice in Farmington Hills, Michigan. Whenever she touches her ear in public, or yawns or runs her finger along her throat, that means, "I can't wait to get you home in bed." It's a way of beginning foreplay hours before your bodies even touch.

Several of our *Men's Health* magazine survey respondents know all about this. "I love it when my girlfriend puts on sexy lingerie and covers it with a sexy silk blouse and a short miniskirt," one guy told us. "Sometimes we'll go see a movie or go out for a romantic dinner, and for several hours I can't stop thinking about her lace panties and bra as well as her thigh-high stockings. It drives me crazy for the whole night, just knowing what's underneath her clothes."

Another man, a 47-year-old academic librarian, told us that he and his wife "make love" three or four times a week, but just as importantly, "we are erotic and loving with each other when we aren't having sex. Many mornings, for instance, I enjoy just sitting on the bed and watching my wife dress. Or she will wash the dishes while nude, or close to it."

If that's not foreplay, what is?

Setting the Scene

One thing about foreplay that men tend to neglect, says Dr. Zussman, is the fact that it often takes women longer to get "in the mood." Men, she says, "can move more-or-less directly from watching football to having sex, but women are much more aware of the setting, the surroundings, the mood. She's more inclined to hold onto her anger that he has not been paying attention to her, and then suddenly he wants to have sex. She needs to be romanced a little; she needs a little more transition time."

And when he begins to touch her, Dr. Zussman says, "women seem to require more overall, nongenital, whole-body touching" before escalating things to intercourse. "Gentle touching is evidence to her that he cares about her as a person. She needs that before she can become aroused."

Tell Me How, Tell Me When

Typically (especially in women's magazines) the whole subject of foreplay is portrayed as a problem caused almost entirely by men. We're too impatient, too clumsy, too self-ish, too orgasm-oriented. But it really takes two to tango, and women are as much at fault for not communicating their own needs during foreplay as men are, Dr. Zussman says. "Many women still have a great deal of difficulty in communicating what they want and need sexually—and if he doesn't know what she wants, his chances of satisfying her are greatly reduced."

Many women, for instance, just assume that he knows when she's ready for penetration—but he doesn't, because vaginal lubrication is a much subtler sign of arousal (and much more easily misinterpreted) than a robust erection.

"Women don't seem to understand that we really want to please them," one 28-year-old theater manager complained. "I would rather have a woman move my hand or mouth or whatever to where she wants it than to lie back and think of England. Tell us what you want—don't expect that we are going to know, and then get mad when we don't!"

> Oh, you men! See that you frolic before copulation. Prepare her for the enjoyment and let nothing be neglected to attain this end.
>
> —The Perfumed Garden
> by Sheikh Nefzawi

Asking her to guide your hand—and in this way show you where to touch her, and how—is a technique frequently recommended by sex therapists. Because when a woman simply tells you what to do, guys are inclined to feel hurt or criticized or unflatteringly compared to some other lover, lingering over the bed like a ghost. Also, adds Dr. Zussman, sexual communication is not just a one-time deal—you can't expect to ask for something once and forever afterward be irritated if he doesn't give it to you. "Once is not enough," she says.

Expert Advice

In our magazine survey we asked a question we felt almost all men would be interested in: "Have you discovered anything that consistently enables your partner to reach orgasm?" Among the responses we received were many from men who were clearly devoted, attentive and skillful lovers. We've come to think of these guys as the expert advisers who've guided us throughout this whole book. And these men mentioned the importance of foreplay over and over again.

"What enhances our sex life the most is lots and lots of foreplay," a young attorney said. "We drive each other nuts before we actually have sex. It leads to incredible orgasms . . . foreplay gets her in such a frenzy that she is halfway to orgasm before we even have sex."

"Foreplay, foreplay and more foreplay," said another. "Touching, caressing, snuggling, sucking, licking and kissing. All this is fun and sensuous, and the more time for it makes for better sex. If we can make the time to enjoy great foreplay, I can almost always give her as many orgasms as she can take."

Or: "Foreplay is a major contributor to orgasm. I will normally begin to stimulate my girlfriend by touching her around the vaginal opening (labia, clitoris, anus) and this causes her to become lubricated. After that, she really enjoys oral sex."

Or: "Sometimes we'll lie in bed and just tell each other fantasies and talk about what we would either want to do or what we would want done to us, and that's foreplay before we attack each other."

And: "I have found that while lying on my side next to her, I can fondle her body while my erect penis is just at the entrance or about an inch inside, and by talking sweet things to her, she will orgasm usually before I penetrate. After that, it really gets good."

We were amazed at how many men mentioned oral sex as an essential part of these sweet rituals.

"I find that, usually, oral sex works wonders and consistently produces intense orgasms when time is taken to properly stimulate both the vaginal and clitoral areas, paying special attention to the G-spot," a 30-year-old network engineer told us. "Thirty to 45 minutes of oral sex during foreplay is not out of the ordinary." For more information on oral sex, see Cunnilingus on page 250.

Aging: The Great Equalizer

As men get older, their sexual responses slow down a bit. The old instantaneous, rock-hard erections of your youth begin showing up a little more reluctantly. They need more coaxing. Over time, says Dr. Zussman, "older men need more direct genital stimulation in order to become erect."

Which means that, as you get older, it's you who starts to need more foreplay. The lightbulb starts turning into an iron. Your hair gets grayer, your stock portfolio gets fatter and the difference between your sexual responses and that of your lover gradually begin to diminish. Which may be partly why so many of our older respondents told us that sex just keeps getting better and better the more time passes under the bridge.

At least you have that to look forward to!

KISSING
The Passion of the Lips

To hear women tell it, guys tend to think of kissing as little more than an impediment to intercourse, like that last, stubborn button. For instance, San Francisco sex therapist and author Lonnie Barbach, Ph.D., writes that "men learn, while growing up, that touching, holding, hugging and kissing are feminine needs and that 'real men' only like intercourse."

Well, we're getting a little tired of hearing this sort of thing. One thing women don't understand about men, one 25-year-old restaurant manager told us in our *Men's Health* magazine survey, is that "men are also concerned about giving pleasure or pleasing their partners in the true sense of the word—I think men are a lot more sensitive than most women give us credit for."

Even so, it's probably true that both men and women, especially in long-standing marriages or relationships, tend to forget how delicious and meaningful the little things like kissing can be. And when lovers gradually forget to kiss and touch each other except when they want sex, touch begins to seem "more like a demand rather than an expression of love," Dr. Barbach says. A kiss becomes "I want to make love now."

> Granted, the sexual revolution went too far, information-wise. When you find phrases like 'suck face' as a euphemism for 'kiss,' it sort of takes the zing out of intimate personal contact.
>
> —Ian Shoales, comedian

Then a downward spiral begins. One or both partners begin limiting the casual kiss or any other physical affection for fear that they'll be interpreted by the other as an invitation to sex. Which winds up being a big drag all the way around—like gradually removing all the appetizers, the soup, the first course and dessert from the feast of sex.

The High School Time Machine

Just to make sure you're not taking her for granted sexually, and to reexperience the joy of kissing and other sensuous, undemanding touches, consider the following exercise. It's quite simple. Don't have intercourse for three weeks. Instead, restrict yourself to any other physical contact— kissing, touching, hugging or manual and oral stimulation. Just don't "go all the way." If you can do it, this exercise will be a sort of time machine, transporting you back to high school and the days before "doing it" was allowed, and you and she were left to discover, and rediscover, the exquisite pleasures of the mouth.

"Nearly all the ancient books (on the subject of sex) emphasize the importance of deep, erotic kissing. They place it second only to the actual act of coition (intercourse)," writes Jolan Chang in a book called *The Tao of the Loving Couple* (about ancient Chinese sexual techniques). If you think about it, he goes on, "in the lips and tongue we have erotic organs with the characteristics of both the vulva and the phallus." The mouth is an invitingly warm, wet, soft interior space; the tongue, a voluntary muscle that can be hard and reckless and penetrating like a penis. A really erotic French kiss (if you don't know, that's when you use your tongues) can sometimes be about as close to intercourse as you get without actually doing it.

In fact, the range of possibilities is amazing—the dry, gentle lip-brush; the probing kiss, more like a question than a touch; the deep, wet, yearning, "soul" kiss; the rough, almost cannibalistic kiss that leaves a bruise. The 2,000-year-old love manual *Kama Sutra*, which can sometimes be as preachy and doctrinaire as the Boy Scouts' manual, goes on at some length about kissing, describing everything from the "kiss that kindles love" (when a woman kisses a man while he's sleeping) to the "kiss that turns away" (when she kisses him while he's engaged in business or they're quarreling). But forget about the *Kama Sutra* and make up something brand-new yourself.

Unfortunately, AIDS seems to raise its ugly head everywhere these days, and there's one small warning that goes with kissing. "Dry" kissing, on unbroken skin, is completely safe because there's no transfer of bodily fluids. But deep, wet French kissing is considerably "possibly" unsafe, according to the physician-authors of *Contraceptive Technology*, because of the very slim chance that HIV virus in her saliva might enter your body if you have a cut on the inside of your mouth. So if you don't know her HIV status, be careful.

How to Be a Great Kisser

In a tongue-in-cheek book called *Art of Kissing*, writer William Cane reports on the results of a kissing questionnaire he distributed to a group of men and women. A few practical suggestions for becoming a better kisser emerged from their comments.

Soften up. Relaxed lips and facial muscles are soft and sensuous; kissing tense, tight lips is like smooching with a lamppost. One young woman said, "I feel like telling guys, 'Soften those lips or you get no kiss!' " Another also complained that the boys she kissed had wooden lips. "They need to practice movement in their lips. I don't know how else to describe it."

Brush your teeth, boy. When asked what they didn't like about kissing, many of the women mentioned bad breath. In his autobiography Bertrand Russell tells how his own bad breath nearly wrecked a promising relationship with a beautiful young girl. The big problem: He simply wasn't aware of it, and she was too shy to mention it, until after he'd discovered it and solved the problem. To be safe, brush your teeth before kissing encounters. Breath fresheners provide a short-term solution but aren't a substitute for a clean mouth.

> I wasn't kissing her, I was whispering in her mouth.
>
> —Chico Marx

Be kissed. There is a subtle difference between kissing and being kissed—and just because you're a guy doesn't mean you always have to be the lip-aggressor. Try being the kissee sometimes, not leading the kiss, just passively receiving the pleasure. "You know what's really fun?" one woman wrote. "When you kiss a guy and you tell him not to kiss you back, so that you're doing everything, guiding the entire kiss. It's such a sexy thing to do!"

"Listen" to her kiss. Great kissers, like great lovers, are sensitive to how their partners are feeling and responsive to what they're trying to communicate with their mouths, Cane says. Take a deep breath, relax and just try to imagine what she's feeling while she kisses you.

Try kissing like a gangster. Sometimes it's fun to play a fantasy role while you're kissing, several of the respondents reported. Some couples got off on playing the role of slave and master while they kissed. Or a bored housewife and the mailman. Or Antony and Cleopatra. One big favorite: The guy pretends to be a crime boss or a gangster, generous and ruthless, sweeping her off her feet as if he's got a pistol in his pocket. One woman said she even liked to wear "a really trashy dress" while kissing her gangster, who'd wear a 1930s-style gray felt hat, like a bank robber.

LASTING LONGER
Techniques to Control Yourself

One of the respondents to our *Men's Health* magazine survey, describing the experience of having exotically naughty sex with his wife while driving a car one hot summer night, concluded his story by saying, "How long this went on I have no idea, but it may have been the most alive I have ever been."

Yeah! That feeling of being absolutely awake in the moment is one of the reasons we go to such ridiculous lengths in search of sexual pleasure. By the same token, it stands to reason that if you could learn to delay ejaculation and thus extend the pleasure even longer, you'd be squeezing that much more life out of your sex life. And who doesn't want to be more alive?

Unfortunately, millions of men just can't seem to control their ejaculations; those moments of hyperaliveness are over all too quickly. In fact, William H. Masters, M.D., and Virginia E. Johnson, of the former Masters and Johnson Institute in St. Louis, speculated that lack of ejaculatory control is probably the most common sexual problem, affecting 15 to 20 percent of all men, especially men younger than age 35.

Such men are sometimes called premature or rapid ejaculators, which sounds as if they have a communicable disease. Actually, therapists have never been able to agree on a precise definition. (It used to be said that a man was a rapid ejaculator if he was unable to keep his penis inside his lover's vagina for a certain length of time—a minute, say—before ejaculation, or if he was unable to last a certain number of strokes—say, 50.)

But rather than get stuck on semantics, let's just say that you're a rapid ejaculator if you lack voluntary control over your ejaculations and you come before you'd really like to. Which, no doubt, is why you're reading this chapter. The good news is that rapid ejaculation is one of the most easily treated of all sex problems. Ninety percent of men who ejaculate too rapidly can be "cured" in an average of 14 weeks by devoting themselves to the techniques described below, according to the late Helen Singer Kaplan, M.D., Ph.D., former director of the human sexuality program at New York Hospital—Cornell Medical Center in New York City. One other bit of good news is that as men get older, their hair-trigger sexual responses tend to slow down, and the task of controlling their ejaculations usually gets easier.

Who says it's all downhill from 40?

Learning to Last

You've undoubtedly tried it yourself . . . to keep from ejaculating, you wore three condoms, smeared yourself with anesthetizing cream or devoted your thoughts to figuring out the square root of 17. But because all these techniques are just attempts to reduce your sexual awareness, they're precisely the opposite of what you need to be doing. Instead, the

---

THREE AND THREE: A GAME OF CONTROL

A 44-year-old executive described a game he and his partner discovered by happy accident during a particularly wild lovemaking session. He calls the game three and three.

"After an undetermined amount of time passes during lovemaking, with my partner on her back, I pull back so only the head of my penis is stroking the first two or three inches of her vagina. This continues until I'm very close to orgasm. Then upon pulling out (very slowly), it produces a 'mini-orgasm,' actually producing several droplets of semen, which I direct on her clitoris. My partner says what turns her on is the hot, wet feeling—and knowing we can continue. The challenge (and the ultimate turn-on) is to accomplish this three times. The intensity is difficult to speak about and enhances the grand finish to excruciating proportions!"

first step toward learning ejaculatory control is to become more aware of your own arousal patterns, according to Barbara Keesling, Ph.D., a California sex therapist and author of *How to Make Love All Night*.

"Arousal is much more than a 'yes' or 'no' experience—there are many levels of arousal, each having its own distinct sensations and types of intensity," she explains. To increase your awareness of these different sensations, rate them on a scale of one to ten, she suggests. Something like this:

1. No arousal. You're doing your taxes.
2-3. Slightly aroused. Fleeting memories of an old girlfriend.
4. Steady arousal. You're turned on, but you could easily turn it off.
5-6. Solid arousal. You could turn it off, but it's beginning to feel so good who'd want to?
7-8. Peaking arousal. Your heart's pounding, face is flushed, you're breathing heavy. This is great!
9. Peak arousal. You're at the brink of orgasm.
10. Orgasm.

The next step is to practice bringing yourself to various levels of arousal, then backing off before ejaculation. Start by masturbating with a dry hand, working yourself up to about a five, then backing off to a two, then up to a six. Try to last 15 minutes without ejaculating. While doing these exercises, take deep, easy, relaxed breaths, breathing from your belly. This helps forestall ejaculation.

It sounds simple, and it is. But this technique, known as the stop-start method, is the basis of nearly all professional treatments for rapid ejaculation. (If you prefer, you can try the squeeze method—instead of merely stopping just before ejaculation, you can firmly squeeze the tip of your penis just behind the head with thumb and forefingers. Hold the squeeze for ten seconds, or until the urge to ejaculate passes.)

When you need only one or two stops in order to last the whole 15 minutes, move on to the next stage—doing it with a lubricated hand. Practice this until you can last 15 minutes with one or two stops. Then move to the next stage: Masturbating with a dry hand for 15 minutes without ejaculating and without stopping. Then do this with lubrication. Eventually, you'll be able to shift your newly learned control to intercourse, which is generally the biggest challenge of all.

Two Other Methods

Hit the brakes. Another way to reduce the urge to ejaculate is to give your pubococcygeus, or PC, muscles a squeeze. (You can identify your PC muscles by trying to shut off the flow of urine in midstream.) "Strong PC muscles work like a good set of brakes in your car—you can use the contraction of the PC muscles to control your arousal the same way you use your brakes to control speed," Dr. Keesling explains. Some guys prefer one big, hard squeeze, others use a series of short, light ones. Whichever you use, take a long, deep breath after each one. For more information, see Kegels on page 171.

Assume the position. Experiment with different positions during intercourse to find one that allows you maximum control. Dr. Keesling says that in her work with men one position seems to work best for ejaculatory control: a kind of modified missionary position. The woman lies on her back, perhaps with a small pillow under her back for comfort. Her legs are raised in the air, knees bent, and the man is on his knees between her legs. "The key to this position is that the man uses his knees instead of his arms to support most of his weight," she explains. By minimizing muscle tension in this way, he's able to use his PC muscles better. "Most men tell me this is the position with which they have their greatest success," she says.

Tantric and Taoist Traditions

The whole idea of delaying ejaculation in order to prolong pleasure is not some invention of twentieth-century TV talk shows. In fact, 2,000 years ago, Tantric and Taoist masters of China, Japan, Tibet and Indonesia taught that "men can-

FIVE TANTRIC EXPLORATIONS

By taking the pressure off "performance" and enhancing a sense of sexual intimacy, ancient Hindu and Buddhist Tantric sex rituals have a great deal to offer modern couples, according to Harrison Voigt, Ph.D., of the California Institute of Integral Studies in San Francisco. He suggests these five "explorations," based on this 2,000-year-old body of erotic wisdom.

Ritual. Create a meaningful personal ritual to "simultaneously celebrate and sanctify the sexual exchange." This can involve candles, colored lights, flowers, perfumes or a special room or bed. Also, consider expressions of affection like sensual massage, reciting poetry or chanting. Make it personal; make it yours.

Synchronized breathing. Touching your partner in some way, bring your breathing into synch in order to create a feeling of relaxation and togetherness. "Best is a 'soft focus' wherein, through a combination of intention, attention and relaxed physical contact, the breathing patterns of partners are simply allowed to come together," Dr. Voigt says. Don't try too hard.

Sustained eye contact. "Sustained, steady eye contact has an almost unlimited potential for generating profound change in sexual experiencing," he says. It will probably feel awkward at first; start out by doing it for brief periods, then extend as your comfort level increases.

Motionless intercourse. After you've penetrated her and you're at a point of peak sexual arousal, become completely still. Start out by doing this for a couple of minutes; then continue for longer periods.

Refrain from orgasm. To take the focus off performance completely, try lovemaking without orgasm at all. "In Tantric practice the purpose of avoiding or refraining from orgasm is to intensify the sexual-spiritual energy," he says. This may help you open up a whole new world of sensuous feeling, without the big O.

not experience true sexual ecstasy unless they develop the ability to control their ejaculations," according to Robert T. Francoeur, Ph.D., professor of embryology and sexuality at Fairleigh Dickinson University in Rutherford, New Jersey, in a paper about the relevance of Eastern erotic traditions.

These ancient traditions, so different from our own sex-obsessed yet sex-negative culture, "celebrate the naturalness of sexual pleasure and the spiritual potential of sexual relations. Tantric and Taoist sexual union is viewed as a way to spiritual liberation, a consciousness of and identification with the divine," he observes.

In their quest to sustain and prolong sexual joy, these masters developed techniques very similar to the stop-start technique mentioned above, foreshadowing Masters and Johnson by 2,000 years. Some of the more extreme of these teachers, believing that semen was a sort of highly distilled life force that should never be wasted, actually recommended that men ejaculate only once every tenth, or even hundredth, time they made love.

No, we're not going to recommend that you try that. But to our surprise, a fair number of our survey respondents said they'd studied these ancient traditions, with pleasing results.

"For several years I've been studying the centuries-old practices of Tantra and Taoist esoteric yoga," wrote one 45-year-old investment banker. "These differentiate orgasm from ejaculation, making it possible for not only women but also men to experience repeated peaks of pleasure. I've learned that sex isn't just about inserting tab A into opening B; for me it isn't just an event relegated to what goes on between the legs. It's a total sensual experience—sight, sound, smell, taste and touch, the latter involving not just manual contact but every accessible nerve ending."

A Thousand Loving Thrusts

In his book *The Tao of the Loving Couple*, a practical discussion of Taoist erotic philosophy and methods, author Jolan Chang says it boils down to three key points—regulation of ejaculation, the importance of female satisfaction and the understanding that male orgasm and ejaculation are not necessarily the same thing.

The oldest and probably the best and simplest method for learning ejaculatory control is called the locking method, Chang says. When you feel that you're becoming too excited, you simply withdraw your penis from her vagina or pull back so that only the head of your penis remains inside her and remain motionless for 10 to 30 seconds. You'll begin to lose your erection, but if you wait until the urge to ejaculate begins to subside before entering her again, you'll also begin to learn ejaculatory control. You can do this as often as you like, until you begin needing to withdraw less and less often.

Taoist masters also advised novices to practice "a thousand loving thrusts," in a variety of styles. For instance, the master Wu Hsien suggested that beginners thrust in a pattern of three slow and shallow, then one fast and deep. If you start getting too excited, just withdraw and wait for it to pass, then resume thrusting. Once you've mastered this, move on to five shallow and one deep, then nine shallow, one deep.

Eventually, writes Dr. Francoeur, men who learn to master their desires may experience the great goal of Taoism: *Yabyum*, a Tibetan term for "the mystical experience of oneness and wholeness men and women can achieve through sexual intercourse."

Which doesn't sound half bad.

RESOURCES

- For more on Taoist techniques, try *The Tao of Love and Sex: The Ancient Chinese Way to Ecstasy* by Jolan Chang.
- A useful videotape that demonstrates the stop-start and squeeze techniques, called *You Can Last Longer: Solutions for Ejaculatory Control*, is available from the Focus International catalog. For a free catalog, call 1-800-843-0305.

LOCATION
Amazing Places Couples Have Done It

In this chapter, we're just going to pass the soapbox to the respondents to our *Men's Health* magazine survey, who, when we asked "Where is the most bizarre place you ever had sex?" came up with some answers that we found just flat-out amazing.

It's not that we're suggesting you run right out and do it on the neighbor's lawn or on the seventh green at the country club. It's simply that when confronted by a couple with a real snoozer of a sex life, sex therapists invariably suggest changing the place they make love. Try doing it in the guest bedroom. Try a motel room. Try the living-room couch after the kids have gone to bed. Just try something different. "I can't tell you how many people have fantasies of making love in the living room in front of a roaring fire but don't do it," says Oakland, California, sex therapist Bernie Zilbergeld, Ph.D., author of *The New Male Sexuality*. "It takes a little effort, but it's worth it."

Consider these truly mind-boggling possibilities.

- "The most bizarre place I ever made love was in an old cemetery at night right on the grave of a guy who died in 1849," said a 38-year-old sales manager. "I figured he could use a lift."
- "Back of station wagon while chaperoning the senior prom. My wife wore open-crotch panty hose just for the purpose."
- "On a driveway with freshly laid cement."
- "In the torture chamber at the Hohensalzburg Castle in Austria."
- "In my college classroom, on the professor's desk."
- "The most bizarre place I ever made love was in the middle of a raging river. We walked out into the river on submerged rocks and sat with our backs against the current. The water flowed over our heads and we were immersed in a huge bubble. It was incredibly intense. She stripped

off her bikini and backed into me. Both of us had the most intense orgasms."

- A 35-year-old engineer said, "On the cold concrete floor of a particle physics lab. One of those moments of youthful passion when location and circumstance did not mean as much as obeying one of the basic laws of nature."

- "I would say it's a toss-up between an elevator at a hotel and the haunted house during a carnival."

- A 40-year-old woman told us, "In my ex-husband's driveway."

- An ad agency president said, "Sitting on the stands during a college football game surrounded by a blanket. She was sitting on my lap and would bounce up and down when our team made a good play!"

- "American Airlines flight 984 from Dallas to Indy!" (Airplanes were a particularly popular site among respondents. The "Mile-High Club" lives on.)

- A 28-year-old theater manager said, "Center stage in the theater-in-the-round I ran in college. She came to see me after rehearsal of a play I was in. She had programmed the light board earlier and did a striptease in the middle of the stage. . . . The stagehands stumbled over us the next morning."

- "On our dining-room table early one Thanksgiving morning." (Take that, Norman Rockwell.)

- "On a ride at Disney World. Truth!"

- "I made love at Fort Walton Beach, Florida, in the water with my girlfriend while another couple was making love not fifteen feet away. Come to find out later, all four of us were extremely turned on not only by the fact that we were having sex during broad daylight with hundreds of other people around but that we could watch one another having sex. Very intense."

- A 28-year-old marketing director for a nursing home said, "My current partner . . . is amazingly open and fun to be with. I mean, we've had sex in closets at friends' parties. Ever get pulled into a closet by an arm coming out of the closet and make love trying not to make a sound?" Also: "In a theater that was an old converted barn, while a performance was going on—40 feet in the air on a plank that was about a foot and a half wide! The crazy things you do in college. . . . "

Lots of guys mentioned the thrill of doing it someplace where there was a risk of being caught, or at least seen.

- "In the dressing room in a department store at the mall. The other was in the driver's seat of our car when we parked two streets away in a residential, wealthy neighborhood in the middle of the summer. I can't believe we haven't been arrested yet."
- "In a park right next to a busy freeway. We drove away from a party in a sexual fury and laid out on a blanket at 6:00 A.M. We had to hurry to beat the sun or risk being seen!"
- A 60-year-old astrologer said, "The most bizarre place I ever made love was in a restaurant kitchen while she was cooking some food for a customer. It was very quick!"
- One guy said he did it in the backseat of his girlfriend's car while her sister was driving down the freeway to Daytona Beach. "What was bizarre was watching all the National Guard soldiers hanging out of the troop trucks we were passing—I just knew after the second truck that they were radioing ahead to alert their fellow troopers. As I was on my back, I knew it was going on but my girlfriend didn't.
- "Christmas Eve, following a big family dinner—a trip out to the garage to store some leftovers led to a very hot time on top of the hood of my father's car. We may have been gone a while, but no one was the wiser."
- A 29-year-old "homemaker/mom" remembered stopping by the dorm room of a friend who was fluent in French, in hopes of getting some help with an upcoming French test. "It was quite late, and his roommate was sleeping. We sat down on his bed and were conversing softly about my test when I took his hand in mine and began to stroke his palm. I then put his fingers on my lips and

licked them. We then started to kiss passionately and gradually undid buttons and removed some of our clothes. We had to be very quiet so as not to awaken the roommate, although I suspected that he was very aware of what was going on, which turned me on even more. The sexual energy between us was irresistible and we were quickly consumed by it. I think the exhibitionism of it really turned me on. Also, he was speaking to me only in French, and I really had no idea what he was saying (but it sounded delicious!)."

Then there were the romantics.

- "How about on the hood of a white Mercedes under a full August moon in an open field of wildflowers?" said a 45-year-old police officer.
- "In the Appalachian Mountains on a 300-foot cliff under a full moon."
- "On the seventh green on a golf course at sunset."
- "On the rocks jutting out into a churning ocean during a thunder and lightning storm at night."

Our favorite, though, was this one, related by a 55-year-old high school biology teacher. "During our university years, on a train from Amsterdam to Copenhagen the urge came over us—but we were in a compartment with four other people, a condition not really conducive to overt sex. My wife happened to be wearing a full skirt and in the darkness, as the other passengers dozed off, she slipped off her panties and we snuggled in together, spooned and comfortable. We thought we were quite discreet, but when we got off the train in Copenhagen an elderly gentleman came up to us and solemnly shook our hands. Never said a thing. Just shook our hands."

Life is short, boys. You have to steal a few breathless moments from death while you still can.

LUBRICANTS
The Right Kind of Slippery

"Wow! I have told so many people how great Albolene cream is and how much I love it as a slow, comfortable lubrication," raved one guy on a computer bulletin board devoted to all things sexual. "What makes it so great is the fact that it doesn't get sticky, it liquefies with body heat and stays slick for a long time. And since it is officially a facial cleanser (you can find it in the beauty section of your local grocery or drugstore), you can just wipe it off with a towel—no need to use soap and water." One other big plus, the slippery cybersurfer adds: "I've been using the same container of Albolene for the last 4½ years and I haven't finished half of it yet."

Obviously, some guys tend to get fairly worked up about their favorite "personal lubricants"—which really are personal, being the only thing that comes between your partner's skin and your own in a moment of supreme nakedness. Couples in training for the Triathlon of Sex may need to use them because prolonged intercourse can chafe the delicate vaginal walls and irritate the urethra, sometimes leading to bladder infections.

An 18-year-old student who responded to our *Men's Health* magazine survey says he likes lubricants because of "the possibility of climaxing at the same time, the possibility of giving her multiple orgasms and the possibility of her wanting it tomorrow, too." (If you've forgotten, that's what it's like to be 18.)

In the age of AIDS, though, the most important thing to remember about sexual lubricants is this: Never use an oil-based cream or jelly (like baby oil, shortening or petroleum jelly) except for solo sex, for two reasons. First, and most important: Oil-based lubricants will destroy a latex condom with alarming speed, opening holes big enough to allow HIV virus to pass through within 60 seconds, and big enough for sperm within minutes. Second, oil-based lubricants tend to cling to the inner walls of her vagina for days after your conjugal visit, encouraging yeast and bacterial growth. You really don't want her to remember you as a yeast infection.

Still, there are some times—for instance, during solo sex or massage—when oil-based lubricants are appropriate. One of them, coconut oil, is generally available in health food stores and some grocery stores; a 14-ounce jar will probably cost less than five bucks and will last practically forever. And its dreamy, tropical odor can send you off to some mental Tahiti. "It's perfect—doesn't need water or any other lubricant, lasts a long time and cleans up easily," enthused another guy on the computer bulletin board.

Cool Water-Based Lubes

Water-based lubricants, on the other hand, have a lot more going for them: They're condom-safe, relatively tasteless (though often faintly sweet, because of the presence of glycerine), nonstaining, not irritating to genital tissue and easily washed out of sheets and clothes.

One of the biggest customer complaints about water-based lubricants, according to the folks at the San Francisco sex-accessory store Good Vibrations, is that they get used up too quickly and you have to keep applying more during the action. Actually, though, you can get more mileage out of them by adding a little more water or saliva—try keeping a glass of water or even a water gun or a plant mister by the bed, they suggest. ("Let me mist your plant, mister," she said.)

Some other water-based goodies:

Astroglide: Plenty of people swear by Astroglide, a space-age synthetic invented by a NASA subcontractor who started out, oddly enough, experimenting with low-viscosity rocket engine coolants. (Since the stuff definitely heats things up, we suppose the experiment was a failure.) Astroglide is fairly expensive, but you only need a couple of drops at a time. It's clear, nonstaining, amazingly slippery and faintly sweet-tasting. Unlike other water-soluble gels, it doesn't dry out on contact with air.

K-Y Jelly, Ortho Jelly: For years these were the old stand-bys, and the only thing readily available in supermarkets and drugstores. They tend to be a little heavy and greasy, though, because they were originally designed for medical use (to help the doc with that old rectal exam).

Spermicides: Some people simply use spermicidal cream, jelly or foam, which are condom-safe and noxious to both sperm and HIV. But since the active ingredient in most of them, nonoxynol-9, is actually a mild detergent, it may taste slightly soapy. Some people also find it's irritating to the skin.

Saliva: Quite a few people (including *The Joy of Sex* author Alex Comfort, M.D., D.Sc.) consider this the all-time greatest sexual lubricant. It's also politically correct: Totally natural, nontoxic and not cruel to animals. It's also free.

Nature's STP

All of these products, whether oil-based or water-based, are manmade imitations of the "real stuff"—the slippery secretions that women (and, to a much lesser extent, men) produce during sexual arousal. The first really noticeable sign that a woman is getting aroused (besides that glint in her eye) is vaginal wetness, as men have known for thousands of years. But it wasn't until the 1960s, when William H. Masters, M.D., and Virginia E. Johnson, of the former Masters and Johnson Institute in St. Louis, began a series of amazing experiments in which they actually peered inside women's aroused vaginas with penis-shaped cameras, that it was discovered this "sexual sweating" begins 10 to 30 seconds after stimulation begins. First, beadlike droplets appear on the vaginal walls; then, very quickly, the droplets coalesce into a smooth, glistening coating—nature's STP. (It's still not entirely clear where this wonderful stuff, which the ancients called water of life or dew of ecstasy, actually comes from.)

One thing lots of guys don't understand, though, is that vaginal wetness is not a reliable indicator of whether a woman is turned on. We tend to think that if she's wet, she's turned on; if she's not wet, we're doing something wrong.

But female lubrication is linked to estrogen (a female sex hormone) levels, and fluctuations in these hormones can sometimes make it difficult for a woman to get wet naturally, even if she's sexually aroused. Women who've recently given birth or are breastfeeding, or older women who've passed menopause or have had a hysterectomy, may be troubled by vaginal dryness. (Women generally reach menopause sometime between age 45 and 55, but occasionally women will experience the first stages, or perimenopause, in their late thirties, according to Judith Seifer, Ph.D., a certified sex therapist in West Virginia and president of the American Association of Sex Educators, Counselors and Therapists. And vaginal dryness is often one of the first signs.) Alcohol, sinus-drying cold medications and stress can also cause vaginal dryness.

There are so many things that can cause problems, in fact, that close to 20 percent of the women surveyed in the 1994 *Sex in America* survey reported having trouble lubricating during sex, according to researchers at the University of Chicago.

One thing that may help, especially for older women: A fairly new class of products called therapeutic vaginal moisturizers, available without a prescription at drugstores. Gyne-Moistrin or Replens are inserted into the vagina once or twice a week, where they cling to the vaginal walls and simulate natural lubrication.

MALE G-SPOT
Be Glad You Have a Prostate

When it happens, you feel like a first-class idiot.

You go into the doctor's office for a physical, and because you're past age 40, he decides to do a digital rectal exam to check out your prostate gland. The prostate is a walnut-size gland that lies just below your bladder, at the base of your penis, whose main job is to produce the milky fluid that's one of the main components of semen. Its other main job is to make your life miserable by swelling up and blocking off the flow of urine (an incredibly common condition called benign prostatic hyperplasia, or BPH) or, worse, to become cancerous.

By slipping a gloved, lubricated finger through the rectum and probing the rounded back wall of your prostate, a physician can tell a lot about your prostate's health. But on this particular occasion, standing there bent ignominiously over the examining table, you begin getting an enormous erection. You can't seem to help it. The doctor's finger alternately makes you feel as if you have to pee or as if you're becoming seriously aroused. You try thinking about horrible car crashes or your jerk of a boss, but no dice. The old boy just stands up and salutes.

Well, don't worry—your doctor has probably encountered that a hundred times before.

"We see this sort of thing a lot and we generally just ignore it," says Joseph E. Oesterling, M.D., professor and chairman of urology at the University of Michigan Medical School and director of the Michigan Prostate Institute, both in Ann Arbor. "It's a completely normal physiological response. There's nothing negative about it. It certainly doesn't mean that you're sexually attracted to the doctor or homosexually inclined."

Why It Happens

So . . . what does it mean?

Simply that numerous nerve bundles pass by the prostate on their way to the penis, and pressing on those nerves is pleasurable, Dr. Oesterling says. For a lot of men the prostate is very erotic.

The prostate plays a small but crucial role in the drama of male arousal and orgasm. For one thing, owing to its location at the base of the penis, a man's erection is more-or-less anchored upon the prostate, says retired sexologist John D. Perry, Ph.D., co-author of the 1980s bestseller *The G Spot*. "When males batter and ram with their penises (during intercourse), it's not to hurt anybody, it's because a stiff penis will transmit vibrations down into the prostate, which is highly pleasurable," he says.

William H. Masters, M.D., and Virginia E. Johnson, of the former Masters and Johnson Institute in St. Louis, also reported on the prostate's role in orgasm. In men, they found, orgasm occurs in a fairly predictable, two-stage process: emission and ejaculation. In the emission stage the various fluids that make up your semen are pumped into a sort of staging area (called the prostatic urethra) in readiness for firing—rather like pumping a shotgun shell into the chamber. In order to release their cargo (a milky, protein-rich fluid) the prostate, seminal vesicles and other ducts go into a series of "regularly recurring expulsive contractions," pumping away like mad in order to fill the firing chamber. At the same time, the vas deferens dumps a load of fresh sperm cells into the chamber, in the process mixing up the great Milkshake of Life.

> Love is the answer; but while you're waiting for the answer, sex raises some pretty interesting questions.
>
> —Woody Allen

It's during this two-to three-second emission phase, when the prostate is having spasms like mad, that men are blessed with one of life's sweetest sensations: What sexologists call the moment of ejaculatory inevitability, when you feel like you're about to come and no force on heaven or earth can stop you. Dr. Masters, never one to hold back, actually monitored these internal events by keeping a finger inside men's rectums at the very moment of orgasm. In young men, he reported, he could clearly feel these rhythmic prostatic contractions (in guys over age 60 or so, he could not).

In the second stage of male orgasm, ejaculation, a sphincter muscle snaps shut so semen won't back up into your bladder. Then a series of muscular contractions drives the semen up your urethra and out the tip of your penis, bound for glory.

THE PROSTATE

The prostate's job is to make fluid for your semen. Some call it the male G-spot because it is highly sensitive (it can be stimulated through the rectum).

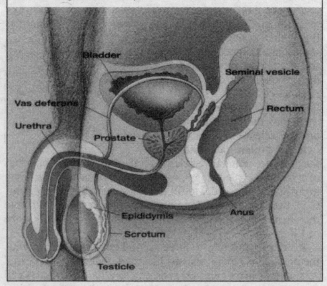

What the Sexes Have in Common

The prostate's erotic potential has been discovered and rediscovered throughout history. One of our survey respondents wrote that "the men of the turn of this century knew the value of prostate massage. There was a steel device marketed for the wife to manually massage her husband's prostate while the two were having intercourse."

During World War II, soldiers and sailors who hadn't been with a woman in months or years were commonly given prostate massages by military medics, as a treatment for "pelvic congestion" (unbearable horniness), Dr. Perry says.

Dr. Perry and his colleagues, Beverly Whipple, Ph.D., and Alice K. Ladas, Ph.D., point out in their book that the male prostate and the female G-spot—a dime-size erogenous zone on the top front wall of the vagina—have a good deal in common because they originate from the very same embryonic tissue. Both produce ejaculate (in all men and in some women) and both are highly erotic, they say. When stimulated, they often trigger a feeling that one needs to urinate. They're both located in roughly the same place. And both are best reached in the same way: through the back door. Most women who respond to G-spot stimulation say the best way for a man to reach it is through rear-entry, "doggie-style" intercourse. In the same way, Dr. Perry says, the big "reward" of anal intercourse for homosexual males is that the tip of the penis is directly stimulating the prostate gland.

This Works for All Guys

Many homosexuals know all about the pleasures of the prostate, Dr. Perry adds. But it's precisely because prostate stimulation is so much associated with homosexuality that so few heterosexual men have ever experienced it (except for the inadvertent examining-room erection). In fact, he says, "It's my theory that it would be easier for a straight man to turn gay in this culture than for a straight man to convince his wife or girlfriend to massage his prostate."

Nevertheless, if you're one of the brave ones, consider the following suggestions.

Internal stimulation: The prostate can be stimulated in two different ways—internally or externally. To stimulate it internally, have your wife or girlfriend slip a lubricated finger (covered with a latex glove or condom, if you wish) into your anus and press toward the front of your body. (Because of its location, it's quite difficult for you to do this yourself.) She should feel a firm, rounded, walnut-or chestnut-size lump, which can be gently stroked.

One of our gay survey respondents told us that "my partner is consistently brought to orgasm when I manually massage his prostate gland." Once the well-lubricated anus is gently penetrated by a finger, "the finger is then moved slowly in and almost out of the anus repeatedly. After a few moments, I find the prostate gland and start massaging very gently," while at the same time manually or orally stimulating the penis.

Strictly speaking, there's no reason she couldn't do the same.

External stimulation: Ask her to press the ball of her thumb into your perineum (the spot you'd sit on if you straddled a fence, between the anus and scrotum). Whether you'll like this or not is quite an individual matter—some men like it only when they're fully aroused, others don't like it at all, according to Patricia Love, Ed.D., a marriage and family therapist in Austin, Texas, in the book *Hot Monogamy*. Some men say it helps them regain or maintain an erection.

Ancient Chinese erotic texts describe a very similar technique to delay ejaculation; one difference is that the man does it to himself. Just at the brink of ejaculation, using the fore and middle fingers of his left hand, he presses on the perineum for three or four seconds while taking a deep breath. This is supposed to delay ejaculation but not orgasm.

Which is great work if you can get it.

MULTIPLE ORGASMS
How to Be a Repeat Performer

One day back in 1970 a young student walked into the office of sex researcher William Hartman, M.D., who was then teaching at California State University, Long Beach. This unassuming young fellow, it turned out, was a sort of philanthropist of love: He said he was able to climax again and again during a single session of lovemaking, and he was interested in teaching other men how to do it.

"At that time, we were not really aware of this phenomenon, but it piqued our interest, so we got him wired up in a laboratory," Dr. Hartman recalls. And the graphs and gauges confirmed the guy's story: Over about an hour, through masturbation, he was able to climax 16 times.

This, of course, is a bit different from most guy's experiences. Lots of men have learned to delay ejaculation, and occasionally may ejaculate a second time if they're able to stay aroused (and awake) long enough. But as a regular thing, "usually one round at a time is all I'm good for," as one respondent to our *Men's Health* magazine survey put it, rather disconsolately.

Two Key Points

The two main differences between male and female orgasms, William H. Masters, M.D., and Virginia E. Johnson, of the former Masters and Johnson Institute in St. Louis, point out, are that males expel seminal fluid and there's a so-called refractory period, or rest stop, after men ejaculate.

Actually, the first point is wrong, but in a small way: There's increasing evidence that some women also ejaculate a small amount of fluid during orgasm. For more information, see G-spot on page 119.

Clearer to most men is that while they need a rest after climaxing, women are instantly ready for more after they orgasm. That's because women have no refractory period; a fairly high percentage of women are able to hit the high note time after time. The female capacity for multiple orgasms far exceeds even the most prolific male. Masters and Johnson found women who were able to reach 50 consecutive orgasms using a vibrator.

It's these two differences—ejaculation mechanics and the need for a refractory period—that puts such a damper on a male's capacity for multiple orgasms. Or, so science once thought.

Of course, it's not quite that simple. One key point, probably discovered and rediscovered millions of times by amorous male adventurers all over the world, is this: Ejaculation and orgasm are not the same thing. "It's now widely acknowledged that there is a difference between the pleasurable sensations of orgasm and the physical event of ejaculation, Dr. Hartman explains. You can have an orgasm without ejaculating, and you can ejaculate without having an orgasm. Which means that your capacity to repeatedly reach orgasm is not limited by your capacity to repeatedly ejaculate (which is fairly limited).

This is one of the sexual secrets multiorgasmic men have learned: to "unhitch" orgasm from ejaculation, Essentially, they've learned to take themselves to the very brink of ejaculation, then stop and relax, allowing the rush of orgasm to sweep over them; then they do it again. The orgasmic pattern seems to vary, according to the few studies that have been conducted on the subject. These men may have a series of "dry" orgasms, without ejaculating at all, then ejaculate explosively; they may ejaculate in a series, each time releasing an increasingly smaller amount of ejaculate; or in some other pattern. But they're always able to distinguish between the two.

The second point, that men need a refractory period after orgasm, also has its exceptions, it turns out. For one thing, the refractory period is not merely a "reloading the gun" process.

The physiological purpose of the refractory period is not entirely clear, Dr. Hartman admits. Sure, once you've ejaculated, it takes a certain amount of time for the prostate, seminal vesicles and other ducts to refill with fluid. But to fully refill these ducts takes hours, sometimes even overnight; the refractory period is far shorter, suggesting it is not merely a break for refilling.

Some men seem to have only a brief or partial refractory period, Dr. Hartman points out. These guys often don't lose their erections before they rise to the occasion a second, third or fourth time. "Their heart rates (a key indicator of orgasm) may top out at 150 during orgasm, but they never fall back to a resting state of, say, 70; they drop back to 120, then bounce right back up to 150 when they have another orgasm," he says.

How'd He Do That?

This phenomenon is not unknown in the sexological literature. The late Dr. Alfred C. Kinsey reported that among his 12,000 male subjects, he found 380 "who had a history of regular, multiple ejaculation at some period in adolescent or adult years." Masters and Johnson report that "many males below the age of 30, but relatively few thereafter," have the ability to ejaculate frequently with only very short refractory periods. One of their male study subjects ejaculated three times within ten minutes.

When we asked a random sample of *Men's Health* magazine readers, "Have you ever had more than one orgasm in a single session of lovemaking?" an amazing 67 percent said yes. (Our question, we admit, was a little vague—these orgasms may have occurred over a period of many hours, during drowsy, long-sustained, start-and-stop lovemaking, or they could have occurred in fairly rapid succession. But we didn't really care to define the term "multiple orgasm" too narrowly; we just wanted these gentlemen to share their tips and techniques with you.)

Many were mystified by how they did it. One 60-year-old executive vice-president told us he'd experienced repeated orgasms "only once 25 years ago, by accident, not by design. I've been trying ever since, but no luck!" Another said, "A couple of times I had an orgasm, maintained my erection and continued on to have a second orgasm before having to stop for essentials (air, water, a back brace). I wish I knew how I'd done this."

A 73-year-old retired machinist gave us the saddest, most succinct answer. "Ever have more than one orgasm?" we asked. "Yes," he said. "How'd you do it?" "Youth," he replied.

Any Man Can

Inspired by his first subject, Dr. Hartman eventually located 32 other multiorgasmic males. For the benefit of science these men agreed to repeatedly bring themselves to orgasm by hand, in a small, dimly lit room in a laboratory, while wired up to a heart monitor and other devices. In 1984 he and his wife, Marian Fithian, co-directors of the Center for Marital and Sexual Studies in Long Beach, California, published a book called *Any Man Can*. It reported their laboratory findings about these remarkable men—and described the simple techniques by which, they claimed, any man can learn to become multiorgasmic.

What was it, exactly, they were practicing? Dr. Hartman and Fithian say it boils down to three simple techniques.

The Stop-Start or Squeeze Technique

Back in 1955 a urologist at Duke University Medical School in Durham, North Carolina, named James Semans, M.D., described a technique for treating premature ejaculation that he originally learned from a prostitute-turned-sexual-surrogate. Over the years it's proven so effective that it's now used by sex therapists all over the country as a way of teaching ejaculatory control. Basically, you simply masturbate to the brink of ejaculation, then stop; do it again, then stop until your body learns to gain control over what is wrongly perceived as one of the most uncontrollable of impulses. Eventually, with any luck you'll begin to have the amazing experience of reaching orgasm without ejaculating.

Some therapists recommend that you squeeze the tip of the penis tightly just before ejaculation, with two fingers underneath and the thumb on top. (This method is called the squeeze technique.) But other therapists say simply stopping, then starting again (the stop-start technique) works just as well.

Dr. Hartman and Fithian recommend these specifics. First, lay on your back while doing this, to get used to the female-superior position during intercourse (they say most multiorgasmic males prefer the female-on-top position). Using a light touch, stimulate yourself right up to near ejaculation, then squeeze or stop. Hold still for 15 or 20 seconds (not too long), until the urge to ejaculate begins to ebb. Then go to work again. Learn to bring yourself to the brink of ejaculation three or four times before letting go. (You can do this same drill with a partner; just get her to squeeze or stop.)

"We've found that learning the squeeze technique is the quickest way for men to become multiorgasmic," Dr. Hartman says. "Many men can achieve adequate control through the squeeze method in a couple of weeks."

Other things to remember: Most therapists recommend that while you're learning this technique, you abstain from other kinds of masturbation or intercourse. You're trying to retrain your body, and reverting to the old way will erase your newfound gains. Also, you should "practice" for several weeks, three to five times a week.

All this was apparently old news to several of our respondents. A 31-year-old teacher said, "Yes, I have had more than one orgasm in a single session of lovemaking. I learned to achieve this by masturbation. When I am ready to ejaculate, I squeeze the tip of my penis. I repeat this several times. When we are making love, I can be inside her thrusting for anywhere from 15 to 30 minutes. When I've achieved one orgasm, I rest and we fondle each other. I perform oral sex on her, and we just go on and on for one to two hours until I have another erection. Then we make love again, and 98 percent of the time I have another orgasm. The key is slow, slow, slow."

Kegel Exercises

A group of deep pelvic muscles called the pubococcygeus, or PC muscles, are known to have a profound effect on men's and women's enjoyment of sex. The PC muscles, which are slung between your legs to provide a sort of floor for the pelvis, are the same muscles you use to shut off the flow of urine in midstream. So that's your first task: Get acquainted with your PC muscles by shutting off the flow of urine. That squeezing, sometimes called a pelvic quickie, is better known as a Kegel exercise, after the gynecologist who began teaching them to women with stress incontinence back in the 1950s.

Kegels are such good exercises that we've devoted a

whole chapter to them in part three of this book. The bottom line: Squeeze often during the day, everyday, with the goal of truly strengthening the muscles. The great thing about Kegels is that no one ever knows you are doing them.

Again, our respondents were onto the concept. A 27-year-old sales rep told us, "I have experienced what might be called multiple orgasms myself many times during a single session of lovemaking. When I feel that I am going to ejaculate, I hold back by slowing down or stopping by pulling out just after ejaculation begins. In order for this to work, however, it is necessary to use the Kegel exercise that everybody talks about. By squeezing these muscles at the point of ejaculation, you will experience what I call miniorgasms that feel quite amazing and also enable you to continue making love for an extended period of time. I have learned to have my 'full orgasm,' or final ejaculation, almost on command, which is always the most intense."

Keep Your Testicles Down

You've probably never noticed this before, but just before ejaculation, your usually pendulous testicles raise up very close to the body, like a pair of helium balloons floating up to the ceiling. "The phenomenon of testicular elevation is of extreme physiological importance," Masters and Johnson reported. "If the testes do not undergo at least partial elevation, the human male will not experience a full ejaculatory sequence."

So these men have learned to keep their testicles pulled down to delay ejaculation, either by holding them between their legs or by gently tugging them down with one hand (or getting her to tug them down).

All of this may strike a reasonable person as a whole lot of trouble for uncertain gains. (Two hundred Kegels a day?) Yet Dr. Hartman claims that "we have never yet had a man who could not learn to become multi-orgasmic using the techniques we describe." And, he adds, he's also never heard of any harmful effects from any of this, so "the worst that can happen is nothing."

Studying the "Superstars of Sex"

Despite its innate fascination, there are few serious studies of male multiple orgasms. But one of the few studies provides some useful additional insights. Researchers managed to locate and question 21 "multiply orgasmic" men whose amorous experiences fit this definition: "two or more orgasms with or without ejaculation and without, or with only very limited, detumescence (loss of erection) during one and the same sexual encounter." These guys lasted from 15 minutes to two hours without noticeable detumescence between orgasms. Most reported from 2 to 9 orgasms per lovemaking session; one guy had 16. (Lest you conclude these guys were just the same liars and blowhards you can find at any corner bar, the researchers also interviewed their wives and lovers, who confirmed their stories.)

Interestingly enough, they ranged in age from 25 to 69; the majority were over 43. "I see a lot of men wanting to learn how to have multiple orgasms in their forties, fifties and sixties—and frankly, they're usually more satisfied than their younger counterparts," says Barbara Keesling, Ph.D., a California sex therapist and author of *How to Make Love All Night*. There is, she adds, one non-obvious benefit to this whole deal: If the man is capable of coming more than once, it tends to make the woman less anxious that he's going to ejaculate before she's ready and spoil it all. "The woman can relax more because she knows her needs are going to be fulfilled," she says.

Another key thing about these guys is that they were pretty laid-back dudes. Their main goal wasn't to have multiple orgasms. It was to please their partners—and if their partners had no interest in repeated orgasms, they gave it up. They liked emotional closeness, a leisurely, undemanding atmosphere and a familiar lover.

As one of our multiorgasmic respondents put it, "Never make the orgasm the goal, just enjoy the fun of each other all night. If it's meant to be, it will happen."

Learned or Innate?

The researchers found that these multiorgasmic males fell into two groups. The largest group had always been able to climax repeatedly and had no idea this was unusual until a (probably glassy-eyed) lover brought it to their attention. One said, "It never occurred to him to stop after one orgasm, and he believed that it was natural to continue." A second, smaller group consisted of men who'd learned how past the age of 35. They either stumbled on it by some happy accident even they didn't understand, or they taught themselves how by mastering the techniques we've just described.

One 59-year-old guy said he'd never climaxed more than once until he was nearly 40. Then one night, after reaching orgasm with his wife, he kept thrusting without losing his erection, and came again. "Doublee!" he shouted gleefully (a term used when skeet shooters bag two clay pigeons with one shot). After that, he was frequently able to repeat the performance (though we certainly hope he stopped shouting).

The two men who'd deliberately taught themselves to become multiorgasmic, the researchers reported, "practiced coming to the brink of orgasm and inhibiting ejaculation until they could separate the sensation of orgasm and the experience of ejaculation. Both of these men used techniques such as the squeeze or the stop-start method in their initial practice."

They also used the technique of building to a peak, stopping and then deeply relaxing, and "the sensation of orgasm followed the deep relaxation." Three of the men reported they used Kegel exercises, clamping down just before ejaculation.

Afterward, the men said, they needed continued penile stimulation and warmth to stay erect; if they withdrew for only a short period, they'd lose their erections. Some said their penises were painfully sensitive after orgasm, but if they re-entered her, or were manually stimulated, they could overcome this momentary hypersensitivity and resume thrusting again in a few minutes.

One of our survey respondents described this experience: "I masturbated frequently during my youth (and still do when my partner is absent) and learned quickly that to postpone ejaculation was to prolong pleasure. In lovemaking I discovered that if I began thrusting again shortly after the initial high of orgasm passed, I could not only maintain an erection but I could also renew the entire sexual enthusiasm."

Being able to climax more than once is potentially a more useful and interesting skill than being able to change the oil in your car. But again, it's a big mistake to set it up as just another desperate male goal, another hoop to jump through during lovemaking.

"The end product is intimacy, not orgasm," Dr. Hartman says. "I mean, if you focus on trying to enter some kind of Olympics of Orgasm, you're liable to have a pretty sad sex life. It's like income: If you focus on money, you never make enough, and if you focus on orgasms, you never have enough. The goal of lovemaking is to become intimate with another person."

NOONER
The Allure of the Midday Tryst

From time immemorial, we suppose, guys have had a special warm spot in their hearts for the quickie daytime tryst, the roll in the hay at high noon, the stander-upper, the nooner.

"Sex is a great stress reliever, and there is no better time I've found to relieve a little job stress than over the noon hour," a 25-year-old attorney who responded to our *Men's Health* magazine survey told us.

Sometimes women have a little trouble understanding this about us. As another guy explained it, "Women need to understand that sometimes men want quick, powerful sex for the physical relief and sudden pleasure. This type of sex does not mean that men do not love their partners or are trying to take advantage of them."

There's at least one other reason we love nooners that has more to do with biology than romance (or the lack of it). Testosterone levels in adult males are subject to circadian rhythms, researchers have found, meaning that they rise and fall in 24-hour cycles—and they tend to peak shortly before noon. In one Japanese study researchers took blood samples from five healthy young males every hour for 24 hours to study fluctuations in circulating testosterone and other substances. Testosterone levels, they found, bottomed out from around 10:00 P.M. to 3:00 A.M., began to rise at around 4:00 A.M. and reached their daytime high just after 10:00 A.M. Then they fell, bottoming out again during midafternoon and reaching a second, slightly lower peak around 7:00 P.M.

Older men, especially, might do well to take advantage of this daily ebb and flow of the hormonal tides. At midday you tend to be well-rested and your sap is at its daytime peak.

One young advertising executive recalled one such particularly memorable midday, in the heat of August, when he and a young goddess climbed up into a hayloft and "for no particular reason just looked at each other, ripped off each other's clothes and went at it like animals. It was really great because it was so completely spontaneous. I mean, we were in love and everything, but what we had that day was just plain, good old-fashioned sex without all the trimmings. And it was this episode that taught me it's okay to just have a consensual 'quickie' with a partner. Not every sexual encounter has to be an hour-long, extended romantic interlude."

Besides, if you waited for that to happen, half the time, it never would.

OLDER MEN, YOUNGER WOMEN
Truths and Myths of "Cradle Robbing"

Back in 1943, when 54-year-old Charlie Chaplin announced his intention to marry a 17-year-old debutante named Oona

O'Neill, it caused an international sensation. That a man his age (who was already three times divorced) would stoop to "robbing the cradle" for a bride was considered scandalous, almost criminal. But despite what the world might have thought, this May–December relationship turned out to be an "extraordinary, perfect love affair," according to one biographer, and it later became a rich and long-lasting marriage.

In our society, old guys who become enamored of much younger women generally have to live with being considered "dirty old men," or with accusations that they're merely interested in scoring a "trophy wife." We're in no position here to argue the moral issues involved in old-young relationships. If you think a 50-year-old man shouldn't be with a 20-year-old woman, it's probably for lots of deep-rooted reasons. But one thing we *can* say is that sexually speaking, there are some legitimate benefits to this type of relationship.

In ancient China there was no such social censure involved in these age-unbalanced unions. In fact, Taoist erotic texts from the Chinese middle ages not only do not frown on these relationships, they actually recommend them.

In his book *The Tao of Love and Sex*, writer Jolan Chang points out that these ancient masters recognized that there were a variety of reasons, both

> There is a quarrelsome couple on the east side of the street with a husband who is young and impressively handsome. There is a loving, harmonious couple on the west side of the street with a husband who is old and nothing to look at. Why? It is simply that the unimpressive old man knows how to satisfy his woman and the good-looking young one does not.
>
> —Taoist master

sexual and psychological, why an older man and a younger woman can often be a "superb combination." For one thing, the whole "problem" of human sexuality is that men tend to become aroused and reach orgasm much more quickly than women do. But as men age, their sexual responses begin to slow. It takes him longer to get an erection. He requires more manual stimulation, more foreplay, to become aroused. In other words, the difference between his sexual responses and hers begins to narrow; a kind of sexual harmony begins to emerge at midlife, for no other reason than the passage of time.

Additionally, younger women produce copious amounts of vaginal lubrication when they're aroused, which is a real blessing for an older guy. It means, among other things, that he can enter her without being fully erect. Older women not only require lots of foreplay to produce sufficient lubrication, their lubrication doesn't last as long as a young woman's (and artificial lubricants bought in a drugstore are never quite as good as the real thing). A young woman's longer-lasting lubrication is another advantage, because he's slower to become erect and slower to ejaculate (in fact, many older men do not always ejaculate at all).

Her youthful body excites him over and over again. Her vagina tends to be tighter than an older woman's, which excites him even more. And for his part, the older man contributes calmness, confidence and skill to their lovemaking, something younger guys have not yet learned (or earned). That is, perhaps, why young women sometimes prefer a graybeard to an impatient young firebrand. "These are men who have had ample experience in both the joys and sorrow of loving and have thus learned through the years the true meaning of tenderness," says Chang.

Reports from the Front

Fair enough. But frankly, we wouldn't have believed all this if we had not heard similar things from the old guys among our survey respondents. We were amazed at how many said that sex gets better as you get older—whether your partner is dramatically younger or not. One 70-year-old lawyer reported that the best sex he ever had was "with a woman 40 years younger over the past two years. It was a fling that had no failure." Another 64-year-old guy said, "I totally believe that sex gets better with age because we don't have the hang-ups and pressures of the young. The children are gone. We are there for each other. We respect each other and we are able to talk about sex openly and freely . . . and we're also willing to experiment."

And a 70-year-old retired journalist told us, "My wife, my grade-school sweetheart, is the only person I've had sex with, except for a brief encounter with a hooker (far and away my worst sexual experience, and a strange way to cel-ebrate ten years of marriage). My orgasm with the prostitute was equivalent to a sneeze; with my love it's a strident, explosive, wall-banging seizure beyond description. No letup in intensity in 50 years. I could be the most envied man on the planet—I should spoil this?"

Indeed. If you've discovered love with some sweetie three decades your junior, cheers. We'll send you roses. But like the Taoist master said, the most important thing is to learn to "satisfy your woman"—no matter what her age (or yours).

PHONE SEX
Getting Your Bell Rung

Anybody who has ever had one of those steamy, late-night heart-to-hearts with a sweetie in a different time zone knows how easily a telephone can turn into a sex toy.

One respondent to our *Men's Health* magazine survey, a 32-year-old corporate trainer, swears that he once helped a girlfriend reach orgasm over long distance, and we believe him. Ever since the advent of 900 numbers, which made credit card billing a simple matter, telephone sex has become a huge—nay, awesome—business in the United States.

According to the 1994 *Sex in America* survey conducted by University of Chicago researchers, 1 percent of American men have called one of those 900 numbers you see adver-tised by girls with pouty lips on late-night TV and in the back of men's magazines. Since there are about 89 million males over age 18 in the United States, according to the Census Bureau, that means roughly 900,000 guys have tried it—maybe even you.

"It's a billion-dollar-a-year business now, involving about 40 companies," says William Kelly, a sex therapist in Rochester, New York, who also works as a consultant to the industry. The company he works for employs 700 "agents" (telephone answerers), who work eight-hour shifts in which they answer anywhere from 60 to 80 calls, usually lasting three to five minutes apiece, at rates ranging from $2.50 to $4.50 a minute. You do the math.

Why You Gonna Call?

Phone sex, like using computer adult bulletin boards, is a sport played mainly by men—99 percent of callers are male, says Kelly, and 99 percent of agents are female. This is something of an oddity, he says, because according to sexo-logical research, it's actually women who are more respon-sive to "talking dirty" than men.

Why do guys call?

"The anonymity allows them to shed their sexual inhibi-tions," says "Nicole," a phone-sex veteran with one of those deliciously sultry-sophisticated British accents. "Women are more likely to open up and reveal their true selves to other people, but men can't seem to allow themselves to do that, especially when it comes to their sexual wants and needs. Often they'd rather reveal their true sexual selves only to a strange woman in some far-off city on the phone than to their mates."

Sometimes guys use phone sex as a kind of "great equal-izer"—they want to stay married (or maintain a long-term relationship), but they have lustier sexual appetites than their mates. They call just to blow off a little sexual steam. In the age of AIDS, of course, phone sex has the added advantage of being 100 percent sanitary. But the biggest reason guys dial 900—the thing that's behind 60 to 70 percent of all calls—is that "they're looking to have adult fantasies ful-filled that would be difficult in real life," Kelly says. "They may want to express strong same-sex feelings, or the desire to be dominated, or cross-dressing, or fetishes or whatever."

Harboring some secret, "specialized sex interest," something a little off the beaten path, something you're ashamed to confess to your partner? Well, if that sounds like you, then you have plenty of company. The *Sex in America* researchers found that "after vaginal sex, watching a partner undress and oral sex, the remainder of our list of sexual behaviors (including anal sex, group sex, and same-sex encounters) appealed only to small minorities of people and were rejected as not at all appealing by most." Which means that, if your sexual tastes deviate at all from the standard menu—and if, on top of that, you happen to live in Dubuque, you're likely to feel lonely.

Which is where phone sex comes in.

Ask for Cheyenne

There are a couple of different ways to turn your phone into a sex toy that generates a credit card bill. You can dial up a sexually explicit recorded message. You can hook up to a "party line"—a sort of erotic conference call—in which you and several other strangers engage in sexy conversation. Or you can talk directly to a live person (almost always a woman) who will indulge you in an erotic fantasy tailored to your specifications.

The way it generally works is that, when you dial a 900 number, you get a recorded "menu" of fantasies. You can have a "hot girl" fantasy, meet a mistress who will dominate you, meet a transvestite, a transsexual or whatever. You can even request a two-on-one fantasy in which you get two dream girls instead of one (for $4.50 a minute instead of $3.50, of course).

At the other end of the line, in an orderly office that looks much like a telemarketing firm, hundreds of women are answering the phones. They range in age from college students to grandmothers; many, says Kelly, are unemployed actresses or psychology majors. The main thing is that they "are able to emote, able to lose themselves in a fantasy," explains Nicole. Each of these women has undergone two to three days of intensive training in which they're taught to develop at least four fantasy characters (straight, transvestite, dominant mistress, transsexual) with names, measurements, personal histories and sexual inclinations. (Hair colors and names go together, Nicole says—blondes tend to be "Barbie" or "Amanda," a brunette might be "Cheyenne," a redhead, "Bianca.")

When you choose dominant mistress from the recorded menu, the woman at the other end knows to pick up the phone in the character of "Iron Maiden" (or whatever her dominant mistress character is called). Then you both take it from there.

Agents not only have to be able to lose themselves in a fantasy, they also need a bit of a literary streak; the Federal Communications Commission (FCC) strictly regulates what they can and cannot say. Raunchy or explicitly sexual words (even "breast") are forbidden, so poetic substitutes have to be used. "I'll say, 'Come into my garden and have a peach—it's soft and fuzzy and I know you'd love to lick it,' " says Nicole in such a way that there's little doubt what she means. Agents are also forbidden to indulge a caller in fantasies that involve bestiality (sex with animals), necrophilia (sex with the dead), rape or any violence against women, a religious person or object, anyone under 18 or incest, including mother-in-law fantasies (a fair number of guys really have the hots for their mother-in-law). Kelly makes 50 test calls a month to see that agents stay within the FCC guidelines.

Also, in case you were wondering, most companies strictly prohibit callers from meeting phone-sex dream girls in the flesh (otherwise the companies could be charged with prostitution). And though you can call and ask for Cheyenne, don't call her more than three times a day. "We don't want a man to become obsessive," Nicole says, "so three's the daily limit."

Of course, there's a way of avoiding all these legal and linguistic restrictions—and the credit card bill, too. Don't call a 900 number at all; just call your wife or girlfriend. Phone sex, after all, is really just a form of fantasizing, and fantasizing with a real-life lover can be lots more fun than doing it with a stranger.

Lots of guys who responded to our survey described in glorious detail the joys of acting out fantasy sex scenes with their mates—and doing it over the phone just adds a delicious new twist. Pretend she's a bored, randy housewife ordering a pizza, for instance; you're the delivery boy getting ready to go out to her house. Or she's a bored housewife calling a plumber (which provides a particularly rich metaphor to work with).

One of the biggest advantages of having phone sex with a friend: When you call Bianca on a 900 line, there's no chance the relationship will go anywhere. But with somebody you know and love, things can go anywhere you want.

POSITIONS
How to Be a Sexual Dancer

> Certainly nothing is unnatural that is not physically impossible.
>
> —Richard Brinsley Sheridan, Irish playwright

There were supposed to have been Arabian women who could, during intercourse, raise one of their feet into the air and balance a lighted lamp on the sole of their foot without spilling the oil or putting out the lamp.

Of course, the main point of trying new positions is not to qualify for the Olympics of Sex but to keep things interesting. And to figure out new and fun ways to delay ejaculation. Like dancing, you should think of positions in a sequence and figure out a series that doesn't involve a lot of climbing over legs or turning your partner around. Here's a menu of maneuvers.

Woman on Top

The oldest known painting of human sexual intercourse, dating back to 3200 B.C. and found in the Ur excavations of

Mesopotamia, shows a woman on top. Which doesn't mean feminists are always right, just that it's a very old position with lots of practical advantages.

"Only the female-superior and lateral (side-by-side) coital positions allow direct or primary stimulation of the clitoris to be achieved with ease," report William H. Masters, M.D., and Virginia E. Johnson, of the former Masters and Johnson Institute in St. Louis, in *Human Sexual Response*. "Clitoral response may develop more rapidly and with greater intensity in the female-superior coition than in any other female coital position."

Many men also find that the stimulation is less intense in this position, so you can delay ejaculation longer. Your hands are free to stimulate her clitoris or breasts. And since you're lying down, you don't get tired as quickly. (The medieval Indian love manual *Ananga-Ranga* says this position "is especially useful when he, being exhausted, is no longer capable of muscular exertion, and when she is ungratified, being still full of the water of love.")

"In our culture another thing that makes the female-superior position so desirable is that she's always been told to just lay there—but by getting on top, she has much more freedom to initiate the action, to explore her own sexuality," adds William Hartman, M.D., co-director of the Center for Marital and Sexual Studies in Long Beach, California. "It allows her to control the movement, depth and pacing of things. She can move around and adjust the angle of his penis, getting it into areas that he would never be able to if he were on top." (See Illustration 1.)

Some guys have trouble with the whole idea of a woman being in the "superior" position. But sexual politics has

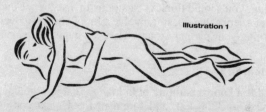

Illustration 1

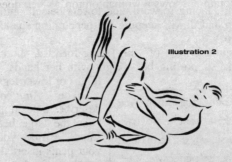

Illustration 2

always gotten in the way of good sex—it's pleasure that should be in the superior position, and if both of you enjoy it, so much the better.

Variations

• Facing you, she can kneel, sit or squat on top of your erect penis. (See Illustration 2.) "When she sits on my penis, it penetrates very deeply and she always has an orgasm in that position," reports a 50-year-old college professor who responded to our *Men's Health* magazine survey.

• She can sit on you, facing your feet, using her hands to push herself up and down. (See Illustration 3.) She can even lie down flat with her back on your chest, with her legs together to keep your penis inside.

• In *The Art of Sexual Ecstasy* Margo Anand describes the Swooping Shakti position. The woman squats over the man's

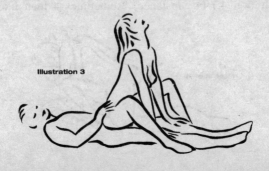

Illustration 3

erect penis, facing forward, and lowers herself onto it. She moves up and down, keeping the penetration shallow, then goes deep.

• Kneeling on top of you, facing forward, she can lean way back, supporting her weight with her hands on your thighs or lower legs.

• The *Ananga-Ranga* describes a position that is "like the large bee": She squats astride you, with your penis inserted, closes her legs firmly and then begins moving her hips in a churning, circular motion until she is satisfied. When she's through, she's supposed to say to you, "Oh, my dear! Oh, thou rogue! This day hast thou come under my control and hast become subjected to me, being totally defeated in the battle of love!"

Nowadays, you won't have any trouble finding a woman who's just dying to say that.

> If whoever invented it, you know, didn't want us to have intercourse, why did he make us fit together so perfectly?
>
> —15-year-old girl quoted in "Adolescent Sexuality in Contemporary America,"
> Robert C. Samuelson

Man on Top

Some may consider it boring, but the missionary position is still the most commonly used position in the world, and it still has lots of advantages for both men and women. (See Illustration 4.) For instance, "sometimes a man likes to

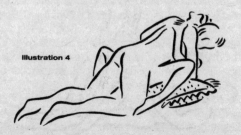

Illustration 4

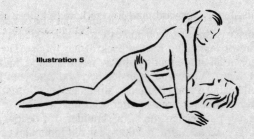

Illustration 5

dominate a woman; there are some times when a woman likes to be 'taken' by a man," says Jude Cotter, Ph.D., a psychologist and sex therapist in private practice in Farmington Hills, Michigan. And if your goal is pregnancy, in this position the vagina is like an upright cup and tends to retain semen.

On the other hand, if he's much heavier than she is, he tends to squash her. And because he's supporting his weight with his smallest, weakest muscles (back and shoulders), it's tiring. Worst of all, in this position he tends to ejaculate rapidly.

Variations

• She can keep her legs down straight, between yours, narrowing the vaginal opening and increasing the friction on your penis. This position also tends to increase the friction on her clitoris.

• One of our *Men's Health* respondents, a 26-year-old student, swears by this "modified missionary position": She is on her back and he is upright on his knees, but with his knees widely spread. Her legs lay over his thighs so that he's lifting her pelvis up a little. "While the penetration is improved, I think just the placement of my penis against the front wall of her vagina is the key," he says. "After about five minutes she is tearing the sheets off . . . every time!"

• Another survey respondent, a 32-year-old customer support specialist who says he's been told he's a wonderful lover, likes the "modified spoon position." Basically, he explains, she lies on her back, he on top—but one of her legs is drawn across his stomach and extended to the side (that is, he's more or less lying on the back of her thigh). Then he enters her at an angle that's halfway from the side, halfway from the rear. "While you're inside her, you take your hand and, while using a good lubricant, stimulate her clitoris. This dual action produces orgasm after orgasm," he says.

• She can put her legs on your shoulders for deeper penetration. The *Kama Sutra*, a 2,000-year-old Indian love manual, calls this the yawning position. (See Illustration 5.)

• She can spread her legs and bend her knees, allowing for deeper penetration.

• She can bend her legs so that her knees are laying against your chest. Or she can have one leg bent on your chest and the other to the side, stretched out straight.

• Put a pillow beneath her bottom to raise your angle of entry. Her legs may either be spread wide or her knees bent with the soles of her feet touching. "This is an admirable form of congress and is greatly enjoyed by both," says the *Ananga-Ranga*.

• Margo Anand suggests what she calls the Rolling Tickle. (See Illustration 6.) The man is sitting or kneeling, with his penis inside her. The woman has her knees pulled

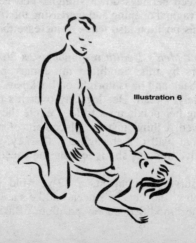

Illustration 6

up to her chest, with her feet flat on his chest. Then the man moves in and out while she "rolls" her hips up and down. If the G-spot exists, this position would be good at reaching it, Anand says, and can "give a sense of power to a man and a sweet taste of surrender to a woman."

Standing Up: The Gangster Position

Among the thousands of men the late Dr. Alfred C. Kinsey interviewed for his famous books were 81 genuine lowlifes—gangsters, pimps, stickup artists and con men. As a group these men were almost unbelievably oversexed and for some reason, they also had a thing for making love standing up, according to researchers who studied unpublished Kinsey data. (Remember the scene in *The Godfather* where Sonny Corleone does it standing up with a bridesmaid at a wedding?)

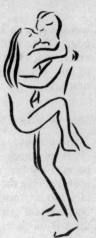

Illustration 7

Maybe that's because standing-up intercourse has always been associated with brief, illicit trysts—less "making love" to her than "having your way" with her. (See Illustration 7.)

Variations

• If you're strong and she's light, try what the *Kama Sutra* calls suspended congress. While you're leaning with your back against a wall, the woman faces you, sitting on your joined-together hands (perhaps with fingers laced), with her arms around your neck. She can move herself by extending her legs and putting her feet against the wall.

• To extend the pleasure and lighten the load, try doing it in water.

• The Standing Shiva position, suggested by Anand, is another way to reach the G-spot, that controversial sensitive spot on the top wall of the vagina a few inches in. The

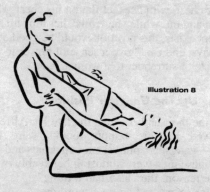

Illustration 8

woman lies on her back on a table, with her vagina at the edge of the table, and he stands between her thighs and enters her while she hooks her feet over his shoulders and in this way adjusts the position of his penis. (See Illustration 8.)

Side by Side

There's a nice, easygoing feel to this, almost like dancing cheek to cheek. (See Illustration 9.) Also, it's not tiring, because neither partner has to support the other's weight. It's useful during the last months of pregnancy and for two people who are mismatched in height or weight. Women like it because you can fall asleep together afterward, which some think is the nicest part of making love.

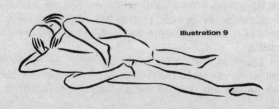

Illustration 9

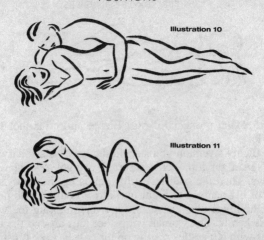

Illustration 10

Illustration 11

Variations

• You can either face each other or face the same direction, in the "spoons" position. (See Illustration 10.)

• Try the "scissors" position where she lies on her back and you lie beside her on your side. If you're right-handed, lie on your left side. She raises her right leg and you pass your right leg between her, making a kind of scissors with your legs and entering her vagina from the side. (See Illustration 11.) "This is one of the best positions," Dr. Hartman says, "because it's not tiring and the weight of your thigh gives extra clitoral pressure."

Skinning the CAT

Old marriage manuals describe something called the riding-high technique, where the man "rides high" on his partner's pelvis during intercourse, using his pubic bone (the hard lump at the base of your penis) to apply direct, continuous pressure on her clitoris.

A variation on this old method, called the coital alignment technique (CAT), was described a few years ago in a book called *The Perfect Fit* by psychoanalyst and self-

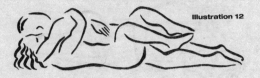

Illustration 12

styled sexual pioneer Edward Eichel and co-author Philip Nobile.

In Eichel's version you start in the basic missionary position—man on top, penis inserted, weight resting on his elbows. Then the man raises his pelvis up over hers so the base of his penis is brought into direct contact with her clitoris; he lowers his chest onto her torso, taking the weight off his hands. The woman wraps her legs around the man's thighs with her ankles resting on his calves. (See Illustration 12.) In this position they both start doing a slow rocking, up and down (not in and out), in strokes about two inches long, while maintaining full body contact and continuous pressure on the clitoris.

"The pattern of movement and stimulation must be held constant throughout the entire buildup and release of the orgasm," he explains. All of this sounds a little difficult, and it is. In fact, when a group of sex therapists led by the late sexologist Helen Singer Kaplan gave CAT a try with their own partners, only one found that it really made the earth move. Still, Dr. Kaplan concluded, the consensus of the group was that the CAT technique "is arousing, erotic and intimate, and an interesting addition to our repertoire of sexual techniques."

The CAT method is described more fully in *Perfect Fit: How to Achieve Mutual Fulfillment and Monogamous Passion through the New Intercourse* by Edward Eichel and Philip Nobile.

Rear Entry

In *The Perfumed Garden* Tunisian poet Sheikh Nefzawi calls rear-entry intercourse after the fashion of a ram or coitus of

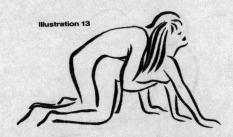

Illustration 13

the sheep. Sometimes it's just called doggie style. (See Illustration 13.) Anyhow, all the animal imagery is appropriate because it's almost universal among mammals, reptiles and birds.

One disadvantage is that it's sometimes a little difficult for the guy to keep his penis inside her in this position. And there's no direct clitoral stimulation (unless she uses her hands). On the other hand, because of the angle and the depth of penetration, it's a good way to reach the G-spot.

Variations

· She can be entered while you're both standing up or laying down flat, kneeling or sitting. Or, of course, you can do it while lying side by side. (See Illustration 14.)

· She can get down on hands and knees on the edge of the bed and you approach her from a standing position.

· In the Piercing Tiger position she gets down on her knees and forearms so that her buttocks are raised, and he kneels

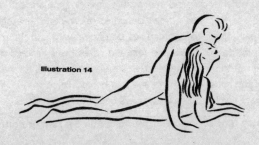

Illustration 14

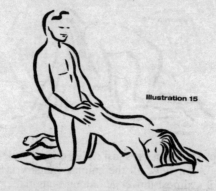

Illustration 15

behind her, controlling the action by moving her waist and hips. A very animalistic position. (See Illustration 15.)

Sitting

Ancient Chinese artists loved to depict the frowsy sensuousness of making love in a chair. Alex Comfort, M.D., D.Sc., in *The Joy of Sex*, writes that an upholstered chair without arms is best. Sitting positions are good for the male because it's not too strenuous and it can help him delay ejaculation.

DON'T TRY THIS AT HOME

Among other exotic and improbable positions, the ancient love manual *The Perfumed Garden* describes one called the hanging posture, in which the woman lies face downward and the man fixes cords to her hands and feet and raises her by means of a pulley fixed to the ceiling. He then lies under her, holds the other end of the rope in his hand and lets her down so that he can penetrate her. He raises and lowers her until he ejaculates.

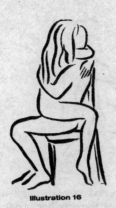

Illustration 16

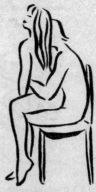

Illustration 17

Variations

• Sit on a chair with your partner straddling your legs, facing you. (See Illustration 16.) Good for pregnancy and women who want to control depth of penetration.

• Try having her sit facing away from you. (See Illustration 17.) She sets the pace by raising and lowering with her feet.

• Try having her sit across your lap, with her legs dangling to the side. You can reach her clitoris easily this way, and she gets an odd sideways angle of your penis.

• An "inverted" position can be especially strange and arousing: She's straddling him, face to face, in a chair—then she falls all the way back, putting her head on a pillow on the floor.

X Position

Popularized in the 1970s by Dr. Comfort, this position is remarkable because it allows you to sustain intercourse for such a long time. Sit facing each other, with your penis inserted. Both you and she have the legs extended. (See Illus-

Illustration 18

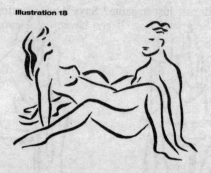

tration 18.) Clasp your hands in hers and move them out to the sides of your bodies. Now both lay all the way back so you're both looking up at the ceiling (or the sky) and are joined only at the hands and genitals. In this way, with little wrigglings, you can sustain pleasure for what seems like forever.

SEX GAMES
The Role of Play in Love

Most of us learned about sex by playing games. First we played doctor. Then later, we played spin the bottle, strip poker and a few other things. So how come that element of play, of laughter and lightness, even silliness, has so often slipped out of sex?

In her book *Hot Monogamy*, Patricia Love, Ed.D., a marriage and family therapist in Austin, Texas, points out that when people want to spice up their love lives, they usually just try a few new positions or do the same old thing in a new location. But she suggests it's also a good idea to develop four or five different lovemaking styles. Sometimes you can do it long, slow, sensuous and full of feeling. Sometimes it's more fun to do it hard, quick and dirty. But why not also sometimes have a lovemaking session that's just pure playfulness, just a game? Says Alex Comfort, M.D., D.Sc., in *The Joy of Sex*: "If you haven't yet learned to be childish in your lovemaking, you should go home and learn, because it's important."

Do-It-Yourself Games

Probably the best sex games are those you make up yourself—homemade erotica, like homemade chocolate, always tastes best.

• Fantasy games. Acting out a shared fantasy with a lover is probably the world's oldest sex game. "I find it entertaining to find my lover in a bar, looking much different from her normal appearance, and picking her up like a new lover," a 37-year-old data analyst told us. "She can be easy or play hard-to-get, and you are never quite sure you will get her in the end."

> Sex is the poor man's opera.
>
> —Italian proverb

Some other popular favorites: doctor and patient, ship's captain and high-class passenger and strict schoolteacher and naughty student. For more information, see Fantasies on page 260.

• Sexual tennis. You can add a sort of sensuous subtext to almost any game—tennis, chess, Monopoly, whatever. Says one of our *Men's Health* survey respondents: "Sometimes it's fun to find some game, a board game or sport, that you are both equally good at, and then to play each other for control of the evening, winner gets everything. This adds some drama to the game."

Indeed.

• "Look, Ma, one hand!" Try making things more interesting by making them more difficult. "I think it is occasionally fun to limit sex to a particular set of behaviors beforehand; for example, hand stimulation only for one night," suggests another survey respondent.

Store-Bought Games

If you're running out of ideas for an anniversary gift, you
can always go out and buy a sex game in a box. Most of
these commercial games, we've found, are astonishingly
tasteless and profoundly unsexy, the cardboard equivalent of
knock-knock jokes. Others (like those listed below) we
thought might actually spark something interesting. Often
they're sold in game, gift or lingerie stores, sometimes packaged with a black lacy bra and panties and marketed as
Valentine's Day gifts. We found these at Spencer Gifts (a
national chain of gift stores), right there among the corny
T-shirts, lava lamps and sperm-shaped soap-on-a-rope.

• The Erogenous Zone Game. This is a board game for
two. The object is to move your player all the way around
the board and in the process have a sensuous and perhaps
even meaningful encounter with your partner. If you land on
a space marked by a question mark, you pick an "intimacy"
card, which poses a probing personal question you have to
answer honestly. If you land on an "action" space, you're
directed to perform some action on your partner for a certain
amount of time—lick her belly button for 40 seconds, say.
To jazz things up a little, these actions are performed using
the "Hot Stuff" oils (in cinnamon, chocolate and other flavors) provided with the game. From TLC, P.O. Box 4428,
North Hollywood, CA 91607.

• Foreplay Dart Game. It's simple: You just hang up this
dartboard on a wall about seven feet from a bed and take
turns chucking darts at all the salacious suggestions written
in each ring. They range from "rub my neck" to "remove
bra/undershirt." The bull's eye: "You're my slave!"

• More Foreplay Game. The game claims it provides
players with over 700,000 erotic possibilities. That's
because it's played by twirling each of four spinners: One
for the part of your body you'll use (finger, tongue, belly),
another for the action you'll perform (kiss, lick, rub), the
part of your partner's body you'll perform the action upon
(breast, lips, thigh) and how you'll go about it ("teasingly,"

"lewdly," "coyly," etc.). Lest she quibble about definitions, lewdly is defined as "indecent, immoral, earthy, erotic and vulgar." (We always liked girls like that.) From Relationship Enrichment Systems, 4845 South Rainbow Boulevard, Las Vegas, NV 89103.

• An Enchanting Evening Game. A tasteful, low-key board game for two. It begins with each partner writing down a "secret wish" that can be shared with the other that evening. Then the two players move around the board, drawing cards that either elicit verbal responses ("First impressions often last. If you saw your partner for the first time at a party, what might attract you?") or actions ("The 'How Much Feeling Can You Put into a Kiss' contest has begun. You are a contestant. Give your partner the winning kiss."). The first partner to make it around the board gets his or her wish fulfilled. From Games Partnership Limited, 116 New Montgomery, Suite 500, San Francisco, CA 94105.

SEX MANUALS
Some of Our Personal Favorites

If you are reading this, then you likely accept the fact that books can be good tools toward a healthier, better sex life. Smart assumption. We think this book is pretty darn good and complete, if we may say so. But if you have a hankering for more advice, here are the best of the bunch.

General

The New Joy of Sex: A Gourmet Guide to Lovemaking for the Nineties by Alex Comfort, M.D., D.Sc. (Pocket Books, 1992). Freshly re-edited for the age of AIDS, this old classic is still the wittiest, most explicit, most useful guide to sex we know of.

The Illustrated Kama Sutra, Ananga-Ranga and *Perfumed Garden* (Park Street Press, 1987). The Richard Burton and F. F. Arbuthnot translations of these classic Eastern love manuals, sumptuously illustrated. Though some of the positions described here are bound to give you back problems, the richness of language and feeling in these "aphorisms of love" take sexuality to a new depth.

The Good Vibrations Guide to Sex: How to Have Safe, Fun Sex in the Nineties by Anne Semans and Cathy Winks (Cleis Press, 1994). This is a compendium of answers to questions about sex toys and techniques asked by customers at Good Vibrations, a San Francisco sex accessory shop where the two authors work. Extremely candid, practical and accepting of all sexual persuasions.

The Tao of Love and Sex: The Ancient Chinese Way to Ecstasy by Jolan Chang (Arkana; Penguin Books imprint, 1977). A wonderful guide to Taoist sexual techniques of male restraint and female pleasure, fusing the sensual and the spiritual. In plain English: How to last longer.

Fantasex: A Book of Erotic Games for the Adult Couple by Rolf Milonas (Perigee Books, 1983). Nice little book, tastefully illustrated.

The Magic of Sex by Miriam Stoppard, M.D. (Dorling Kindersley, 1991). "Sex manuals" used to be "marriage manuals": This one is written with the presumption that sex is most magical within a loving, enduring relationship. Everything is described from his and her viewpoints, with 100 soft-focus color photos.

> All too many men still seem to believe, in a rather naive and egocentric way, that what feels good to them automatically feels good to women.
>
> —Shere Hite, sex researcher

The Art of Sexual Ecstasy: Paths of Sacred Sexuality for Western Lovers by Margo Anand (Jeremy P. Tarcher, 1989). Anand calls her book "a unique path to sexual ecstasy that I call High Sex," based on her explorations of esoteric traditions from both East and West. It is, she says, a way of "bringing the spirit back into sex, of honoring sexual union as a bridge between body and soul."

The Kinsey Institute New Report on Sex by June M.

Reinisch, Ph.D., with Ruth Beasley (St. Martin's Press, 1990). Written in question-and-answer format by the former director of the Kinsey Institute for Research in Sex, Gender and Reproduction in Bloomington, Indiana, this fat, useful (though somewhat clinical) book covers all the bases.

For Men Only

The New Male Sexuality by Bernie Zilbergeld, Ph.D. (Bantam Books, 1992). A practical, sensible, reassuring guide to all sorts of male sexual questions, by a psychologist who specializes in human sexuality.

The Male Body: A Physician's Guide to What Every Man Should Know about His Sexual Health by Abraham Morgenthaler, M.D. (Simon and Schuster, 1993). All about prostate problems, male genital infections and injuries, infertility and other sexual difficulties.

How to Overcome Premature Ejaculation by Helen Singer Kaplan, M.D., Ph.D. (Brunner Mazel, 1989). This book explains a simple, effective method so well you may not need a therapist at all.

Men in Love by Nancy Friday (Laurel, 1980). Based on responses from over 3,000 men, this collection of male sexual fantasies makes for riveting reading. Love, lust, fear, aggression: an unexpurgated journey into maleness and self-acceptance.

The Advanced Course

Human Sexual Response by William H. Masters, M.D., and Virginia E. Johnson (Little, Brown and Company, 1966). This classic text was once called the worst-written bestseller of the century. Though it's written in indigestible medicalese, and some of the research has since been discredited, the subject is never dull.

Sexual Behavior in the Human Male (W. B. Saunders, 1948) and *Sexual Behavior in the Human Female* (W. B. Saunders, 1953) by Alfred C. Kinsey, D.Sc., and colleagues. Based on personal interviews in the 1940s with 18,000 men and women from all walks of life, these books are the most definitive and endlessly interesting body of sex data ever compiled. If you can find them (try a graduate school library or a used bookshop), there is hardly a page that won't amaze you.

SEX TOYS
What's in the Play Chest of Love

You usually associate sex toys with things you buy in places with names like The Pink Pussycat Boutique. But that ignores all the stuff you already have lying around the house. Even, by George, your washing machine.

A 42-year-old public service administrator who responded to our *Men's Health* magazine survey told us that "my wife had a fantasy about being 'taken' on the washing machine during the spin cycle. So we did . . . and have many times. I am six feet tall, so I simply stand in front of my wife and she wraps her legs around my hips. We make love while the cycle is spinning, and when it ends, I just reach behind her and start it back up again. It's like a giant external vibrator. It's great fun!"

A woman might be tempted to use a towel or blanket laid over the top of the machine, just for comfort, he adds—but the towel shouldn't be a very thick one, because "that would diminish the vibratory effect."

It's a Guy Thing

Though we didn't really have household appliances in mind when we asked the question, we did ask about sex toys and accessories in our formal survey of *Men's Health* subscribers. Fifty-five percent of respondents said they'd used steamy videos, 46 percent said they were connoisseurs of lingerie and 27 percent said they'd used some kind of sex toy or accessory. (We've devoted separate chapters to lingerie and videos.) Almost two-thirds of respondents also said that it was the male partner who was more likely to suggest the use of erotic accessories; only 20 percent said women were more likely to suggest it.

Researchers from the University of Chicago who conducted the 1994 *Sex in America* survey (and who also found that men were much more likely than women to buy erotic books, videos and sex toys) discovered something else. The guys who buy and use this stuff are generally not geeks and loners with an unnatural attachment to life-size latex dolls, "not the sexual loners that popular imagery depicts." Instead, they found, the people who use sex accessories "are the people most interested in sex and the most sexually active." They're the ones with the most sex partners, the lustiest sexual appetites and the ones who are most open to the widest array of sexual practices.

In other words, the ones most likely to have that blissed-out look in their eyes at the watercooler Monday morning.

Vibrators

Vibrators are probably the most legendary of sex toys. They've been around a long time, and their phallic shape can't help but spark the imagination. And yet, few couples use them.

"Vibrators are the best-kept secret of the twentieth century," claim Anne Semans and Cathy Winks, co-authors of *The Good Vibrations Guide to Sex: How to Have Safe, Fun Sex in the Nineties*, who spent many years working at the San Francisco sex shop of the same name. Vibrators came into wide use in the late nineteenth century, they say, mainly as a medical treatment for female "hysteria," a common health complaint thought to be caused by sexual deprivation. Vibrators were great medicine, doctors discovered, because they often triggered what was then known as hysterical paroxysm. Yup: orgasm.

A vibrator is not necessarily a dildo, by the way. Sure, some vibrators are shaped like a penis and are meant to be inserted. But others are strapped onto the hand and are used for massaging the entire body.

Semans and Winks maintain that, though vibrators are usually associated with female masturbation, a few guys use and enjoy them, too, and they can also be used as a pleasant adjunct to partner sex. Another of our magazine survey respondents, a 33-year-old certified public accountant, adds, "I think at least one vibrator is essential. Women do love them, but it is important not to use them so much that she becomes desensitized, and normal sex no longer satisfies her. . . . A good vibrating massager (as opposed to a penis-shaped vibrator) is excellent for massage, which is a good prelude to languid sex."

And our survey respondent went on to say that "I have also used vibrating dildos on several occasions if the woman is amenable to it. I have found that inserting a vibration device into the woman's anus prior to intercourse can have a profound effect on her ability to quickly achieve vaginal orgasms. I have recently experimented with a vibrating dildo in my own anus. I especially enjoy the added sensations during fellatio. Some women even seem to like manipulating the vibrator placement and speed while they perform fellatio on me, which I find extremely erotic."

> There are a number of mechanical devices that increase sexual arousal, particularly in women. Chief among these is the Mercedes-Benz 380SL convertible.
>
> —P. J. O'Rourke

Indeed.

One of the most popular kinds sold at Good Vibrations, Semans and Winks say, is the "wand type"—usually about a foot long with a soft rubber tennis-ball-size attachment. Other kinds look like small handheld mixers with various attachments; another type is the "Swedish massager," which is attached to the back of the hand and which transmits sensations through your fingertips. Though you can find an amazing variety of vibrating sex toys in adult catalogs, you can also find vibrators in your handy neighborhood department store.

A Few More Tasteful Suggestions

Here are a few other items you might want to consider for your play chest, many of them household items.

Old T-shirts: "When a T-shirt gets old I like to wear it during lovemaking and let my wife rip it off me," says a 52-year-old account executive. "That's been a ball-boiler since I first lost my virginity. In fact, rags of all kinds figure pretty prominently in our lovemaking. Ripping off clothing is great!"

Food: "Bringing food into the bedroom is not only erotic, it creates a more open and playful atmosphere," says one

---

WHERE TO BUY

If the idea of going downtown to the seedy district to buy a vibrator leaves you cold, here are a few reliable and discreet catalog companies that let you buy in privacy.

Blowfish: This is a new catalog, mainly of erotic books, magazines, videos and lubricants. For a catalog send $3 to Blowfish, 2261 Market Street #284, San Francisco, CA 94114; (415) 864-0880; e-mail address: blowfish@canetcom.com.

Good Vibrations: This San Francisco-based outfit calls itself a "clean, well-lighted place" to shop for sex toys, books and videos. Nice selection of vibrators, lubricants, "safer sex supplies" and a few things you probably didn't know existed. The catalog arrives in plain packaging with "Open Enterprises" as the return address, and the company pledges not to rent your name to anybody else. Good Vibrations, 938 Howard Street, Suite 101, San Francisco, CA 94103; 1-800-289-8423; e-mail address: goodvibe@cawell.sf.ca.us.

Eve's Garden: A catalog produced by "pro-sex feminists" and meant mainly for women, this catalog offers a nice selection of vibrators, dildos, videos and books. For a catalog send $3 to Eve's Garden, 119 West 57th Street, Suite 420, New York, NY 10019; 1-800-848-3837.

survey respondent. "But do something unusual. A banana is too obvious—try orange slices or melon balls."

Others suggested chocolate ice cream, honey, jelly, whipped cream, olive oil, "lots of strawberries," cherries or kiwifruit. One guy said, "I find barbecue sauce adds some 'spice' to our lovemaking." And a 30-year-old copywriter said simply: "One word: Molasses."

Weird light: Another ingenious respondent mentioned that "a black light near the bed helps, because it gives us both a pleasant-looking tan without having to destroy our skins in the sun."

Now that's an intriguing idea—faces and bodies bathed in colored light take on an exotic, disembodied aura, loosening your inhibitions, almost "taking you out of yourself," like mask-wearing. They're also cheap: You can buy a black light at a novelty shop for a couple of bucks. There might be something more profound to it, too: Ancient Oriental Tantric texts claim that violet or ultraviolet is the color of female sexual energy, which is why "violet light should be included in the lighting arrangement for a ritual union," according to Rufus Camphausen's *Encyclopedia of Erotic Wisdom*.

Actually, any kind of colored light (especially red) might add some exotica to your bedroom. After all, how come sex is always associated with "red light districts"?

Rings: Crude and uncomfortable as they may sound, "cock rings" can sometimes help extend sexual pleasure (especially for older men) by keeping an erection from wilting quite so soon. A metal or latex ring, or a leather strap that fastens with snaps or Velcro, is simply slipped over the base of the penis in order to slow down the outflow of blood. Since they cut off circulation, don't fasten them too tightly or wear them for more than half an hour or so. Still, some guys find them worth the trouble.

"I occasionally employ a cock ring to help maintain my erection," a 33-year-old certified public accountant told us. "I find that it helps retain my erection even after I've had an orgasm and with a little experience, I have become virtually multiorgasmic. . . . After achieving an orgasm, usually vaginally, I cease thrusting until the most intense sensations have subsided (but before I lose my erection . . . this is where the ring is of the greatest help). Then, slowly, I begin thrusting again . . . after a little while, the physical response is much the same as before I had my first orgasm, except that is usually takes progressively longer to have the next orgasm (but not always!). I usually have three orgasms this way without exiting the vagina or losing my erection . . . I have had up to eight orgasms this way (but that does take time, not to mention a willing partner)."

Another respondent, a 37-year-old data analyst, adds, "Cock rings are helpful at times, especially for the older man; since it is sometimes difficult to maintain an erection without direct stimulation, they can be used when more elaborate sex is in the offing. They produce a slightly thicker erection, which most women find pleasurable."

Blindfolds: "They take enormous trust but are very exciting," one guy said.

Feathers and fur: Anything that reawakens your skin is wonderful—like silk scarves or sheets, turkey feathers, sheepskin, leather or, one guy said, "clean sheets and pillows hot out of the dryer."

Chocolate body paint: We don't really have to tell you what sorts of things you can be done with a jar of syrupy chocolate body paint—but a friend of ours says it feels like doing it in silky mud. Body paint by Tom and Sally's Handmade Chocolates can be ordered through the *What on Earth* catalog. Free catalog from 2451 Enterprise East Parkway, Twinsburg, Ohio 44087.

SIMULTANEOUS ORGASM
It's Nice, but Not Necessary

Two lovers falling off the brink of ecstasy at precisely the same moment: It's an idea that's enchanted and misguided people for centuries.

Hundreds of years ago, the Tunisian poet Sheikh Nefzawi

advised lovers in *The Perfumed Garden*: "Try then by all means to make the ejaculations simultaneous, for that is the secret of love."

In the 1930s Wilhelm Reich, the nutty Austrian psychologist and self-styled sexual pioneer, wrote that in both sexes, "orgasm is more intense if the peaks of genital excitation coincide. This frequently occurs in individuals who are able to concentrate their tender as well as their sensual feelings on a partner."

Even the late Dr. Alfred C. Kinsey himself acknowledged that simultaneous orgasm "represents, for many persons, the maximum achievement that is possible in a sexual relationship."

And anybody who has experienced it knows what these guys are talking about. In some ways, simultaneous orgasm is the ideal solution to the "problem" of human sexuality: The fact that men and women are running on unsynchronized watches. Men tend to be easily and quickly aroused; women tend to be slowly and intricately aroused; and the whole sweet task of loving is to slow him down and speed her up so you meet somewhere in the middle. When you both explode in the same shared moment, it's truly a kind of bliss.

The trouble begins when you start turning simultaneous orgasm into just another desperately sought-after goal, just another trophy to achieve (or fail to achieve). What you can wind up with is a situation like this one, described rather piteously by one of our *Men's Health* magazine survey respondents: "I can hold back (thinking about walking in the woods helps) but I still can't time my orgasms to hers. I'm early sometimes, late sometimes and seldom on time. I've been practicing since I was a bit shy of 15, and I doubt if I'll ever get it right."

Man, oh, man. Think of all that this poor guy—and his lover—are missing! By focusing on "being on time" (what, is he trying to catch a plane?), he's tuning out a large world of sensuous pleasure. And we really doubt if he'll ever quite succeed in pleasuring his partner either. As the late Helen Singer Kaplan, M.D., Ph.D., former director of the human sexuality program at New York Hospital-Cornell Medical Center in New York City, observed: "Actually, simultaneous coital orgasms are the exception rather than the rule . . . the myth of the mutual orgasm is extremely harmful."

A better way: Make sure she has an orgasm before you go for yours. That way the pressure's off, both of you are relaxed, and if she comes again when you do, fine. If not, that's fine, too.

Because there's a Zen-like paradox at the heart of both sex and love: You get there by not trying to get there. You achieve by not trying to achieve. You are most abundantly rewarded by giving everything away.

SKIN FLICKS
Offensive Is in the Eye of the Beholder

The consensus view of male sexuality is that guys are more visually oriented than women: We respond mightily to imagery. Which is why men watch skin flicks so much more than women do. In one national survey, University of Chicago researchers reported that 23 percent of American men said they'd watched an X-rated movie or video in the past year, while less than half as many women (11 percent) said they'd done so. Guys were also four times as likely as women to have ogled a sexually explicit book or magazine.

But consider this study, described by Patricia Love, Ed.D., a marriage and family therapist in Austin, Texas, in her book *Hot Monogamy*. Researchers got together a group of 40 men and women, wired them up with probes and gauges to monitor their sexual responses and showed them all a couple of steamy videos. The resulting data, the researchers discovered, showed "strikingly similar male-female response patterns." Their conclusion: "The commonly held view that males show a greater sexual responsivity to visual erotic stimuli than do females is not supported."

Personally, it's our theory that men tend to be more "visually oriented" when it comes to sex simply because women are a whole lot more interesting to look at than we are. The real difference between the sexes, reflected in our differing tastes in celluloid erotica, is in the nature of what turns us on. As a whole slew of studies on the difference between men's and women's sexual fantasies have shown, what men desire in the secret sanctum of their hearts just isn't the same thing women desire. Just consider the difference between pornography (almost always produced by and for men) and romance fiction (almost always written by and for women).

"The basic themes in male pornography have remained amazingly stable since at least Victorian times: The main character taking an active role as seducer, anonymous sex, multiple partners, a primary focus on genitalia, a swift progression to sexual acts," says Joseph Matyas, who coauthored a study of gender differences in sex fantasy at San Francisco State University. "Romance fiction—as well as women's erotic fantasies—tend to be concerned mainly with a loving relationship that develops, typically involves only one partner and builds to erotic excitement only very slowly."

Or as novelist Guy Garcia observed in the *Washington Post* in an article about men's and women's sexual preferences at the movies: "While women's tastes tend to meander into romance-novel territory: flirtatious glances, smoldering passions, a steamy kiss in the rain . . . male sexual fantasy on screen can be pretty well summed up by the words 'nude blonde.' "

What the Guys Say

As a practical matter, this tends to be a problem. As one respondent to our *Men's Health* magazine survey phrased it, summing up the dilemma that confronts lots of couples at the video rental shop: "It takes a lot of searching to find a video that has enough sensuality for her and enough explicitness for me."

Many other respondents told us that though they often or occasionally use erotic videos to enhance their lovemaking rituals, women are inclined to find them demeaning to women, offensive, unarousing or just plain dumb.

"I don't know (past or present) any women who isn't turned off by erotic videos," a 45-year-old biologist told us. "At best, I have found them to be very exciting for about five minutes. After that, they're boring. At worst, I find them disgusting. My wife and I once went to an erotic movie and walked out after five minutes demanding our money back. On the other hand, some tame movies that are on prime TV have aroused me so much that I have dragged my wife up to the bedroom for immediate sex."

Another guy said: "My wife is more aroused by strong R-rated videos with an emphasis on eroticism and slow development of relationships into sexual arousal. She finds the X-rated videos more boring and laughable than offensive. She can't relate to the quickness with which the men and women seem to become so wildly aroused."

Not So Simple

Still, women's attitudes toward sexy movies aren't universally scornful.

One respondent observed that "women say they are offended, yet I found my ex-wife and her sisters viewing them in private—then our lovemaking was much more intense and erotic. I believe they definitely turn women on."

And a 54-year-old police officer told us an amazing story. One time he rented a sexy video, brought it home and tried to get his wife to watch it. She adamantly refused. Then, in the middle of the night, she woke him up—after she had gone downstairs and watched the thing all by herself. "We had one of the best sessions of aggressive intercourse we've ever had," he recalled. But that, alas, was that. After that one incident, she refused to ever watch another. (Kind of reminds us of the comment of one other respondent, a guy in his seventies, who told us: "Any man who thinks he understands women is in big trouble.")

We also heard from a couple of women in our survey, several of whom had as lusty an appetite for erotic movies as any of the men. "I love erotic videos," said one 29-year-old self-described homemaker/mom. "My husband and I watch them about once a month. I find that they allow me to lose all inhibitions and really improve my 'technique.' I do not find them offensive at all." Said another: "Watching people turn each other on and gorge on their own sensuousness is a definite turn-on. We prefer movies with the three Rs: realistic sex, relationships you can care about and eRoticism (okay, so we fudged that one)."

A Few Helpful Hints

If you've been having trouble finding skin flicks that are "sensuous enough for her but explicit enough for you," here are a few hints. The following are titles suggested by Laura Miller, a spokesperson for the San Francisco-based sex accessory shop Good Vibrations, who says her job is to "sort through the dreck" and find the good stuff.

- Anything produced by Candida Royalle, whose Femme Productions takes a "feminist approach to heterosexual love and lust." In practice, says Miller, that means "more focus on women's experiences and pleasure in orgasm, no rough sex, no demeaning of women." Two of her favorites: *Sensual Escape* and *Revelations*. Other titles: *Christine's Secret, Rites of Passion, A Taste of Ambrosia, Her Fantasy Love Scenes, Cabin Fever*.
- "One thing women don't like is cheap, tacky, low-class productions," Miller says. A pioneer in classy, high-quality, explicit-but-not-offensive videos for couples is Andrew Blake, whose videos are filled with beautiful people, beautiful settings—and minimal dialogue or story. Titles: *Night Trips, House of Dreams, Secrets, Femmes Erotiques, Hidden Obsessions*.
- A couple of other picks from Laura Miller: *The Masseuse, Cat and Mouse, The Dancers* and the classic *Behind the Green Door*.
- Several of our *Men's Health* survey respondents mentioned Showtime's *Red Shoe Diaries*, a series originally

produced for cable TV. Another suggested the Playboy "Erotic" videos, especially the ones with dream sequences, because "those allow us to get in the mood more easily." Another said that "recently, I have found that the newer 'hard R' movies (such as those made by Erotic Escapades) are better made, more interesting and less offensive."

- Of course, you don't have to go all the way to "X" to find steamy videos suitable for bedroom viewing. Some of our personal R-rated favorites: *Basic Instinct, The Fabulous Baker Boys, Last Tango in Paris, Fatal Attraction, Risky Business, Body Double, Body Heat, The Year of Living Dangerously, The Postman Always Rings Twice.*

- In fact, you don't have to go to the video store at all—it's easy enough to make your own erotic movie with you as the star. All you need is a camcorder, a partner and some privacy. One of our survey respondents, a motorcycle mechanic, told us that "I've never used videos as part of our lovemaking beforehand, but taping our lovemaking sessions and then watching them afterward and many more times helps us to become more open with one another, with no inhibitions at all." But *always* make sure your partner is a willing party to the taping. No hidden cameras allowed.

- And consider this ingenious concept, suggested by a 32-year-old business owner who's figured out a way to use his sex drive to lose weight and build fab abs: "I always

---

MORE RESOURCES

For a free, tasteful catalog of sexually explicit videos and books, including those mentioned here, call 1-800-289-8423 and ask for the *Sexuality Library* catalog. Or write Good Vibrations, 938 Howard Street, Suite 101, San Francisco, CA 94103. For older, more obscure titles, try contacting Great Pictures Mail Order, 150-50 Coolidge Avenue, Jamaica, NY 11432, 1-800-445-6662. They have a mail-order catalog and search service.

became bored during a workout, even with good music playing. Then I discovered that watching a favorite 'smut' tape—that's an 'erotic adult video' for you politically correct types—not only keeps me from feeling like Captain Kirk in the thought-sucking chamber, but I get considerable extra stamina and enjoyment from my own exertions because it feels like the same kind of repetitive effort expended in a marathon lovemaking session. Every exercise from curls to bench presses to sit-ups have a close analog in a creative sexual bout. I've even come up with a few new surprises for my lover. Imagination is a powerful tool!"

TALKING DIRTY
The Erotic Potential of Words

To hear our survey respondents tell it, about the only thing most guys love more than when she wears a black, lacy body stocking is when she talks dirty in bed.

"I think most men are extremely stimulated by the sounds women make," said one. "If they sound like they are being satisfied and, even better, say they are during lovemaking, most of us could go much, much longer and more creatively."

A 25-year-old attorney said, "When she is physical and also talks about how much she loves me, or how aroused I make her, or other erotic things, I always become aroused."

A paramedic said the best way for him to help his lover reach orgasm is "slow, deep thrusting with verbal stimulation."

A 26-year-old woman seemed to confirm what these guys were saying: "He likes me to talk dirty about what we're doing; my moans and my climax take him over the edge every time."

Unfortunately, another guy told us about the down side of sexy talk: "I used to tell my girlfriend stories about her with other guys as I fondled her. That technique did wonders for our sex life until she went ahead and acted it out with another guy while I was 500 miles away."

Talk Dirty to Me

Good communication is the mantra of sex therapists. In one *Redbook* magazine survey of 100,000 married women, the strongest indicator of sexual and marital satisfaction among them was "the ability to express sexual feelings to their husbands. The more they talked, the better they rated their sex lives, their marriages and their overall happiness."

But "talking dirty," though closely related to good sexual communication, is not precisely the same thing. What we mean here is verbalizing sexual acts, or sexual fantasies, while you're in the process of acting them out—usually using words that are rude, crude and naughty. (The naughtier the better, in fact, because the big turn-on is the fact that you're breaking a strict social taboo.) In a way, this is advanced sexual communication: You've gotten past the point where you still feel awkward talking about sex, and you're just exploring the power of words to arouse. You're not asking questions or criticizing or giving directions—you're just narrating.

Though women have traditionally felt a bit more uncomfortable with raunchy talk than men, this has begun to change in recent years, according to Samuel S. Janus, Ph.D., and Cynthia L. Janus, M.D., co-authors of *Janus Report on Sexual Behavior*, a national sex survey. The survey showed that by the early 1990s men and women were almost equally accepting of talking dirty during sex (58 percent of men and 57 percent of women said it was "very normal" or "all right"). "Women no longer swoon at obscenity," the authors say. "It represents a great change for relationships that women can feel free to express intimate sexual feelings explicitly."

Defusing the Land Mines

Even so, any kind of communication between men and women is fraught with peril, and talking dirty can be especially explosive. She may find coarse language offensive or demeaning—so that it has precisely the opposite of its intended effect, turning her off instead of on. Or she may find it arousing—but only after she's really turned on. If she's not aroused when you start talking like a sailor on shore leave, she may kick you out of bed. Other women (and men) would really rather not talk at all during lovemaking, because it "spoils the mood."

Patricia Love, Ed.D., a marriage and family therapist in Austin, Texas, in her book *Hot Monogamy*, says that people typically have four sets of terms to talk about sex—clinical terms ("sexual intercourse"), dirty talk ("screwing"), slang terms ("doing it") and romantic terms ("making love"). There's a huge difference between these words—and there's also a huge difference between the acts they describe. Sometimes you feel like "making love" and sometimes you'd rather just "screw"; describing it that way is both arousing and accurate. Your English teacher was right: Language really does matter.

But to help defuse some of the potential land mines of sexy talk, Dr. Love suggests the following exercise: Make two copies of a list of clinical terms for various sex acts (intercourse, fellatio, cunnilingus) and male and female body parts (breasts, nipples, clitoris, penis). Then, beside each of these terms, both you and your partner write down your preferred "dirty" terms for each thing. Now exchange the lists and talk about them. Tell each other which words you find really erotic, which ones you find more-or-less neutral and which you don't like at all.

If that sounds like something you would never actually do in a million years, you can always just ask her. But do it carefully. "Don't bring it up too early in the relationship—don't do it the first time you're in bed together," says Oakland, California, sex therapist Bernie Zilbergeld, Ph.D., author of *The New Male Sexuality*. "When you do, you can phrase it as a fantasy, or as something you read or as something you used to enjoy with a previous partner: Say, 'I read about people talking real plain English when they were having sex, and that really turned me on. How do you feel about that?' "

"Sure, some women do find it offensive, and that has to be respected," he adds. "But as long as there is safety and trust in the relationship, almost anything can be worked out."

YOUNGER MEN, OLDER WOMEN
Why Age Doesn't Really Matter

Ever since Dustin Hoffman got seduced by Mrs. Robinson in the 1967 movie *The Graduate*, lots of guys have had the fantasy of being introduced to sex by an older woman with terrific legs. One of the respondents to our *Men's Health* magazine survey, a 52-year-old account executive, still vividly remembers his seduction by an older woman one sultry summer afternoon in the 1950s when he was a teenager.

"She was in her midthirties, a widow of four years, a pillar of the community, and she had a very fine body," he recalls. "I mowed her lawn. She'd planned my seduction to the last detail. It was high summer. I'd finished mowing the front and came around to the back, a yard surrounded by high, thick bushes and hedges, where I found her sunbathing on a chaise longue, wearing a bikini. Today it would be a pretty modest suit, but in the late 1950s any bikini was the equivalent of a woman wearing a thong and pasties to a beach today. It gave me a raging erection. Then she rolled over on her stomach and undid the straps to avoid white lines. I was in a lather thinking about what was under that top! And she knew it. When I came up to tell her I was done and to collect my pay, she rose up and held the bikini top a little askew, exposing a nipple. I seriously thought I was going to pass out."

That's when she invited him up onto the porch for cookies.

Differences in Sexual Aging

In some ways, relationships between younger men and older women would seem to be a neat fit, sexually speaking, because of the widely accepted notion that men tend to reach a sexual "peak" in their late teens, while women peak later, in their early thirties. But it turns out that that notion really isn't true.

There are some differences in the "sexual aging" of men and women—but this business of sexual peaks is really just a misunderstanding of the late Dr. Alfred C. Kinsey's incidence data on orgasmic frequency, explains Ira Reiss, Ph.D., professor of sociology at the University of Minnesota in Minneapolis, who has written widely about sex.

Dr. Kinsey simply reported that in their late teens, males were likely to have more orgasms than at any other time in their lives; women tended to have the most orgasms when they were a little older. But this really had more to do with social mores of the 1940s (when the Kinsey studies were done) than with some innate ability to respond sexually. Men felt free to explore their sexuality at an earlier age than women did at that time, "but today, women are raised in a much more sexualized way than they were in the 1940s—so they tend to reach this orgasmic peak much earlier than they once did," he says.

There are things about May–December relationships that younger men may have to adjust to, though. An older woman is inclined to produce vaginal lubrication more slowly than a younger woman, for instance—so she'll require more foreplay, and perhaps some store-bought lubricants to help as well. The younger man, of course, is inclined to have more trouble delaying his ejaculation until she's satisfied than an older man might. On the up side, she's likely to be more aroused, more quickly, by a firm, young male body than the body of a man her own age.

But all in all, these sexual differences are relatively minor, and nothing that can't be overcome. In fact, the most important thing about these "intergenerational" relationships is not sex at all. After all, "if your relationship is based on sex and nothing else, you're in trouble to begin with," says Dr. Reiss. "What really matters is, what else besides sex have you two got going?"

Overcoming the Social Stigma

What may be harder to overcome than physical differences is the social stigma attached to the relationship. Society tends to be considerably more skeptical of a younger man who develops a thing for an older woman than the other way around. An older guy who snags a "trophy wife" two decades his junior is thought to have added a new conquest to his career, and in the process rejuvenated his sex life and himself. But a young guy who falls in love with a woman old enough to be his aunt—well, people just can't quite figure it out.

"Traditionally, the way societies have worked is that the dominant group has the 'pick of the litter'—and since most societies are male-dominant, almost all societies favor older men and younger women," Dr. Reiss says. "To go against this challenges the power differential between men and women."

As a practical matter, an older woman in our society—whether widowed, divorced, married or single—is likely to have little wealth or power. She might have kids. If she's past her fertile years, however, she can't offer him kids of his own. Toss into the equation the huge premium society places on female youth and beauty, and it's just plain hard for the world to understand how he made such a bargain.

Nevertheless, in modern-day America it's likely that unions between younger men and older women will become more common (and, perhaps, more accepted) because of simple demographics. As women get older, they have an increasingly difficult time finding a mate, because guys start dying off in significant numbers in their forties, say the University of Chicago researchers who released the *Sex in America* survey in 1994. Looking solely at the numbers, they point out, the only time when there are more men than women is when people are in their twenties; then, there are 105 men for every 100 women. But by ages 40 to 44, there are only 98 men for every 100 women. By age 50, 22 percent of women report they had no sexual partner in the past year, compared to only 8 percent of men; and after that, the "man shortage" just keeps increasing. (Naturally, if you're a guy with a thing for older women, this represents a delicious and ever-expanding opportunity.)

The Rest of Our Story

Which brings us back to the rest of our account executive's story.

"She led me up onto the screened porch and went to get the money," our narrator went on. "On the table was an art book of some kind. I picked it up and opened it across my lap to cover the bulge in my shorts, but unfortunately (by her plan), the book was no help at all. It was full of pictures of nudes."

When she returned with a plate of cookies and his pay, she told him she had a better book inside, in the study. And when he got there, she gently pushed him down onto a couch. "That push got through to me that she didn't have art in mind. . . . I could hear my breathing, my heart beating, felt everything touching my body." She picked up another art book, this one even more explicit, and sat down next to him on the arm of the couch. "With her leaning over, her breast was right at my mouth and then the bikini just wasn't there any more." He made a two-handed grab for her and before long "she was mewing and groaning and kept encouraging me while she ripped my T-shirt to shreds and yanked down my shorts and underwear. When she steered me inside her, I was so excited I came immediately, but, since I had heard that sex took hours, it never occurred to me to stop.

"I 'mowed her lawn' nearly five years until she remarried and moved away," he recalled. "I always thought it was an advantage to be taught by an experienced woman."

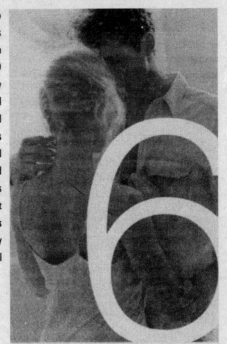

6

FAMILY PLANNING

CERVICAL CAP
Call It a New, Improved Diaphragm

The cervical cap is a miniature diaphragm. It looks like a toy rubber top hat that is inserted to the back of the vagina, where it fits over the cervix and seals off the uterus from invading sperm. Like any barrier method, it's used in conjunction with sperm-killing chemicals called spermicides.

It's better than its first cousin, the diaphragm, in that a woman can leave it in for 48 hours without taking it out, cleaning it up, putting in more spermicide and putting it back in. That makes it the perfect accompaniment to a romantic weekend. But she should take it out after 48 hours to avoid any risk of toxic shock syndrome—a rare but serious disorder marked by sudden high fever, rash, vomiting, dizziness and achiness. The main advantage to the cervical cap is its simplicity. Its chief disadvantage is its relative ineffectiveness, as you can see by the percentages below. The higher failure rates are for women who've had children; the lower, for women who've never delivered. Cervical caps are not forgiving of user failure. But even if used perfectly, one study shows that women who make love more than three times a week are at more than twice the risk of failure. Also, caps don't fit 6 to 10 percent of women, even though they come in four sizes.

> The reproduction of mankind is a great marvel and mystery. Had God consulted me in the matter, I should have advised him to continue the generation of the species by fashioning them of clay.
>
> —Martin Luther, German theologian

Although the Food and Drug Administration didn't approve the cervical cap for use in this country until 1988, it's been around, in one form or another, for centuries. That rake Casanova, in his memoirs, promoted the use of a

CERVICAL CAP: THE NUMBERS	
Theoretical Effectiveness	74–91%
Real-World Effectiveness	64–82%
Popularity	1%

squeezed-out lemon half to cover the cervix. Today's models are not all that different from those developed in 1838 by a German gynecologist.

Men might get involved in the insertion. If a woman ever hands you a spermicide-smeared cap and says, "Here, why don't you put this in?" fold its edges together and slide it in along the vaginal floor up to the cervix, which is the dome-like entrance to the uterus located in back. Move your finger around the cap to make sure it's in place, then depress the top to feel the cervix through the rubber.

CONDOMS
The Not-So-Ugly Truth about Latex

Can we talk man-to-man here? Let's drop the public health administrator pose and admit, right up front, that condoms are the cod-liver oil of contraception. About the only thing to be said on their behalf is that they're good for you.

Of course, this is a terrible, horrible, irresponsible statement to make in print. Everyone knows that sexually active people should be wearing them. Especially teenagers. Condoms are the only method of birth control that will also prevent the spread of deadly diseases. Condoms are good medicine.

But most men feel they do not make for good sex, which is why they are used so haphazardly. The reigning cliché is that it's like taking a shower with a raincoat on—and a lot of guys are leaving their raincoats off. Of the men who should be using them the most—men who've had sex with

CONDOMS: THE NUMBERS	
Theoretical Effectiveness:	97%
Real-World Effectiveness:	88%
Popularity:	19%

three or more partners in the last 12 months—nearly half say they never use a condom, according to the 1994 *Sex in America* survey conducted by University of Chicago researchers. Other surveys show that between one-fifth and one-third of sexually active gay men engage in unprotected sex. And even among people who have HIV, the virus that causes AIDS, one eight-nation study showed that the majority do not use condoms consistently when having sex with their uninfected partners. If those people won't use condoms, who will? Everybody knows why condoms should be worn. We'll skip the rest of the sermonette. Instead, let's get right down to business and tell you about the best condoms on the market today. Our hope is that you try them and discover that the raincoat analogy just isn't true any more.

Ultrathin latex: This is one more area where the Japanese have whupped our butts. Their condoms are paper-thin, so they transmit more warmth. When you're in the bathroom afterward, taking it off, stretch it over a finger and admire its close-to-nothingness. They come in designer colors—sea green, a rather colonial blue, that sort of thing. Look for names like Sagami Type E, Kimono MicroThin, Beyond Seven and Crown. Don't be put off by a lame name. They are more expensive—at least a dollar apiece.

Nonlatex: Are you ready for the polyurethane condom? Made by the company that also produces Ramses and sold under the Avanti label, they are thinner than latex condoms, making them more sensitive, yet they're twice as strong. They're also twice as expensive, often costing more than $20 a dozen. (We paid $6 for a three-pack.) Avanti has a fuller cut and a definitely different texture than latex. It's a little crinkly—like the look of that table your dad tried to refinish with polyurethane varnish. Don't let that dissuade you. Try 'em. We liked 'em. Avanti was the only brand available to us, but others are in the pipeline.

There are two added benefits: Polyurethane condoms are safe with any lubricant, including oil-based products, like petroleum jelly or baby oil, and they're the only alternative if you or your partner is allergic to latex. Don't laugh—up to 2.5 percent of the population gets an allergic reaction.

Baggy-pants style: As you start to unroll the Pleasure Plus over yourself, your first reaction might be, "Honey, I shrunk the penis!" That's because the condom is baggy up top, where it counts (the most sensitive area of your penis is the tip), and snug along the shaft of your penis, so it stays on. "World's only dynamic-action condom," brags the box. It moves. You're moved. Made by Reddy Labs. We paid $5 for a three-pack.

> Contraceptives should be used on all conceivable occasions.
>
> —Spike Mulligan, British comedian and writer

If you cannot find these brands in your local drugstore and there's no condom specialty store nearby, call Condomania's mail-order division at 1-800-926-6366. Or call Mile High Condoms at 1-800-664-5344.

Burning Rubber

Condoms have been around since the vulcanization of rubber in the 1840s. Some guys complain their rubbers *feel* like they were made in the 1840s. But others, especially young men whose girlfriends are starting to call them Speedy, may appreciate the loss of sensation and delay in orgasm. Besides, they allow us to take responsibility for contraception. And they're still ideal for the single gentleman who hopes a lovely surprise is out there, somewhere, waiting for him. Condoms are mainly for the young and the restless: Most users are under age 30.

THE FEMALE CONDOM

Since a woman is three times as likely to get a disease from one act of intercourse as a man, and 100 percent likely to be the pregnant partner if an egg is fertilized, there's a built-in demand for a female condom.

Such a product was approved by the Food and Drug Administration in 1992. Marketed under the brand name Reality, it's an extended diaphragm, in a way—a flexible ring at the closed end of the sheath fits loosely around her cervix; another flexible ring at the open end hangs just outside the vagina. In between is a polyurethane sheath. Female condoms can be inserted up to eight hours before intercourse. Some women prefer them to the feel of the male condom. Other women find them to be too much of a damned contraption. They are slightly less effective in preventing pregnancy than male condoms. They're not cheap. Last we checked, a three-pack sold for $7.99 at a major pharmacy chain.

To make the most of your condoms:

- Put a drop of lubricant on the head of your penis, *under* the condom—not so much that it slides on and off, but enough to give the tip some free play.
- Don't use petroleum jelly, baby oil, hand lotion or any other petroleum-based product for additional lubrication, inside or out—it can damage the condom. For better products, see Lubricants on page 292.
- Pre-lubricated condoms are less prone to breakage.
- Do not store condoms on the radiator or window sill.
- Do not carry condoms around in your wallet for months. Note the expiration date. Old condoms break.
- Have her put it on you. Instead of letting it be an interruption from sex, incorporate it into sex.

DIAPHRAGM
Why It's Losing Popularity

The nice part about a diaphragm is that when it's placed inside the vagina correctly, neither you nor she will feel it during sex. And there are none of the side effects that you get with hormonal birth control.

The bad part is it's inconvenient, messy and high maintenance. It provides protection for only six hours. If you make love more than once during that time, more spermicide must be injected into the vagina. And it must be left in place six hours afterward. Sheesh. If you enjoy performing cunnilingus, you may enjoy it less—most spermicides made to be used in conjunction with it have an unappealing taste and smell. Also, it may interfere with stimulation of the G-spot.

If its use seems complicated, the device is simplicity itself: a round, soft latex dome with a flexible spring encased in the rim. It needs to be sized by a doctor to fit a woman's cervix correctly. Like its smaller cousin the cervical cap, it acts as a barrier to sperm in their mad rush to swim up the uterus.

Some women get repeated urinary tract infections when using a diaphragm. Switching to a different size or brand sometimes solves the problem.

The diaphragm predates the Pill. Indeed, many women abandoned it when the Pill came along in the 1960s. During the 1980s its use declined further, especially among unmarried women and women under age 30. During that time new and improved low-dose formulations of the Pill came on the market, attracting many women who had been put off by the side effects of the earlier, higher doses. But even today's lower dosages are intolerable to some women, who might turn to the diaphragm as an inexpensive, nonhormonal method. Its ideal user is the less sexually active monogamous woman who needs some temporary birth control between kids. (One study shows that women who make love more than three times a week are at more than twice the risk of failure.)

DIAPHRAGM: THE NUMBERS	
Theoretical Effectiveness:	94%
Real-World Effectiveness:	82%
Popularity:	2%

IUD
Popularity Is Down, but Why?

It remains a mystery why a woman doesn't get pregnant when a foreign object is placed in her uterus. But prehistoric women knew it worked as well as doctors today; they would insert pebbles into their uteri for birth control.

Intrauterine contraceptive devices, or IUDs, are far cleaner, safer and more effective than pebbles, but work on the same principle: A device is inserted into the uterus to prevent pregnancy. The device is left there for months or years, meaning once it's in, your birth-control concerns are pretty much done with for a good, long while.

IUD use peaks among women in their thirties and forties, and with good reason. The ideal IUD user is faithfully married with children (a key reason: In childless women the device is more likely to be spontaneously expelled). Her family is complete, but neither she nor her husband want to take that big step off the cliff and get sterilized. If all that describes your wife and your life, consider getting rid of those rubber devices in your bedside drawer. IUDs offer all the protection of the Pill, but with few to no side effects.

There are other benefits. Because the IUD is up in the uterus, it does not interfere with the sexual pleasure of either partner. And because it's always there, you're ready for sex whenever you want: no tearing, inserting, mixing, fussing.

Depending on your perspective, it's either a plus or a minus that a doctor must prescribe an IUD and be the one to insert it.

Among the brands the ParaGard Copper-T IUD is most

IUD: THE NUMBERS	
Theoretical Effectiveness:	99.4% (Copper-T)
	98.5% (Progestasert)
Real-World Effectiveness:	99.2% (Copper-T)
	98.0% (Progestasert)
Popularity:	1%

popular because it keeps working for ten years, though, as mentioned, doctors aren't sure what it does exactly.

The Progestasert IUD, which operates on a slightly different principle, needs to be replaced annually. It works by releasing synthetic progestin, just like Norplant or Depo-Provera. Progestin inhibits ovulation and thickens mucus so that sperm have a harder time getting through.

An IUD costs $200 to $300 when inserted at a family planning clinic. There may be some pain and cramping for 10 to 15 minutes following insertion. It can be removed at any time.

The biggest risk is a slight chance of pelvic infection mostly within the first month after insertion, and perhaps caused by contamination during the insertion process. But a woman remains at risk for PID (pelvic inflammatory disease, a general term referring to infections that invade the female reproductive system) if she gets a sexually transmitted disease. If your partner just had one inserted, be on the lookout for a late period, pain, fever, discharges, anemia or spotting.

There's also a slight risk that the device will pop out. From 2 to 10 percent of users spontaneously expel their IUDs during the first year. But usually she'll see it come out, say, on her tampon during a period.

In general, as long as a woman is properly screened by her doctor to be an appropriate user, IUDs are extremely safe. There was a world of problems with IUDs in the 1960s and 1970s, most notably with the Dalkon Shield. Several products were withdrawn from the market after lawsuits charged that they caused infections, infertility and death. In some cases the suits were successfully defended, but the legal costs became prohibitive. Now the World Health Organization and the American Medical Association consider IUDs to be among the safest and most effective birth control methods.

MALE INFERTILITY
Increasing the Chances of Fatherhood

About 10 to 15 percent of couples are infertile. If they seek treatment, about four in ten couples will be told that the man is either the sole cause or a contributing cause of their inability to have children.

Male infertility is addressed with lots of fancy terms, but it all comes down to one thing. Sperm. They're lacking. In quantity or quality, but probably both. The standard way to determine whether you have a fertility problem is to order up a semen analysis. For a full description, see Semen on page 69. In an hour you'll get a rough idea what's right and wrong, and whether or not you can go forth and be fruitful and multiply.

The word "infertility" is often an exaggeration, as most fertility experts will tell you when reviewing the results of your semen analysis. Rarely is a man totally spermless. Rather, we all fit somewhere on a big spectrum. We have 50,000 sperm in our lovin' spoonful or 500 million. They're straight-ahead swimmers or lollygaggers. If you're highly fertile and your wife is not, or vice versa, she'll probably get pregnant eventually. But when both of you have problems, you're much more likely to wind up in a waiting room. In most cases infertility is really a "couple" problem.

When you find yourselves in that waiting room together, here's something to bear in mind. Reproductive medicine is an emerging field. In other words, there's a lot they still don't know. For instance, just 20 years ago it was all the rage among doctors to make a diagnosis of "varicocele," which is a varicose vein of the testicle, usually on the left side. A varicocele, they claimed, was probably the most common cause of male infertility. Nobody could explain why so many fertile men also had varicoceles, but no matter. This "problem" had to be corrected with surgery—a varicocelectomy. The widespread practice of that surgery was, and is, a "scandal," says fertility expert Sherman J. Silber, M.D., in his book *How to Get Pregnant with the New Technology*. Basically, he says there are a lot of doctors out there who are dying to operate on your wallet: "The fact is, many urologists who treat male infertility depend heavily on varicocelectomies for their incomes."

Other diagnoses are not really diagnoses at all. They're just more ornate words for your condition. "Why, sir, you have oligospermia." Translation: Uh, hey, you're a little short on sperm. The doctor may have no idea why you're coming up short. At least, not yet. But there's probably a good reason. That there's a reason doesn't mean there's a cure; sometimes nothing can be done for you. Other causes can be treated by modern reproductive medicine. Let's quickly review which is which.

What can't be changed:

Testicular injury or testicular cancer. Either of these in your past can cause infertility. This is particularly true if your injury led to orchitis, which is inflammation of the testicle, and that caused the loss of the germ cells that make sperm. Mumps after puberty has been known to lead to this kind of irreversible loss.

Genetic factors. These include chromosomal abnormalities.

Undescended testicles as a child. This might have resulted in permanent damage to your sperm-generating machinery.

What can be changed:

Hormonal deficiencies. They're rare, but they are the best-understood cause of male infertility and, thus, the most treatable.

Infections. Asymptomatic infections can bring sperm production to a halt. They're simply treated with antibiotics. To what degree infection causes infertility is still controversial.

Prescription drugs. Ulcer drugs, diuretics, high blood pressure drugs and some antidepressants can interfere with your reproductive capability. Anabolic steroids make trouble, too.

Retrograde ejaculation caused by disease or injury. Basically, your semen squirts backward when you ejaculate and goes up into your bladder rather than out your penis. Doctors can treat it by recovering your sperm from your bladder and performing artifical insemination.

Blockages of the ductwork, primarily the epididymis or vas deferens. Sometimes a blockage is caused by a sexually transmitted disease, although in men this is not as big a problem as it is in women. Blockages can also be caused by injury or inadvertently during hernia repair. If your testicles are normal in size and the amount of semen you ejaculate is normal and you have normal follicle-stimulating hormone levels, but your sperm count is very low, you may well have a blockage. It's removed by surgery. "The surgery itself is very successful in overcoming the blockage, but the problem is the blockage can lead to other problems," says James W. Overstreet, M.D., Ph.D., professor at the University of California, Davis, School of Medicine and chairman of the committee on male reproduction of the American Society of Reproductive Medicine. What happens is that your body eventually produces antisperm antibodies—"and those antibodies don't go away when the blockage is reversed," says Dr. Overstreet. Success depends on the length of time a blockage has been present.

Varicocele. Even though it's overdiagnosed, and some doctors believe it's never a factor, most doctors believe it can be a contributing factor in perhaps 30 to 50 percent of the men who have it. "Varicocele happens in many men who have no fertility problems—but it occurs more frequently in infertile men than in fertile men," says Dr. Overstreet.

As you can see, male infertility is an extremely complicated subject. There are no routine cases. If you have a problem, we strongly suggest that you seek out a urologist who has a special interest in fertility and sees a large number of male patients. And because nothing is routine, beware of fast answers.

What You Can Do about It

About 20 percent of all infertile couples are diagnosed with unexplained infertility. Doctors can't find anything wrong. In these cases it can't hurt to apply a little self-help. Here's the most common advice.

Don't smoke. One study found cigarette smoking to be associated with about a 15 percent drop in sperm count. Another five-year study of in vitro fertilization (IVF) patients found a 64 percent increase in miscarriages among couples where either or both smoke. Still another study found that nicotine inhibits the ability of sperm to penetrate the egg.

Maintain your boyish figure. Grossly overweight men subject their testicles (hence their sperm) to more heat than your average Slim Jim. Plus, all that fat metabolizes testosterone into estrogen, which could affect sperm counts.

Keep cool. No clinical study has ever proven this for certain; nonetheless, all fertility specialists, knowing that the scrotum is exquisitely designed to keep your testicles 4°F below your body temperature, will tell you that hot tubs and tight underwear can't be doing you any good.

Volunteer to be a designated driver. Alcohol is a toxin and has a direct toxic effect on sperm. Heavy drinking has been associated with birth defects. Ditto for recreational drugs.

Eat right. A University of California at Berkeley study showed that men who received one-third the recommended dietary allowance of vitamin C suffered so-called free-radical damage to their sperm. Deficiencies of other vitamins and minerals, as well, will show up in sperm health sooner or later.

Don't run yourself down. Several studies have shown the sperm-depleting effects of intense endurance training. In one study of six athletes put on a two-week regimen of running and cycling, the mean sperm count dropped 29 percent.

Get out in the sun. Researchers in San Antonio found that sunlight increased sperm production in men. But we have to give the usual warning: Sun is murder on your skin and can lead to skin cancer, so be sure to put on strong sunscreen if you are soaking up rays for fertility purposes.

Avoid nasty materials. Chemicals, including pesticides, some glycol ethers (used in painting, printing and glues) and heavy metals, like lead, all suppress healthy sperm production. If you work around these chemicals, wear the protective gear.

Take a break. Fertility specialists have plenty of anecdotes about high-power guys with low-power sperm counts. Then these guys take a decent vacation, and presto. More documented is the stress of fertility treatment itself. Some couples who take a break from the regimen conceive shortly after doing so.

More Solutions

If you're trying to conceive without medical help, one of your first tasks is to figure out your wife's ovulation time. Buy one of the predictor kits at your local pharmacy; they have names like Answer, Conceive and Q Test. Use one to get a rough idea of when ovulation occurs—but don't become a slave to it. In fact, having intercourse anytime within five days leading up to ovulation is preferable to getting all stressed out about doing it within some imagined 12-hour time frame.

Second, don't try to "save up sperm." That was the old advice. The new advice is to go for it. Do it twice a day if you want. The more sex the better. Lo and behold, men with low sperm counts come up with as much or more sperm during Act Two, in contrast to men with normal sperm counts, who give their all in Act One.

Many couples delay seeking medical help because they fear its invasiveness. It *is* invasive. And stressful. And expensive. Doctors may switch from one strategy to the next as if they don't know what they're doing. That's because, as Dr. Overstreet says, "almost all therapies are empiric." Which is a fancy way of saying sometimes the magic works, and sometimes it doesn't. If it doesn't, you end up facing some very expensive technology such as IVF or intracytoplasmic sperm injection (ICSI).

Luckily, these high-tech approaches have had remarkable improvements in just the last decade. Basically, the doctor gathers an egg from the woman's fallopian tube and attempts to fertilize it with several of your sperm in a dish in the lab, then places it back into her fallopian tube. Now, for the guy whose sperm can't fertilize the egg plopped down beside them, there's ICSI. The doctor can actually inject one of your sperm right into the middle of her egg. This technique has worked, even for guys with 100 percent misshapen sperm ("100 percent abnormal morphology" are the words a doctor would choose to tell you delicately). At the cutting edge of this technology, some doctors in Europe claim that they are fertilizing over 90 percent of their ICSI patients.

> Rare are they who prefer virtue to the pleasures of sex.
>
> —Confucius

High tech means high cost: $7,800 per cycle, on average, and a couple may go through as many as four cycles before their chances of success begin to dim. But fewer than 5 percent of infertile couples ever get to that point, often because other, less expensive measures end up working for them. Because of all the advances in just the last decade, more than half of all couples who seek fertility treatment now achieve pregnancy. And that's really some of the best news in medicine today.

MALE PILL
The End of Gender Wars?

This is one of those things that's our fault, you know. Sooner or later, wherever a battle of the sexes is being waged, they throw this in our faces: "If more women were scientists, there would be a male pill by now!"

Be warned that women have been known to speak these words just before they decide not to spend the night.

Okay. You got us. It's true. All those male scientists found it easier to stop one egg per month than the production of a million sperm per hour. The chauvinist dimwits. But they're not all bad. They did try a few things, really they did.

In the 1950s, scientists really thought they had something when they tested a group of organic compounds called bis-diamines on a prison population. Worked great. Then they broadened clinical trials to a more general population. Not so great. Combined with alcohol, it caused vomiting, chills and shortness of breath. Forget it.

In the 1970s the Chinese thought they had something with gossypol, a derivative of cottonseed oil. Interest faded once we learned the Chinese were ignoring a few side effects, like kidney damage and permanent sterility.

In the 1980s the World Health Organization (WHO) took our own sex hormone, testosterone, and turned it on us. Produced naturally, it makes us men. Taken in mass quantities, it causes sperm counts to plummet. The WHO did a big, worldwide trial of 271 men. It met with some success. It also ran into problems. For instance, only 157 of the men had their sperm counts drop to zero after six months, for an effectiveness rate of 58 percent. That's abysmal. Administration required weekly injections in the buttocks. And some men began to report irritability, increased aggressiveness, acne and other side effects.

Meanwhile, here at home, the National Institute of Health (NIH) in Bethesda, Maryland, was testing something called a GnRH antagonist—basically, a drug that turns off the production of the two hormones responsible for sperm and testosterone production. (Artificial testosterone is then given to maintain your virility.) "In theory it works," says Nancy Alexander, Ph.D., chief of contraceptive development at NIH. But the problem, again, is that it needed to be injected on a weekly basis. At least. If anyone's going to come out with a widely accepted male contraceptive, they're going to have to do better than that. "Weekly injections are not going to be the ticket," Dr. Alexander says.

Now what? By the time you read this, Dr. Alexander hopes that the WHO and NIH will have started clinical trials of testosterone in a supposedly new-and-improved formulation, testosterone bucyclate. We'll see. It requires one injection every three months—just like the latest female contraceptive, Depo-Provera. For more information on the latest female contraceptives, see New Methods on page 373. As for side effects, time will tell. Lots of time. But if a male pill ever does come along, it would be the biggest breakthrough in contraceptive technology since the Pill. And you won't be seeing it before the year 2000.

Which is a long time to wait before she sleeps over again.

MORNING-AFTER PILL
What to Know about Emergency Contraceptives

When you're young and sex is new, you make mistakes. You're with someone, you take no precautions and the next morning you look at each other and say, "Uh-oh."

If you're older, maybe that happened to you, once. Or maybe it happened last year. Maybe it happened to someone you know and love. But it does happen, all the time. About 800,000 abortions are induced every year on women who were not practicing contraception, period. Another 800,000 abortions are induced on women who failed to use what they had or whose method failed them.

If and when unprotected intercourse occurs, most people chew their fingernails to pieces waiting for her period to arrive. Women who've been forced into sex suffer fear of pregnancy in addition to the trauma of the crime. There is an alternative: Pills you can take, after the fact, that can reduce your risk of pregnancy by 75 percent. Most doctors know about these pills but won't prescribe them unless a woman asks. And millions of women don't know enough to ask—a Harris poll showed that four in ten women had never even heard of such pills, and only 20 percent knew they were effective up to 72 hours after coitus. Apparently, the name is a problem. Perhaps they should be called the three-mornings-after pill.

There are two brands on the market.

Ovral is the brand name of a pill that combines estrogen and progestin, hormones that are also in many birth control pills. Two tablets are taken within 72 hours, and two more are taken 12 hours later.

Danazol is the brand name of danocrine, a synthetic steroid also used to treat endometriosis (a condition in which tissue that normally grows in the uterus begins to grow in the pelvic region). Three tablets are taken within 72 hours, followed by three more 12 hours later.

Both brands temporarily disrupt a woman's hormonal patterns and either prevent fertilization or stop the fertilized egg from implanting. The upheaval exacts a price: nausea in 50 to 70 percent of women, and in fewer cases vomiting and headaches for a day or two. Danazol is reported to have a lower incidence of these side effects.

An even better morning-after pill is in the works. The antiprogestogen mifepristone—better known as RU 486—is 100 percent effective and produces no side effects. It's currently licensed only in France, Britain, Sweden and China. The first U.S. trials of the drug as a morning-after pill began in San Francisco in 1994.

NEW METHODS
Making Contraception Foolproof

At first the Pill seemed so easy. Just take one a day, every day, and women would be all but guaranteed not to get pregnant. Well, that's not so easy. One survey showed that one in four women forgot to take at least one pill during a three-month period. Most users of the Pill are women under age 25, women whose lives are often anything but routine.

Two solutions to that problem came on the market in the early 1990s. These goofproof methods are:

Norplant. Instead of daily pills, a woman receives six matchstick-size implants under the skin on the inside of her upper arm. They release five years' worth of hormonal contraceptive into her system. The $500 cost is covered by Medicaid.

Depo-Provera. Also called the Shot, that's exactly what it is: a shot of hormonal contraceptive that costs $35 to $45 and lasts three months. It's invisible—there are no implants and, needless to say, no pills in an underwear drawer that a little brother might find.

Both methods rely on synthetic progestin rather than a combination of estrogen and progestin, the basic formula in most birth control pills. Progestin works by inhibiting ovulation and thickening the cervical mucus so that it hampers the passage of sperm into the uterus. It also makes the uterus less hospitable to a fertilized egg. These new methods provide long-term, hassle-free birth control for women who don't plan on having a family, or any more family. They do not provide protection against STDs.

Their main disadvantage is that, like any hormonal method, some women experience side effects. These include slight weight gain, headaches and irregular menstrual bleeding. Women may also experience an increased number of "light days" or a complete cessation of their periods. The majority of Depo-Provera users report having no period after two years.

At the time this book was being written, Norplant was the subject of class-action lawsuits by women saying they'd had problems with Norplant rod removal. Many medical experts say this may not be the fault of the product so much as the inexperience of the doctor who removes it. Nonetheless, the Shot seemed to be upstaging Norplant as the long-term contraceptive of choice among the young. Though it was kept off the U.S. market for years by the

NORPLANT: THE NUMBERS	
Theoretical Effectiveness:	99+%
Real-World Effectiveness:	99+%
Popularity:	1–2%

Food and Drug Administration, it enjoys a much more global popularity than Norplant—it's used by more than 15 million women in more than 90 countries around the world.

THE PILL
It's Gotten Older and Better

It's quite an amazing thing when you think about it, that when you say "the Pill," virtually every adult in America knows what you are talking about: oral contraceptives for women. Only something with deep social significance can reach the lofty plateau of being recognizable with such a simple title. Off the top of our head, the only equivalents we could come up with are The King (Elvis Presley) and The Bomb (nuclear weapons).

Among women in their twenties, the Pill is the number-one contraceptive choice. It's highly reliable, if the user is—it needs to be taken every day. And it's no muss, no fuss. It never interferes with sex. The two of you can be completely spontaneous. For women with long, heavy periods, it reduces the flow and duration and may lessen the severity of cramps. Plus, it seems to offer long-term protection against uterine and ovarian cancers. For those who stay on the Pill for ten years, risk of ovarian cancer drops by 80 percent, according to one study.

Luckily for them, today's users have more choices and fewer side effects than their mothers experienced when the Pill was first approved in 1960. And their daughters will have even more choices, as new versions with fewer side effects come on the U.S. market. The Pill may even become available without a prescription someday, as it is in many other countries already and as many birth control experts say it should.

There are some 50 oral contraceptives on the market. They're all loosely called the Pill. Most of them are combinations of the female hormones estrogen and progestin. On average they contain about one-fourth as much estrogen and one-tenth as much progestin as the Pill that was sold when JFK was in the White House.

Since the 1960s there have been two basic refinements. The minipill, containing only progestin, was introduced in 1973. Consistent usage tends to eliminate menstruation, as does the injectible version, Depo-Provera. For more information on Depo-Provera, see New Methods on page 373. The multiphasic or triphasic pill was introduced in 1984. It varies the levels of hormones over the monthly cycle. This allows for lower doses and fewer side effects.

Today's pills are very safe. "In the United States it is safer to use pills than to deliver a baby, unless a woman is over 35 years of age and smokes more than 35 cigarettes a day," states the practitioner's handbook *Contraceptive Technology*. In fact, the Pill only poses one serious risk: cardiovascular problems, including thrombosis, embolisms and strokes. But these complications are extremely rare and usually brought on by a synergy with other risk factors such as being a sedentary, overweight, over age 50 smoker. Any woman with a medical history of blood clots, stroke or heart attack probably should not be on the Pill in the first place, but if she is and smokes, too, the risks of recurrence are increased.

There are other side effects with the Pill. Some women experience slight weight gain, acne, breast tenderness, bleeding or spotting, headaches and slight nausea for the first cycle or so. A woman should report any side effect to her doctor. It's generally recommended that she come back for a visit within three to six months after starting on the Pill. If a woman doesn't react well to one kind of pill, she can try another.

THE PILL: THE NUMBERS	
Theoretical Effectiveness:	99+%
Real-World Effectiveness:	97%
Popularity:	25%

The Two Paths

What Will the Girl Become?

AT 13
BAD LITERATURE

AT 13
STUDY & OBEDIENCE

AT 20
FLIRTING & COQUETTERY

AT 20
VIRTUE & DEVOTION

AT 26
FAST LIFE & DISSIPATION

AT 26
A LOVING MOTHER

AT 40
AN OUTCAST

AT 60
AN HONORED GRANDMOTHER

—*From Safe Counsel by B. G. Jefferis, M.D., and J. L. Nichols, 39th edition, Intext Press*

Some women find the Pill to be a boon to their sex drives—it frees them from worry and allows for sexual enjoyment. Other women find the Pill a bust. It dries up their libidos or quite literally dries up their vaginal lubrication, making intercourse uncomfortable. This may be caused by the Pill's suppression of testosterone production by the ovaries. Another rare side effect, depression, may show up as well.

Older women generally spurn the Pill, and that may be because they're relying on information that is now out-of-date. When the Pill consisted of higher doses of estrogen, women were told to stop taking it at age 35 because of potential health hazards. Now healthy, nonsmoking women can take the Pill until menopause. It may even make the transition to menopause easier by regulating periods and preventing hot flashes.

There's also been controversy over whether the Pill increases a woman's risk of breast cancer. It's still an open question, but the largest studies done to date have shown no evidence of a link.

RHYTHM METHOD
Consider It a Learning Experience

Of all the methods of birth control, this one has the most to teach a woman about her body and herself. It also requires the most patience and self-control. It is not for the young or the young-at-heart.

The rhythm method is also called periodic abstinence and the calendar method, but perhaps the most informative name for it is fertility awareness. Using it, a woman becomes aware of when she's fertile and when she's not. It requires her to figure out the fertile days of her monthly cycle and either abstain from sex then or use barrier methods, such as condoms and diaphragms. Learning about these things may eventually prove helpful if the two of you decide to have children but have a difficult time. If you can pinpoint when one of her ovaries releases an egg, your sperm have a much better chance of fertilizing it.

There are three ways to figure out when ovulation is afoot. First is the measurement of basal body temperature. Every morning before she gets out of bed, she has to take her temperature and record it on a chart or a calendar. That's because from the day after an egg is released until the start of her next period, her temperature rises a little less than 1°F. Do this for a few months and, if she's at all "regular," a pattern will emerge, so that she can pretty much know when she's about to ovulate. On average, ovulation occurs 14 days prior to the arrival of the next period.

Once you identify Ovulation Day, avoid unprotected intercourse for up to seven days beforehand (because your sperm can live for two to seven days in the womb) and three days afterward. That's the no-fire zone.

Unfortunately, all those months of daily temperature-taking and chart-making will not guarantee a result. Some women show no elevation in basal body temperature. Or they do, but their rhythm marches to a different drummer every month. The basal body temperature can also be thrown off by illness, jet lag, stress, fatigue or interrupted sleep. The more irregular her ovulation, the wider you'll have to make the period of periodic abstinence.

Another way to determine ovulation is the Billings method. Just before an egg is released, the mucus on a woman's cervix becomes incredibly elastic. It will look like raw egg white and will actually stretch between your fingertips for a couple of inches—or her fingertips if she's not letting you perform amateur pelvic exams. There's also more

---

RHYTHM METHOD: THE NUMBERS

Theoretical Effectiveness:	91–99%
Real-World Effectiveness:	80%
Popularity:	3–4%

of it. This test is better at confirming than predicting ovulation. And, once again, not every woman's mucus follows the pattern.

An accurate way to confirm ovulation is the LH-dipstick method. It comes in a home test kit and is sold at any pharmacy under brand names like Answer, Conceive, First Response and Q Test. Given three minutes and a little of her urine, it can predict when she's undergoing the hormone surge that accompanies ovulation. It's really made to help couples have a baby, not avoid one. It gives but a day's warning that she's ovulating; by that point, it's way past time to stop having sex if you don't want a baby—and nearly too late if you do.

The rhythm method will be truly effective if you spend months figuring this stuff out and your partner has an extremely regular monthly cycle. Otherwise, you're winging it. And that's where people run into trouble. Some women could even become pregnant from intercourse during their periods—her ovulation might occur soon thereafter, or yours could be the sperm with enough staying power to live inside her womb for a full week. You stud, you.

SPERM BANKS
Are You Top Seed Material?

Care to make $4,000 to $5,000 on the side this year? It's inside work, and you come and go as you please, so to speak. If masturbation is something you do in your free time, perhaps you'd like to do it for remuneration in the "cupping room" of your local sperm bank. Oh yes—you need to be young, bright, healthy and capable of producing fabulous semen samples on demand.

You'll need to be free of communicable diseases, of course, but before you get that first paycheck, you may also need to do some serious geneological research to come up with a complete genetic history. You may be given essays to write and psychological tests to take. Think of it this way: If you pass, you'll have top bragging rights when you go pub crawling on Friday nights . . . although you may not want to mention that you go pub crawling on Friday nights.

That's all it takes to be a highly paid, highly valued sperm donor. "Without them, we don't exist," says Barbara Raboy, the founder and director of the Sperm Bank of California in Berkeley. "We tell them when there are pregnancies, and they appreciate knowing. It renews their commitment to the organization."

When it comes to sperm banks, 'tis better to give than to receive. It's ironic, really—the men who walk in the door either have more sperm than they know what to do with or they have no sperm at all, and this is the last stop on a long road of reproductive medicine that has left them with no place else to go.

Sperm banks are in the fatherhood business. And it is a business. Of the more than 100 sperm banks in America, Raboy says most are for-profit operations. (Hers is not.) She guesses that donor sperm may result in 60,000 pregnancies each year. No wonder this has become a high-tech, highly sophisticated industry. Sperm banks now issue catalogs of their anonymous donors, boasting such traits as profession, IQ, educational achievement, ancestry, eye color, diet, travel history and hobbies. Not that you can inherit, say, a fascination with bowling.

At the Sperm Bank of California the customers who pore over the donor profiles are split about evenly between infertile married couples in need of donor sperm and single women who want a baby. That split is probably not typical, says Raboy; many sperm banks deal more directly with doctors, who tend to get the married-without-children clientele.

There's another kind of customer, too. Men who want to store their own sperm for the future. They could be men about to have a vasectomy or men going off to war. But Raboy says most of the men she sees coming in for "private sperm storage" have some form of cancer. They hope to recover eventually but realize that their sperm-making machinery may not. So they pay about $350 to keep about a dozen units of their sperm in a very deep sleep at a few hundred degrees below zero.

If you're donating, you probably won't be concerned with protocols, but if you're storing or making a withdrawal, you ought to at least inquire into the operations side. Sperm banks are not federally regulated, although the industry feels that some form of oversight is just a matter of time. The major states perform inspections. A trade group, the American Association of Tissue Banks, has accredited a few sperm banks.

In the last couple of years, sperm banks have gotten some bad press. The more designer-genes operations have been teased for reducing parenthood to a shopping spree for aging career women. Aside from that, there's the very idea of single women deciding they don't need a dad to start a family. Surely this is not the sperm banks' fault. Moreover, they help men as much as women. Still, it makes us feel sort of . . . disposable. A lot of us had absent fathers. But has it really come to this?

SPERM COUNT
How Low Can You Go?

Low sperm count—three words no man wants to hear. Regardless of whether he's trying to start a family at the moment, he still wants to have, you know, firepower. And that means numbers. Big numbers. Like salary or SAT scores or RBIs, it gets our competitive juices flowing.

If you're handed a diagnosis of low sperm count, be wary on two fronts. First, don't get insulted. This is not a competitive sport. And second, don't necessarily believe it. The medical definition of low sperm count has been sliding downward for the last few decades—and even under the new guidelines, supposedly infertile men are getting their wives pregnant.

"When I started out in this field, a man had to have 60

million motile sperm per milliliter of ejaculate to be normal," says Jerome H. Check, M.D., a reproductive endocrinologist in the Philadelphia area who runs one of the five largest in vitro fertilization centers in America. "That was 1974. Then it came down and down until today, when 10 million motile sperm of ejaculate is normal."

Is that the bottom? Does that now mean a guy with fewer than ten million actively kicking sperm per milliliter of ejaculate (most of us produce two or three milliliters each time we ejaculate) really and truly can't have children? That's what Dr. Check wondered. "So we did a little study," he says.

It wasn't so little. It involved 281 couples who hadn't been able to conceive for at least a year-and-a-half. All of the women in the study had some factor that would ordinarily inhibit pregnancy. They weren't ovulating or their hormonal cycles were screwed up or their cervical mucus wasn't cooperating. Dr. Check treated all those factors. Then he asked the 281 couples if they'd like to take part in the study by trying to conceive for six more months without any further measures taken. In other words, it was up to the guys now. Could their low sperm counts pull through?

The 281 couples were divided into five groups: guys with less than 2.5 million motile sperm per milliliter of ejaculate, with more than 2.5 million but less than 5 million, with more than 5 million but less than 10 million, with 10 million to 15 million and with greater than 15 million.

"Less than 2.5 million motile sperm is pretty low," says Dr. Check. "And yet, at the end of six months, 22 percent of that group had achieved a pregnancy. I was surprised we got any."

The next group—2.5 million to 5 million—jumped up to a 69 percent pregnancy rate, and the group with 5 million to 10 million, which is still technically subnormal, achieved an 81 percent pregnancy rate—exactly what the two groups with so-called normal sperm counts achieved. (And even they would have been diagnosed as infertile just 20 years ago.)

Dr. Check relates this study by way of saying that low sperm counts have spurred treatments that weren't really necessary. Back in the 1970s men who had motile sperm counts of 40 million per milliliter were undergoing expensive and painful operations to correct a varicocele—a varicose vein in the scrotum. Back then, doctors were convinced it was a leading cause of infertility in men. Some doctors still believe it. If some of the 281 guys with varicoceles in Dr. Check's study had been seeking the aid of reproductive medicine two decades earlier, "they would have been treated for a problem that, really, they didn't have."

The gold standard of sperm health is set forth by the World Health Organization (WHO). As of 1992, the WHO had decided that a total sperm count of 40 million, with 20 million sperm in each milliliter of ejaculate, was normal. Now here's the fine print: If a quarter of them are dead, half of them can't swim so well and up to 70 percent of them are mutants, that's okay. You don't have to bat a thousand.

Fertility specialists now know that sperm count is not all-important. What counts is quality as well as quantity. For more information, see Semen on page 69. Low sperm count is a problem only if your wife also has a fertility problem. True, a very low sperm count (less than 2.5 million motile sperm per milliliter of ejaculate) seems very likely to decrease your chances—but not as much as, say, having sex less than once a week. Look at it this way. Low doesn't mean give up. Low may simply mean try harder.

Where Have All the Sperm Gone?

Certainly, sperm-count standards have been dropping. Have sperm counts themselves been dropping? That is, are all men the world over producing fewer and fewer sperm these days? Study after study has said yes. This is one of the hot issues in the field of male fertility.

The study that got the most attention was done by a group of Danish researchers in the early 1990s. They analyzed 61 previous studies of male sperm count, conducted between

1938 and 1991, and concluded that the global sperm count has dropped 50 percent in the last 50 years. Since then, other scientists have speculated as to the culprit: chemical pollutants in our water and food. Pesticides, plastic, chlorine compounds that bleach your coffee filters white, feeds that fatten up your processed chicken—all these bear a remarkable resemblance to estrogen. The presence of these imposters, albeit minute, may trick our bodies into switching off our sperm-making machinery.

Scientists don't know any of this for sure, but "we know enough to make us worry," wrote the Danish fertility expert Neils E. Skakkebaek, M.D.

Other scientists pooh-pooh these findings. Their chief complaint is that the studies done thus far are not conclusive because they deal only with the men who seek out fertility doctors and not with a truly random sampling. One study re-analyzed the Danish study and said that if other mathematical models are used, sperm counts actually rose slightly in the last 20 years. That paper was authored by three doctors from . . . Dow Chemical Company!

Meanwhile, more studies come to light. Semen collected at a Paris sperm bank during the years 1973 to 1992, for example, showed an average drop in sperm count of 2.1 percent per year during that period.

And what does Dr. Check say of these claims of declining sperm counts? "I do believe I've seen it," he says. "I mean, I've been doing this for 20 years, and I've seen a tremendous difference in the semen. Fortunately, it doesn't seem to matter" because the overall fertility rates have not changed.

At least, not yet.

SPERMICIDES
Sometimes They Can Be So Irritating

Spermicides are sperm-killing chemicals found in contraceptive creams, foams, gels and vaginal suppositories. Most condoms are coated with a spermicide as well. They can be used alone or to provide added protection to the barrier methods of birth control. The good thing about them is that you can get them in drugstores without a prescription. The bad thing is that they ought to be used in conjunction with a latex condom for best results.

The most common active ingredient in spermicides is nonoxynol-9, which can cause minor irritation and soreness, both for her and you. It's not uncommon for such an irritation to cause penile discharge. If so, try switching brands (to a spermicide containing octoxynol) or birth control methods. Condoms can be especially bothersome because of nonoxynol-9's concentration, up to 18 percent. If so, shop around for nonlubricated condoms. About 5 percent of users get a mildly allergic reaction as well.

Spermicides work by destroying the surface membrane of the sperm. Unfortunately, they taste like they're destroying the surface of your tongue. To make them more appealing, you can buy fruit-flavored spermicides at your local erotic emporium or through specialty mail-order catalogs.

The advantages of spermicides for a woman are that there are no serious side effects, they can be used only when needed, they're a backup if she forgets to take her pills and they provide her with some protection against gonorrhea and chlamydia.

If the two of you can get used to using them, spermicides are surprisingly effective, especially when used with a condom. If you're in charge of placement, place it deep inside her and give it time to work. Follow the directions on the box. Use a new application for every act of intercourse.

SPERMICIDES: THE NUMBERS	
Theoretical Effectiveness:	94%
Real-World Effectiveness:	79%
Popularity:	6%

VASECTOMY
Quick, Painless and Permanent

One friend of ours compared his vasectomy with going to a dentist. He walked in, got a shot to muffle the pain and 20 minutes later walked out of the office. "The same out-of-date magazines in the waiting room and everything," he said.

Here's what happens: You lie down, your scrotum is shaved, then you get a shot of local anesthetic in your scrotum. It's called a vasectomy because the doctor then makes a tiny incision or hole near the top of your scrotum, pulls out the vas deferens, clips it, cuts out a small segment and cauterizes the ends. Our friend was not prepared for the sensation at that point—despite the anesthetic, it felt like someone tapped his testicle lightly with a rubber mallet.

The vas is a tube that leads from each testicle to your urethra and serves as the pipeline for the millions of sperm you produce every day. A vasectomy eliminates sperm from the ejaculate—which is 5 percent of it, at most. Once sterilized, you won't notice any difference. And the sperm, having no place to go, simply dissolve inside you.

Yes, you *are* being sterilized. But you are not being neutered—your testosterone production is not being toyed with one little bit. (Your testicles dump testosterone directly into the bloodstream, not into the vas.) The big disadvantage is that it's permanent. Yes, there are operations to reverse the procedure, but the success rate is 50/50 at best. If you must hedge your bets, have some of your sperm frozen in a sperm bank beforehand.

Some studies have shown that men who get vasectomies are about twice as likely to get prostate cancer about 15 years later. Other studies have found no correlation. Scientists concede it's a worrisome matter, but they don't know how to explain it and say there's still not enough evidence to recommend any cessation in vasectomy practice.

As with any surgery, those who are shopping around for a vasectomy should choose a urologist who performs scores

VASECTOMY: THE NUMBERS	
Theoretical Effectiveness:	99+%
Real-World Effectiveness:	99+%
Popularity:	Nearly 500,000 procedures performed annually

of vasectomies a year, rather than a handful. You might ask: Does he do an open-end or closed-end vasectomy? An open-end procedure—in which the testicular end of the vas is left open—reduced subsequent cases of congestive epididymitis from 6 percent to 2 percent in one California study of 6,220 vasectomies. (Congestive epididymitis is the most common postoperative complaint. It involves pain, swelling and tenderness in one testicle during the first year after the procedure and usually goes away within a week.) Some doctors still close both ends because they fear that the open end might enable the severed vas to reconnect—and then you'll sue him for child support.

Women can be sterilized, too. It's called a tubal ligation or, in common parlance, having your tubes tied. A tubal ligation may be slightly easier to reverse but it's a more complicated and more expensive procedure. Sterilization does not reduce sexual satisfaction in either sex. In fact, there's some evidence that satisfaction is improved afterward—since you needn't worry about having a baby.

WITHDRAWAL
Why You Shouldn't Rely on Luck

If you were born before Sputnik went up, you will surely remember "coitus interruptus." You pull out just before coming. Sure you do.

This method has always been popular among teenagers, who begin having sex before they begin to think about its consequences. Teenage boys, as we recall, are the last people to be trusted with perfect timing in this regard. But even if they could be trusted, their Cowper's glands can't be. In most men these two pea-size glands secrete a drop or two of natural lubricating fluid long before orgasm; this fluid may contain a few sperm. And all you need is one.

Nonetheless, your chances of fertility are greater with a full ejaculate containing 100 million sperm. For every 100 couples using this method, about 23 of them will become pregnant within the first year. (As opposed to 85 couples who would become pregnant if nothing were done.) It works about as well as the rhythm method. But the rhythm method is a *lot* less nerve-wracking. And not nearly as messy.

Other Bad Ideas

More than a third of American women douche regularly. Some of them believe that douching after sex has contraceptive benefits. There's even the myth that, contraceptively speaking, Coke is the Real Thing. The problem with this is that sperm start swimming through the cervix within seconds of ejaculation, so that, even if a good squirt of Coke has acidic effects, it may be too late. In truth, douching after sex will have some contraceptive effect, but the failure rate is even higher than withdrawal—about 40 of 100 women using this method alone will become pregnant within a year. And douching with carbonated beverages can be deadly.

Besides, Coke won't work anyway. From the We-Couldn't-Possibly-Make-This-Up Department: A biologist in Nigeria tested the effects of Coke, Pepsi and Krest bitter lemon soft drink by pouring them into semen-filled test tubes. Only the Krest wiped out the sperm. He concluded that Krest would make a good, cheap, Third World, postcoital douche. Sez him.

How about masturbation? Masturbation before intercourse may take the edge off an otherwise hair-trigger ejaculatory response, but it won't blow off all your sperm. "Any man who tried to use multiple ejaculations as a form of birth control would collapse from exhaustion before he ran out of sperm," reports the *Kinsey Institute New Report on Sex*.

Then there's breastfeeding. An item of folk wisdom passed around in La Leche League circles is that breastfeeding naturally suppresses ovulation. Some nursing mothers do note a delay in resumption of their periods, although nearly four out of five nursing mothers don't experience a delay. But eventually, ovulation does resume—and you can never tell when.

Finally, there are folk remedies. Some 450 plant species around the world reportedly contain substances that can interfere with fertilization. At one time or another, women in every culture have tried them all. In parts of Appalachia some women still take a teaspoonful of seeds from the weed Queen Anne's lace after coitus uninterruptus. Pennyroyal supposedly has the same powers—but in 1978 a Colorado woman took pennyroyal oil to end a pregnancy and ended her life instead.

Where plants have been scarce, people have turned to animals. The women of rural New Brunswick, Canada, used to take a dried beaver testicle, soak it in booze and drink the result. Mmm, mmm, good. This represented a slight improvement over the ancient Egyptians, who would fill their vaginas with crocodile dung.

We pass along these solutions solely for their entertainment value. If you get it in your head to make beaver-testicle booze, please do not toast us.

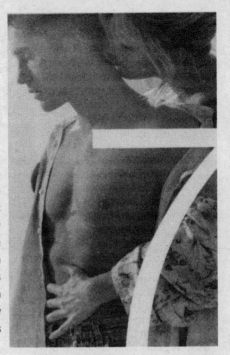

TROUBLE IN PARADISE

ALCOHOL
The Soft Truth about Drinking

In ancient times Bacchus, god of vineyards and wine, was honored in quaint religious ceremonies called bacchanalias. But it wasn't too long before these wine-sodden affairs turned into orgiastic Roman Woodstocks. Bacchus turned into a god of fertility attended by goat-footed satyrs (woodland deities known for their insatiable sexual appetites). The whole thing got so out of hand that Bacchus-worship was outlawed in 186 B.C.

The reputation of alcohol as an aphrodisiac is still widespread today (especially in fraternity houses). As one alcohol researcher observed, "It appears that many males possess a profound belief in the magical abilities of alcohol to reduce their sexual anxiety or guilt and enhance their sexual arousal."

But basically, the problem with alcohol—except in small amounts—is that it doesn't deliver on what it seems to promise. At low levels a bit of bubbly really does lower inhibitions, enhance sexual joy and generally add to the fun. But because it's a depressant, at higher levels it decreases a man's ability to become aroused, get an erection, have an ejaculation or (of course) talk. The porter in *Macbeth* says it all: Drink "provokes and unprovokes. It provokes the desire, but it takes away the performance."

The Scientific Proof

Modern day researchers have merely underlined this shrewd observation. In one study male college students were given various amounts of alcohol and shown erotic movies while strapped into a weird instrument called a penile plethysmograph (which measures the speed with which a guy gets an erection as well as its firmness). Below blood alcohol concentrations (BAC) of .025 percent, a little booze actually increased the speed with which their penises rose and saluted (suggesting that moderate alcohol use may mildly stimulate arousal). But above a BAC of .050, the researchers found, the rate at which these guys got erections decreased rapidly. They may have felt aroused, but their bodies were not responding. (A BAC of .050 is roughly the level a 150-pound man would reach after consuming three mixed drinks in a space of one to two hours.)

The only experiment to evaluate the effect of alcohol on orgasmic response and ejaculation found that the higher the BAC (.03 to .09), the longer the time it took male subjects to ejaculate through masturbation. At the highest levels of drunkenness, some guys couldn't come at all.

The practical result of all this was shown in a study in which 99 men and women kept daily diaries recording their drinking and sexual activities over a period of ten weeks. It was discovered that drinking alcohol was actually associated with a decline in sexual activity.

For older men, whose ability to get it up is often a bit shakier than it once was, heavy drinking can have even more disastrous effects. William H. Masters, M.D., and Virginia E. Johnson, of the former Masters and Johnson Institute in St. Louis, observed that "while under its influence, many a male of any age has failed for the first time to achieve or maintain an erection." But among men in their late forties or early fifties, excessive alcohol consumption is the number-one cause of secondary impotence (impotence caused by outside triggers such as stress or medications).

Effect on Women

In women alcohol seems to have a bit more complicated effect. In one study intoxicated women were shown erotic movies while wired up to a female version of the penile plethysmograph (which monitors vaginal changes indicating arousal). Paradoxically, the researchers found, the more intoxicated the women said they felt (their BACs averaged

04), the less aroused their bodies actually were. Like men, at high doses their bodies became increasingly lethargic, sexually speaking—yet their subjective feelings of arousal increased.

What's to account for this odd mind-body imbalance? Japanese and Finnish researchers have suggested that the explanation may lie in the fact that about two hours after imbibing, women's blood levels of testosterone spike up briefly. (Testosterone has been associated with increased feelings of sexual desire in both men and women). This effect is especially pronounced in women who are ovulating or taking oral contraceptives, they reported. By contrast, they found that "acute alcohol ingestion, if anything, tends to decrease blood testosterone levels in normal healthy men."

> I had a fighter pilot's breakfast—two aspirin, a cup of coffee and a puke.
>
> —Test pilot Chuck Yeager,
> first man to break the sound barrier,
> when asked what he used to have
> for breakfast in the old days

It's Just What You Expect

But, of course, human sexual arousal is not merely a matter of how much sex hormone is circulating in your blood, or even a matter of burgeoning body parts or tingly nerve beds. We're complex social creatures, and what we think or feel has a profound effect also.

In fact, other researchers have suggested that "perhaps feelings of sexual arousal and pleasure are more closely tied to psychological variables than to physiological reactions." And one of the most important of these variables, numerous studies have found, is the expectation, the belief, of what that gin and tonic is going to do to you.

In one study one group of male college students were given what they were told was alcohol (but it was actually tonic water). A second group was given a drink they were

A TOAST TO THE NEW YOU

Heavy-duty alcohol consumption has been linked to an extremely unnerving condition called gynecomastia: an unnatural swelling in one or both of a man's breasts. Gynecomastia is surprisingly common, though generally harmless and shortlived, and is thought to be caused by a hormonal imbalance between estrogens (female hormones), which stimulate breast tissue, and androgens (male hormones), which reduce them. Drinking can alter this hormonal balance, and so can drugs, aging and testicular tumors. That's also why boys going through the hormonal tumults of puberty (especially around age 13 or 14) sometimes develop breast swelling.

Take the bizarre case of Mr. X, a 28-year-old health care worker who returned from a week-long vacation in the Virgin Islands with awesome breasts. He told the doctors who examined him at the Mayo Clinic that the only things he consumed during the entire vacation were mass quantities of beer, vodka, bourbon and grilled chicken. He was often "too drunk to swim," he reported. Basically, the dude boogied till he puked, every day and every night.

The doctors theorized that the man's shapely new figure was the result of off-the-charts alcohol consumption, which reduced his testosterone production and stimulated his estrogens. The grilled chicken might have had something to do with it, too—female hormones are still fed to poultry sometimes as growth stimulators.

Anyhow, the guy's bust disappeared after about ten days. No telling what he did with his Wonderbra.

told was tonic water (but it was actually alcohol), which raised their BAC to .03 or .04. Then the researchers dragged out the old penile plethysmograph and rolled the erotic movies. The guys who were told they were drinking booze got significantly more robust erections than those who thought they were drinking tonic. "The results indicated that alcohol expectancies can play a significant role in sexual arousal," the researchers reported.

There was also a darker side to this: A similar study in which inebriated males were also shown films of sadistic aggression and forcible rape found that the guys got bigger erections when they thought they were drunk.

There is a widespread, popular belief not only that alcohol is an aphrodisiac, but also that it triggers a sort of socially acceptable form of "temporary insanity." Demon rum briefly releases you from the constraints of conscience and the fear of punishment—and these effects are especially powerful, researchers have found, in "subjects who manifest high levels of sexual guilt."

Whatever its actual physiological effect on these poor dudes, its psychological effect is to give them an excuse to do things they normally would not do. Which is not entirely good.

The Wino Effect

If the effects of short-term, occasional drinking are a bit ambiguous, the sexual consequences of heavy, long-term drinking are not. They're disastrous.

Studies of hard-core alcoholics show that alcohol over time permanently destroys the cells in the testicles that manufacture testosterone. Female hormones begin to rise as male hormones fall, ultimately resulting in a hormonal profile that may be similar to your mother's. In the end the old guy chugging something out of a paper bag begins to acquire female secondary sex characteristics. He loses body hair and muscle mass. His testicles shrink. One researcher has estimated that 70 to 80 percent of male alcoholics have decreased sexual desire or potency or both. And, lo and behold, his breasts begin to swell, just like your mother.

Not exactly what you'd call a Top Gun.

BACK PAIN
Don't Strain Your Sex Life

A bad back is a serious thing, and any guy who's had one knows it. Truth is, if your back is aching and a tumble in the hay has the portent of throwing it out completely, you're probably not going to tumble. As one book about back pain puts it, "Do not let your lovemaking distract you from protecting your back."

Of course, there's a big difference between legitimate self-preservation and unfounded fear. Back pain, for most men, needn't equate to abstinence. As we will explain, there's lots you can do to keep your sex life humming even when your back isn't in full support.

It's a common issue. About 58 percent of the population will have back trouble at one time or another, according to the *British Medical Journal*. The big news from back clinics is that the vast majority of these cases—estimates range from 70 to 90 percent—are caused by muscle or ligament problems rather than damage to the spine itself. So the general drift of advice from back specialists these days is that, most of the time, the key to avoiding pain is to regularly stretch and strengthen your back muscles.

Back-Sparing Sex

It's a lot easier to throw out your back by lifting a garbage can than it is by interpreting the *Kama Sutra*, a 2,000-year-old Indian love manual, a bit too literally. So if you're worried about throwing out your back during sex, relax, because it's a pretty rare phenomenon. If you already have a bad back, the guidelines for lovemaking generally involve minimizing the pain you already have, not worrying about throwing it out anew.

What follows are some general guidelines from back specialists and a few sexual positions that have been found to minimize back pain. Just remember, though, that this should be no substitute for your doctor's advice. If you have a genuine spinal injury, like a herniated disc, your doctor is the one to listen to, not us.

Communicate. First of all, you have to talk to each other. Communicate clearly what hurts and what doesn't, what feels good and what doesn't. If intercourse is too painful to attempt, there're plenty of other things you can try. (Back pain could actually become a blessing in disguise, forcing you to expand your sexual repertoire beyond the old in-out.)

Be passive. The person who does not have the pain should do most of the thrusting and, in general, play the more active role. The person with the pain should play the passive role, mainly receiving pleasure. (You may actually find yourself getting back pain quite often.)

Get support. The person with the back pain should be positioned so that the lower back is supported and relaxed. One good way is to lie on your back on a firm surface with pillows under your knees. This position "unloads" the spine and restores a natural curve to the back, experts say. Some people also like a smaller pillow tucked into the small arch under your lower back for added back support. You can also use a beach towel rolled into a long tube.

> Sex is not only a divine and beautiful activity; it's a murderous activity. People kill each other in bed. Some of the greatest crimes ever committed were committed in bed. And no weapons were used.
>
> —Norman Mailer

Stay flat. Try not to arch your lower back during sex; arching puts a lot of stress on the spine.

Get firm. Your mattress doesn't have to be as hard as a rock, but it should be firm enough to give your back plenty of support during sex. Water beds are inclined to be too mushy.

When He's in Pain

If it's the man who's the one in pain, consider these positions.

- He lies on his back on the bed, with pillows under his knees and a smaller pillow under his lower back. She straddles him, either facing forward or backward. She controls the thrusting. She can also use her hands or mouth to drive him crazy. (This is really just the woman-on-top position with minor modifications.)
- She can kneel on the edge of the bed, presenting her rear. He stands upright on the floor, entering her from behind. He remains relatively motionless; she rocks back and forth. She can also lay on her back on the edge of the bed, legs spread. He stands on the floor between her legs. Again, she supplies most of the motion.
- He sits on an armless, straight-back chair and she sits on his lap, facing toward or away from him. It may be more comfortable if he tucks a small pillow or towel roll behind his lower back to maintain its normal arch.
- You're both kneeling on the bed, and he's behind her. He enters from behind.

When She's in Pain

When she's the one with the troubled back, consider these positions.

- She can sit on her partner's lap in an armless chair. She straddles him, either facing toward or away from him, and gently rocks her pelvis.
- She lies on her back with the man on top in the missionary position. It's important for her to keep her legs comfortably bent, out to the sides. She may also wish to have a small pillow under the small of her back.

When Either One Is in Pain

One of the most often recommended positions when either partner is in pain, especially acute pain, is the "spoons" position. You both lay on your sides, the man behind the woman, and he enters her from behind. This way, you're both resting, there's very little muscle strain and it's easy to control the position of your back. For added comfort, pillows can be placed between the knees of either partner.

If you have any other specific questions about lovemaking with a bad back (or any other questions or concerns about back pain, for that matter), call the Back Pain Hotline at the Texas Back Institute at 1-800-247-BACK or see your own doctor.

COCAINE AND MARIJUANA
When Getting High Keeps You Low

Sigmund Freud, one of many well-educated people who used cocaine in the late nineteenth century when it was still a legal ingredient in many medicines, believed that the drug had an aphrodisiac effect. In that polite age, you can almost imagine the old boy imbibing cocaine in his oak-lined study, wearing a smoking jacket, noting with interest the small lump forming in his pants.

But in our gritty, dangerous, impolite century, the sexual allure of cocaine and other illegal drugs has created much nastier images. Smokable crack cocaine is so wildly addictive it has led to the exchange of sex for drugs in seedy crack houses, which in turn has been linked to a huge new surge in syphilis and gonorrhea in the inner cities. In the age of AIDS the disinhibiting effects of drugs have been linked to very unsafe sexual practices, including unprotected anal, vaginal and oral intercourse and multiple sex partners.

And the use of intravenous drugs has turned out to be one of the favorite ways for HIV to gain entry to the bloodstream and thus link drugs and sex in a very direct, very deadly way. After gay males, intravenous drug users are the second largest group at risk for getting AIDS in the United States, according to the Centers for Disease Control and Prevention in Atlanta.

The irony is that despite the sexual mythology that surrounds many of these substances (especially cocaine and pot), they don't deliver what they seem to promise. In the

beginning, in small amounts, cocaine and marijuana sometimes do seem to act as love potions. With low doses of
cocaine, for instance, the libido is stimulated and sexual performance is enhanced by a retardation in ejaculation, one
researcher noted.

But with long-term chronic use, everything gradually
goes wrong. Eventually, nearly all chronic, high-dose
cocaine users become sexually dysfunctional, notes Arnold
M. Washton, Ph.D., executive director of the Washton Institute on Addictions in New York City.

Marijuana: Sperm Stomper

There have been lots of claims made about marijuana's sexual side effects, but they vary so widely it's hard to take any
of them seriously. Some people claim it helps them last
longer or enhances orgasms; others say it has no effect at all
or only works sometimes. In one survey of 251 college students, about half said it increased their sexual desire and
enjoyment. Other surveys suggest that pot's alleged sex-
enhancing effect has mainly to do with the fact that it seems
to make time go slower, and hence (seemingly) makes the
pleasure last longer.

There's better evidence about its effect on fertility. A
number of studies have suggested that smoking pot can disrupt healthy sperm production in men and cause distur-
bances in ovulation (egg production) in women. One study
found that young men who smoked pot at least four days a
week for six months had lower testosterone levels. In addition, 35 percent had lower sperm counts and 10 percent were
impotent, according to pharmacist M. Laurence Lieberman,
author of *The Sexual Pharmacy: The Complete Guide to
Drugs with Side Effects.*

Sure, those dudes were smoking a lot of pot. But the
safest advice for the couple contemplating pregnancy is for
the husband to refrain from marijuana use, says Ernest L.
Abel, Ph.D., professor of obstetrics at Wayne State University in Detroit. If you're looking to get her pregnant, it's
probably best to knock off the pot about two months before

you start trying (since it takes around 70 days to produce a mature sperm cell).

Cocaine: End of the Road

Compared to pot, the evidence of cocaine's effects on sexuality is clear, convincing—and scary. What ultimately happens to long-term cocaine users was laid out in depressing detail in a study by researchers from New York University School of Medicine in New York City, who questioned 50 people (most of them males) who had been heavily using crack cocaine as their drug of choice for anywhere from 14 to 44 months.

• Loss of desire. The results of the investigation revealed that sexual desire decreased significantly with prolonged use of crack, the researchers reported. When the spouses and sex partners of these users were interviewed, they reported that virtually all the cocaine smokers were experiencing periods of sexual disinterest.

Other studies of people who snorted one to four grams of cocaine a month found that they experienced sexual stimulation without significant sexual dysfunction. But the difference, it seems, is dosage: Snorting it delivers lower blood levels than smoking it. The crack users in this study made the same observation: If they smoked two or three vials, they would be sexually aroused and able to have an erection. Any more, and they lost interest and were impotent. Women crack users reported even less interest in sex than the men did. Of course, cocaine is addictive and illegal, so don't even think you can carry on as a "light" user without causing harm to yourself.

• Erection problems. Twenty-four out of 38 male patients said they couldn't get an erection while high on crack. Other investigators have found the same thing. In one study of 32 cocaine freebase smokers, 13 reported no sexual activity during periods of freebase use and 20 of 23 males said they could not get an erection in many situations. Because they were impotent, if these men had sex at all, it was usually oral.

• No satisfaction. Most men complained that they were rendered impotent by crack and that they could hardly feel the orgasms when they climaxed, the researchers reported. What's the point of getting an erection if you can't even enjoy it?

There's at least one other reason to be concerned about coke use (besides the fact that it's dangerous, addictive and illegal): It, too, has been linked to abnormalities in sperm production. In one Yale University study of 775 predominantly white males ages 31 to 35, researchers found that cocaine may be related to male subfertility.

In guys whose semen showed a low sperm count, cocaine use within the past two years was significantly more common than in guys whose sperm counts were normal. And in guys who had been using coke for five years or more, really messed-up semen was considerably more common. (Many of these men were found to have a high number of abnormal sperm cells, low overall sperm count and low motility—a measure, in effect, of the sperm cells' liveliness.) The good part: Guys who had used cocaine in the past but had quit did not seem to have these semen problems, suggesting that the effects may not be permanent.

Other researchers have found that at low doses cocaine boosts testosterone; but at high doses it lowers testosterone. That may explain why it seems to be a love potion only at low doses. And since testosterone is necessary for the formation of sperm and early sperm development is adversely affected by low testosterone, that may also be why it's harmful to fertility, some experts suggest.

How Cocaine Works

Like amphetamines (speed), cocaine is a central nervous system stimulant—it stimulates the sympathetic nervous system, which prepares the body to respond to emergencies by constricting blood vessels, boosting heart rate and blood pressure and raising the body's internal temperature. You feel giddy, alert, anxious. But when the sympathetic nervous system is revved too high or too often, the result can be deadly, resulting in a heart attack or a stroke.

But the brain is the major organ affected by cocaine, a team of psychiatrists from Cornell University Medical College in New York City concluded in a research report. Cocaine triggers the release of the brain's neurotransmitters, like dopamine and norepinephrine. Normally, neurotransmitters are chemicals that allow a spark to jump across the gap, or synapse, between nerve cells. After the spark crosses, the neurotransmitter is re-absorbed into the body. But cocaine blocks the re-absorption of these neurotransmitters, so that neurons just keep on jangling the brain's pleasure centers (in the limbic system), which are central to the enjoyment of food and sex. That's what makes you feel euphoric—and makes the drug so addictive.

Very rapidly, though, users develop a tolerance for the drug, and the high gets weaker and fades out quicker. The half-life of a cocaine high is about an hour, but as tolerance builds, heavy users on a binge will do it as often as every five minutes. Ultimately, the frenetic, repeated jangling of the brain's pleasure centers dulls a person's ability to experience any pleasure, including sex. The libido is depressed and sexual performance is impaired, with impotence in males and inorgasmia (inability to reach orgasm) in females, the psychiatrists observed.

Sounds like a real party, eh?

DEPRESSION
How Mood Affects Love

You may have noticed the connection in your own life: When you feel blue, you're also inclined to feel about as sexy as an old shoe.

Low sexual desire, in fact, is one of the most common

symptoms of depression. That's been documented with depressing regularity in studies of large populations. In one such survey, the Massachusetts Male Aging Study, investigators from the New England Research Institute in Watertown, Massachusetts, surveyed 1,700 men ages 40 to 70. They found a frighteningly clear and powerful link between sexual troubles and depression. In fact, nearly 90 percent of the most severely depressed men reported moderate or complete impotence (inability to get an erection). Among moderately depressed men, 60 percent reported some erection problems. And even among those who reported they were only slightly depressed, fully 25 percent said they had trouble getting an erection.

It's possible these guys were physically capable of getting it up. But if you have no interest in sex in the first place, what's the point?

Depression can penetrate the subconscious so deeply that it impairs your ability to have an erection even when you're asleep. It's long been known that healthy males will have three to five erections every night during periods of rapid-eye-movement sleep. Men who are having erection problems are often asked to wear a snap-gauge device to bed as a way of measuring these nocturnal salutes. The theory was simple: If the guy is having trouble getting erections during sleep, clearly there's something wrong with his underlying physical apparatus (rather than his emotional life), since no psychological state can affect nighttime erections. But no more. It's emerged that severely depressed men, who are otherwise completely healthy, will also have fewer, limper erections in dreamland.

As a cause of sexual dysfunction, depression is as real as diabetes, says C. Norman Shealy, M.D., Ph.D., of the Shealy Institute for Comprehensive Health Care in Springfield, Missouri.

The Trouble with Drugs

There's an obvious connection between depression and loss of sexual interest, because sex is never sex, it's always something else, says Herb Goldberg, Ph.D., a Los Angeles therapist and author of *The Hazards of Being Male* and other books. Sexual response is a kind of barometer that registers many things positive and negative. Among the latter is all the personal sludge in a relationship—unresolved issues, blocked feelings, anger, boredom, feeling trapped. Weak sexual response is a symptom, not a cause.

So though many men would probably prefer to just take a pill for their depression, actually reviving their feelings (and their erections) may involve something more difficult: dealing with the underlying problems in their lives and relationships—the spadework and heavy lifting of the soul. In therapy when he's treating a depressed man with sexual troubles, "I never start out by dealing with the sex; I always deal with the unresolved issues. Where the guilt is. Where the anger is," Dr. Goldberg says.

Going to a psychiatrist and getting a prescription for antidepressant medication, he adds, should be used only as a last resort. The medicinal solution assumes the problem is biochemical or hormonal, which it may not be. In the end, pills are usually just a temporary solution.

Another big problem with antidepressant medications is that they're likely to make your sexual problems worse. That's because these drugs can have a host of sexual side effects. Lithium carbonate, often prescribed for manic depression, has been reported to cause erectile failure in some men; amitriptyline (Elavil) sometimes causes erection problems or impaired ejaculation and imipramine (Tofranil), desipramine (Norpramine) and protriptiline (Vivactil) have been associated with erection problems, loss of sexual desire or impaired ejaculation, according to medical researchers.

Some of the newer antidepressants, like Prozac, lessen genital sensation and in that way lessen the likelihood of orgasm, says James Goldberg, Ph.D., a research pharmacologist in California. When most men lose feeling in their penises, they begin to lose a lot of their drive to have sex.

There is one antidepressant that may boost sex drive, though, and is actually being tested as a treatment for erectile dysfunction: trazodone (Desyrel). In one trial of 33 men,

64 percent experienced an increase in the frequency or quality of erections sufficient for intercourse within one to three weeks of beginning treatment. Given orally three times a day, it proved more effective than yohimbine or topically applied nitroglycerine, the researchers reported. The most serious side effect seems to be drowsiness.

There's one thing you can do immediately that might help you drag yourself up out of your pit: Start working out regularly. Exercise won't solve all your problems, but a growing body of evidence suggests that it can help men clear the cloud of gloom from their hearts—and that can have a profoundly uplifting effect on your love life.

ERECTION PROBLEMS
Ways to Stage a Sexual Comeback

An erection is an absolutely amazing natural event, on a par with the metamorphosis of a caterpillar into a butterfly. One second you have a limp, insignificant wad of flesh, the next, a towering tool. This incredible transformation involves complex hydraulics in which the penis suddenly fills with eight times its normal volume of blood; it also involves hormonal commands, nerve conduction, the mysteries of psychological arousal, the smell of her hair and lots of other things that urologists still don't completely understand and may never understand.

No wonder the doggone thing doesn't work every time!

Almost every adult male has had trouble achieving or maintaining an erection from time to time—that's completely normal. Yet it's something lots of men don't fully understand, says E. Douglas Whitehead, M.D., associate clinical professor of urology at Mount Sinai School of Medicine of the City University of New York and co-director of the Association for Male Sexual Dysfunction, both in New York City.

Many things can cause that rare bout of limpness: physiological reasons, like too much alcohol or an unexpected side effect from a medicine, or psychological reasons, like performance anxiety, anger or exhaustion.

But occasional difficulty getting it up is not what we're talking about in this chapter. What we're talking about here is something that used to be called impotence: The inability to get an erection—and keep it—long enough to have intercourse, all or most of the time.

Just for the record, be careful with that word impotence. It's a loaded and misleading word, which also means powerless, physically helpless, useless, washed up. The truth is that most guys who are having erectile problems are past age 40 and in every other way are likely to be at the top of their careers, at the peak of their earning power and brimming with success. They're hardly impotent—they just have physiological problems getting an erection.

There's a big difference.

Preventing Trouble

How common are male erectile problems?

In one 1994 study of 1,700 men between the ages of 40 and 70, researchers found that an amazing 52 percent complained of having minimal, moderate or severe erection problems. The Massachusetts Male Aging Study, conducted by investigators from the New England Research Institute in Watertown, Massachusetts, found that about 5 percent of 40-year-old men could not get an erection at all; among 70-year-olds, that number tripled to 15 percent. The researchers suggested that somewhere between 10 million and 20 million American men may have genuine erectile dysfunction (no erections at all). If you include men who are just having a few problems, the number increases to 30 million.

So at least there's no reason to feel lonely!

Even so, there was plenty of other more encouraging news in the Massachusetts aging study. Basically, the researchers found, erection problems are strongly associated with aging (big surprise). But that association seems to have more to do with the fact that as men get grayer, they're more inclined to get sick—and that's what increases their chances of having sexual problems. Heart disease, prostate cancer, adult-onset diabetes and a host of other mortal troubles can cause erection problems—in this study the chance of a diabetic man having erection problems was three times higher than a man who was free of the disease.

The implication is that there's no reason a healthy man can't stay sexually active until long after his grandkids get married.

"Our data show that while impotence is strongly associated with age, it has many causes, some of which can be reversed by lifestyle and behavioral changes," says John B. McKinlay, Ph.D., director of the New England Research Institute.

Here are a few reasonable steps you can take to head problems off at the pass.

Eat lean. The researchers found a strong correlation between erection problems and heart disease, high blood pressure and low levels of high-density lipoprotein cholesterol (HDL, the "good" kind). In fact, it's now widely believed that the most common cause of impotence is atherosclerotic plaque forming on the walls of the penile arteries—a possible consequence of high cholesterol in the blood. This narrows the diameter of the vessels that carry blood to the penis. When your body can't deliver enough blood to engorge the penis, it doesn't matter how turned on you are—you won't be able to get or maintain an erection.

In 1992 the National Institutes of Health (NIH) in Bethesda, Maryland, convened a panel of medical experts to develop a consensus statement that would summarize the current knowledge about erection problems. One of their conclusions: Most of the medical disorders associated with erectile dysfunction appear to affect the arterial (blood flow) system. Which means that sticking to a lean, low-fat, high-fiber diet can be one of the best things you ever did for your love life.

Get off your duff. Exercise is known to boost levels of HDL cholesterol, which can also be a boon to your manhood.

Don't smoke. The study on aging found that cigarette

COMING BACK TO LIFE

For more information on erection problems, contact:

Impotents Anonymous, 2020 Pennsylvania Avenue NW, Suite 292, Washington, DC 20006; (410) 715-9605. Send a self-addressed, stamped envelope for free information.

Impotence Information Center, P.O. Box 9, Minneapolis, MN 55440; 1-800-843-4315. Call or write for the free booklet, *Impotence Help in the USA*.

The phone book. E. Douglas Whitehead, M.D., associate clinical professor of urology at Mount Sinai School of Medicine of the City University of New York and co-director of the Association for Male Sexual Dysfunction, both in New York City, suggests looking up urologists and selecting one who advertises treatment of male sexual dysfunction. Or call the urology department of a local hospital or medical school for a referral.

Read up on it. For more information about treatments, here are two good books.

Making Love Again: Regaining Sexual Potency through the New Injection Treatment by J. Francois Eid, M.D., and Carol A. Pearce. A book about injection therapy co-authored by the director of the Erectile Dysfunction Unit at New York Hospital—Cornell Medical Center in New York City.

The Potent Male by Irwin Goldstein, M.D., and Larry Rothstein. A thorough review of all the medical treatments available, co-authored by a leading authority.

smoking, already known to be associated with erectile problems all by itself, can also dramatically amplify the ill effects of heart disease or medications. In men who were being treated for heart disease and who also smoked, the probability of impotence was 56 percent, compared to only 21 percent in men with heart disease who didn't smoke. Twenty percent of guys with high blood pressure who smoked couldn't get an erection; only 8.5 percent of nonsmokers with high blood pressure couldn't get an erection.

"While we can't alter age, race and family history, reducing other risk factors, like smoking, cholesterol, inactivity and high blood pressure, are proven and realistic methods to promote heart health," says Dr. McKinlay.

Watch your medications. Erection problems were also strongly associated with high blood pressure medications, vasodilators (heart medications to dilate blood vessels), low blood sugar medications (for diabetes) and others. For more on this, see Medications on page 444.

Going to See Somebody

If you are encountering erection problems, it's probably time to screw up your courage and seek professional help. Taking that first step is likely to be the most difficult part of the whole deal. In fact, 64 percent of guys with erection troubles put off seeing a doctor for a year or more, and it's not uncommon for men to wait five or ten years to get help, according to a survey of urologists by the Impotence Information Center. Men's biggest worry: Just having to talk about it openly with a doctor. Men's second biggest worry: The solution will require surgery (very unlikely).

In general, men only see a doctor when a problem has become absolutely intolerable, says Kenneth Goldberg, M.D., founder and director of the Male Health Center in Dallas. Women, on the other hand, openly discuss their gynecological problems with their personal physicians as well as with their women friends. They're much more willing to seek help.

As little as 15 years ago, if you'd gone to see a specialist about your sexual problem, he'd almost certainly have told you that it was all in your head. But the big news of the last 10 years is that we've discovered emotional and psychological problems do not cause most cases of impotence, says Dr. Whitehead. Advances in mapping the blood flow of the penis have shown us that approximately 80 or even 90 percent of impotence is organic (physically caused), Dr. White-head says. This is especially likely to be true in men over age 50. To lots of guys, this comes as a real relief: It's probably, in effect, a faulty carburetor, not some twisted Freudian complex involving your mother.

But getting to the bottom of the problem—which may involve hormonal, neurological, vascular and other bodily systems, or side effects of medications, or past surgeries—can be a daunting task. That's why the ideal thing is to find a treatment center that employs a multitude of penis specialists—a urologist, an endocrinologist (hormone specialist), a sex therapist, a psychiatrist.

During the initial meeting, Dr. Whitehead explains, the urologist will take a complete medical and sexual history, which can be highly revealing. Some things that would strongly suggest a psychological explanation.

- The guy can get an erection with one partner or during masturbation, but not with another partner.
- He's going through some heavy-duty life stress, like divorce or job loss.
- There's a history of depression or some other mental illness.
- There's an absence of physical problems—diabetes, heart disease, advanced age and so on.

Of course, nothing in life is quite so simple.

Usually, even if the guy's problem is primarily physical, he has almost always developed some emotional problems to go along with it. Who could blame a diabetic man who frequently has trouble getting erect for having performance anxiety when he makes love to his wife?

"We have found that, no matter what the underlying problem, sex therapy is very important, and very helpful, during this whole process," Dr. Whitehead says.

A variety of screening tests can also help clarify the origin of the problem.

Nocturnal penile tumescence test. Healthy men will normally have three to five rigid erections every night, each lasting 15 minutes to an hour, during periods of rapid-eye-movement sleep. To find out if this is happening—in other words, if your underlying physical machine is working properly—the doctor may send you home with a snap-gauge device that slips over the penis and is worn while you're sleeping. It consists of three bands of increasing strength, which will break under increasing erectile force. There's also a fancier device called the RigiScan, which continuously monitors the night life of your penis, leaving tracings on a paper graph in the morning like a sort of sexual stock market.

Biothesiometry. Basically, this is a kind of sophisticated tuning fork that, when struck and held against the penis, indicates whether or not there's underlying nerve damage.

Trial injection. Again, just to see if the machine is working, some urologists will administer an injection of a drug known to induce erections in healthy men. If a very high dose is required, that's highly suggestive of a physical problem.

A Multitude of Options

If the history and screening tests suggest a psychological problem, you'll be referred to a sex therapist or a psychiatrist. For more on this, see Sex Therapy on page 479 and Performance Anxiety on page 450.

If the doctor suspects a physical problem, you have an amazing array of options—many of which have only become available in the past 15 years or so. In terms of treatments for erectile problems, you're living in the twenty-first century. Very likely, the physician will begin by suggesting the simplest, least invasive therapy. At many clinics that's likely to mean oral medications or testosterone replacement, followed by vacuum constriction devices or injection therapy.

Hormone Treatments

It's possible, especially in older men, that the problem has to do with a hormonal disturbance such as low testosterone. But this is pretty rare—less than 5 percent of cases, according to most authoritative estimates. According to Stanley Korenman, M.D., chief of the endocrinology division at the University of California, Los Angeles, Medical Center, in a survey of his own male patients who were over age 50, 30 to 40 percent of them had low "bioavailable" testosterone. But, he says, that's not likely to be the only cause of their impotence, nor will replacing testosterone necessarily cure it.

Nevertheless, sometimes it will cure it. You either get injections once a month or wear a skin patch on your scrotum, which releases the hormone more steadily than shots do (and, of course, without pain).

Occasionally, men will develop problems with another hormone called prolactin, which has been successfully treated with a drug called bromocriptine.

Still, the NIH consensus statement warns: "For men who have normal testosterone levels, androgen therapy is inappropriate and may carry significant health risks, especially in the situation of unrecognized prostate cancer." (Male hormones stimulate the growth of prostate cancer; treatments for prostate cancer focus on reducing male hormone levels.)

Pills and Potions

Lots of guys will ask their urologists, "Can't I just take a pill?" But of the dozens of oral medications that have been tried, most just don't seem to work very well. Two of the most promising:

Yohimbine: The granddaddy of all love potions and the most popular prescription medication for erectile problems, yohimbine is sold under three brand names: Yocon, Yohimex and Aphrodyne. It's made from the bark of an African tree, which makes it seem kind of exotic.

But clinical studies have also shown that yohimbine helps restore erections, either partially or fully, in about a third of the men with erection problems who try it. (There's no evidence it does anything for guys without erection problems.) Critics say it's nothing more than a placebo—that it works only because men think it's going to work. Still, though it's less effective than more drastic measures (like a vacuum device or injections), it does have certain advantages: It's relatively cheap, noninvasive and has few side effects.

Trazodone: Usually, antidepressant medications cause erection problems, but this antidepressant (brand name: Desyrel) may have the opposite effect. In one trial of 33 men, 64 percent experienced an increase in the frequency or quality of erections sufficient for intercourse within one to three weeks of beginning treatment. Given orally three times a day, it proved more effective than yohimbine or topically applied nitroglycerine, the researchers reported. It has even been found to prolong erections in nonimpotent men, apparently by blocking the nerves that signal blood to drain from the penis. This research has a lot of exciting possibilities, says Sheldon Burman, M.D., director of the Male Sexual Dysfunction Institute in Chicago. Since the most serious side effect seems to be drowsiness, it might be worth asking your doctor if it's worth a try.

Injection Therapy

Here's the basic concept (try not to say ouch!): Shortly before you want to make love, you give yourself an injection at the base of your penis with a tiny needle, which produces a natural-looking erection that lasts anywhere from half an hour to a couple of hours.

Despite its obvious drawbacks, injection therapy is immensely popular—tens of thousands of men are now on injection treatments all over the world, enthuses Drogo K. Montague, M.D., director of the Center for Sexual Function at the Cleveland Clinic Foundation.

Various drugs have been used, but the most effective and well-studied are papaverine, phentolamine and prostaglandin E_1. They all work by causing the blood vessels to dilate, engorging the penis with blood, Dr. Whitehead explains, and they can be administered so that the erection lasts as long as you wish. (Using injections, you shouldn't stay erect more than four hours, and you shouldn't have sex more than eight or ten times a month, he warns.)

Injections seem to work for older men as well as younger

ones. In a study conducted by researchers at Duke University Medical Center in Durham, North Carolina, medical records of two groups were investigated: men ages 35 to 55 and men over 65. Both were getting injections of a papaverine/phentolamine mixture. Though the causes of impotence were quite different among these groups, the injections seemed to work equally well for both, though the older men often needed a higher dose of the drug to get an erection and used the medication less frequently. Complications were few, of minimal consequence and occurred with equal frequency between the two age groups, the researchers added.

The big drawback is having to give yourself a shot in the privates each time. The trouble is that researchers have been unable to figure out a better way to deliver the drug into the two long, narrow chambers of the penis (the corpora cavernosa) that fill with blood during an erection. The chambers are surrounded by a tough, fibrous tissue called the tunica albuginea; it has to be pierced to deliver the drug directly to the chambers. Simply applying a topical medication to the skin, wearing a skin patch or taking a pill just doesn't work.

Another drawback is that injection therapy is fairly expensive. Depending on how often you inject yourself, a two-month supply can cost $100 to $200. (Some health insurance policies will cover part of this.)

In the early days, when papaverine was used alone, men sometimes got prolonged, painful erections that required a (very embarrassing and unfortunate) trip to the hospital emergency room to get the doggone thing to go down. This required the use of drugs that could trigger potentially life-threatening high blood pressure. But this side effect was greatly reduced when phentolamine was added to the mix. And nowadays, Dr. Whitehead says, the most popular drug is prostaglandin E_1, which doesn't produce this side effect at all.

Years of shots may also produce small, hard nodules of scar tissue on the shaft of the penis. In one survey, after eight years about 50 percent of men were still using the injections, but about 22 percent said they'd developed nodules at the injection site, though few said they were really bothersome.

Injecting yourself also takes a fair amount of manual dexterity—so injection therapy is really not appropriate for men with bad eyesight, Parkinson's disease, psychological problems or a big belly.

Taken together, all of these drawbacks have resulted in a fairly high dropout rate, usually early in the treatment. It's unclear whether this is related to side effects, lack of spontaneity or just because lots of guys think it's a drag.

There are a few new improvements. For men who get the heebie-jeebies at the thought of sticking a needle down there, Israeli scientists tried using the Instaject 11, a tiny needle gun used for injecting insulin. The 35 men who used the device described the injections as painless and easy. Other researchers have developed a device that looks like a ballpoint pen; you simply press the button on the top and a tiny needle makes the injection.

Other researchers are developing an intraurethral insertion system in which shots are replaced by inserting a tiny pellet of the drug into the tip of the penis with a small applicator. In preliminary studies pellets seemed to work as well as injections.

Vacuum Devices

Basically, vacuum devices work like this: You slip your limp penis into a plastic cylinder that has a rubber band around the end of it. A short plastic tube connects the cylinder to a lightweight vacuum pump. A sealant is applied between the rim of the cylinder and your skin to create an airtight seal. Then you squeeze the handle of the pump, which reduces air pressure inside the cylinder, creating an erection by drawing blood into the penis. After a few minutes you slip the rubber band down around the base of the penis to trap the outflow of blood. You have an erection that lasts about half an hour (or until you remove the rubber band).

The big advantages of vacuum devices: There are very few complications, no drug side effects and no surgery. It's reversible. And there's only a small one-time cost, which is fairly low.

Unfortunately, vacuum devices are also cumbersome and weirdly unnatural. Sometimes they impair ejaculation, which can be uncomfortable. The erection is a little bit cool and sometimes slightly bluish from the pooling of venous blood. And the stability is not so good, Dr. Whitehead says. It only hardens the outer two-thirds of the penis, the visible part. So it's a wobbly erection, but usually hard enough for penetration.

In one study conducted by urologists at the University of Texas Health Science Center at Houston, 216 men who had used the devices filled out questionnaires during the third month and the twenty-ninth month. Seventy percent of the men said they'd used the device regularly, about 85 percent said they and their partners were satisfied and 90 percent said they were satisfied with the hardness, length and circumference of their erections. Also, 79 percent said their frequency of intercourse had significantly increased during the first year.

There were a couple of problems. Ten percent of the partners said they were bothered by the coolness of their partners' penises. Five percent of the men complained of numbness or bruising, and 12 percent complained that it was a little painful. Nevertheless, despite its limitations, the vacuum constriction device appears to be an effective and durable nonoperative treatment for erectile dysfunction, the researchers concluded.

Surgery

In a very few cases erections can be restored through surgery either by arterial revascularization (increasing blood flow coming in through the arteries) or by venous ligation (decreasing outflowing blood through the veins).

The bottom line, though, is that this is highly specialized surgery, with quite limited long-term success, that is really only useful in a small percentage of men with erection problems (less than 5 percent).

Surgery is mainly for younger men who've sustained a traumatic injury to the arterial blood supply by damage to the perineum (the spot between the scrotum and anus)—like a guy riding a bike who rides over an open manhole cover, Dr. Whitehead explains.

Reported success rates for this kind of surgery have ranged from 12 percent to 80 percent. But it also appears that the surgery's apparent success two to six months after the operation gradually fades over time.

Implants

Surgically implanting a mechanical device that creates an erection is the most extreme, most invasive treatment for erection problems, and they're generally used only after every other treatment has been tried.

There are two basic kinds of implants.

In the semirigid types a pair of bendable rods are surgically implanted into the corpora cavernosa. The rods can be bent by hand. You bend them down close to the body to conceal your penis when dressed; bend them up when ready for action. One problem is that it's always rigid and you can always feel it.

Inflatable implants use a hydraulic device that allows you to pump up an erection whenever you need it and deflate it when you don't. One model has a fluid reservoir and a fillable chamber built into the implant itself. Another, more elaborate model has a separate fluid reservoir hidden in the belly and a pump hidden in the scrotum; when you're ready to make love, you gently squeeze the scrotum and it inflates.

Yeah, that's an awful lot of plumbing, and mechanical failure is one of the biggest drawbacks, though improvements have brought the failure rate down to around 3 percent. The other big drawbacks are infection (around 1 percent) and erosion, where an implant erodes through the skin of the penis (around 3 percent). Nevertheless, success rates are high (about 90 percent, in terms of patient and partner satisfaction) and most implants will last from five to ten years.

Also, says Dr. Whitehead, when there's a malfunction, almost everybody wants them replaced, not removed. "That, to me, shows they were happy with it," he says.

One study looked at 112 patients (average age: 51) who'd gotten a three-piece inflatable prosthesis called the Alpha-1. Seventy-five percent of these men had tried other things first—injections, vacuum devices, hormone therapy, psychotherapy—to no avail. Eighty-three percent reported they were able to have intercourse within eight weeks of surgery. Eighty percent said they could get good erections, and their partners were satisfied. After two years, however, 7 percent of the men had to have a second operation because of various problems, 3 percent developed infections and three of the men's partners were noisily unsatisfied. The partners noted that the prosthesis was too unnatural, too small or caused painful intercourse.

Despite it all, one guy in his sixties who'd had an implant told a *Men's Health* reporter: "I'm not going to tell you that it's exactly like having a 25-year-old penis, but there's no comparison with one that doesn't work at all."

Which is a sentiment that's not hard to understand.

FATIGUE
Knowing When to Have Energy

Guys are forever being accused of falling asleep right after sex. But nowadays, there's an even more common problem, of which both men and women are guilty: falling asleep before sex.

Chronic overscheduling, overwork, stress and fatigue have become a standard part of nearly everyone's life. Even kids are so busy they need appointment calendars. And when push comes to shove in a busy, complicated life, it's often sex that gets left behind.

In your own life, what is the biggest impediment to good sex? Among the respondents to our *Men's Health* mail survey, the most common answer by far (54 percent) was fatigue. The

next most common answer (42 percent) was lack of time—
which, in a roundabout way, amounts to the same thing.

Chronic physical exhaustion can interfere with good sex
in a variety of ways, explains Lonnie Barbach, Ph.D., a San
Francisco sex therapist and author. The sexual response
cycle is a multistep process that's sometimes subdivided into
five parts: desire, arousal, readiness, orgasm and satisfaction
(or resolution). Fatigue and stress are known to interfere
with the desire and arousal phases, Dr. Barbach observes—
sex gets nipped in the bud, so to speak, because you're so tired you just don't feel like it. And if it's your partner who's exhausted, that can be equally problematic, because fatigue has been linked to lack of desire, lack of orgasm and painful intercourse in women, Dr. Barbach says.

> One thing I've learned in all these years is not to make love when you don't really feel like it; there's probably nothing worse you can do to yourself than that.
>
> —Norman Mailer

And it's not just physical exhaustion that's to blame.
William H. Masters, M.D., and Virginia E. Johnson, of the
former Masters and Johnson Institute in St. Louis, report
that mental exhaustion—usually worries about work or
money—is an even greater deterrent to male sexual responsiveness than physical fatigue, especially among older men.
This sensitivity of male sexuality to mental fatigue is one of
the greatest differences between the responsiveness of the
middle-age and the younger male, they write.

The 18-Hour Revitalization Plan

We don't claim to know how you should manage your time.
But here are a few ways therapists suggest you can keep
fatigue from ruining everything.

Put last things first. Usually, when you make love with
your mate, it's the very last thing you do in the day. But
practically speaking, that's likely to be the worst of all pos-

sible times because that's when you're most exhausted (and the older you get, the more of a problem this becomes). So switch your priorities from time to time and make love first thing in the day. Get a babysitter on Saturday morning, lock the bedroom door and then take your time.

Make an appointment. In the movies the greatest sex scenes are the ones that just happen: a spontaneous, button-popping explosion of uncontrollable desire, usually in some odd place like the kitchen. In real life, though, spontaneous sex is more the exception than the rule—and if you sit around waiting for it to happen, it may never. So (unromantic as it sounds) you may just have to schedule it, for a time when both of you are at your best. Ask her to leave Thursday night open (early) or Friday at noon. The anticipation is likely to add spice to things once you finally meet. "A good sex life doesn't fall out of heaven. Sometimes you have to work to make it happen," says Jude Cotter, Ph.D., a psychologist and sex therapist in private practice in Farmington Hills, Michigan.

Don't overindulge. Making love when you're tired, with a heavy meal or a too-happy Happy Hour on top, can be disastrous. (Male erectile failure after such an occasion is sometimes called the martini effect.) Masters and Johnson report that men who have sex after overeating often report a decline in sensual feeling almost approaching anesthesia—and then they fall asleep. So if you're already fatigued, eat light (if at all) before sex.

Call on room service. Frequently, couples find that their sexual interest in one another miraculously resurfaces when they go on vacation. If that happens, it's clear that the only real problem you have is twenty-first century syndrome: overwork, stress and fatigue. Of course, you can't just take the red-eye flight to Honolulu every time your sex life starts to sag. So consider the idea of the 18-hour relationship revitalization plan—tiny little weekend vacations that aren't too long, too expensive or too far from home. Try checking into a local hotel, call room service for supper and see what happens next.

Consider other health problems. Sometimes chronic fatigue is not merely the result of overwork—it's possible there's some other health problem involved. For instance, fatigue is one hallmark of anemia, caused by iron-poor blood (iron is crucial because it helps red blood cells transport oxygen throughout the body; without it, you're chronically tired). Though anemia is most common in women, men may also develop iron deficiencies from gastrointestinal bleeding or other disorders, doctors say.

It could be a drug side effect. Many drugs, including antihistamines, pain relievers, diuretics and high blood pressure medications, may also cause fatigue. Or sometimes a combination of drugs may make you chronically tired (check the package insert to see if fatigue is listed as a side effect). You should never stop a prescription medication on your own, but you might consider asking your doctor to switch you to a different medication, which sometimes takes care of the problem.

There's also the remote possibility that you may be suffering from a mysterious malady known as chronic fatigue syndrome (CFS). Though debate over the exact nature and cause of CFS has been raging for 50 years, it's now generally defined as self-reported persistent fatigue or relapsing fatigue lasting six or more consecutive months, according to David S. Bell, M.D., a CFS researcher and instructor in pediatrics at Harvard Medical School.

Typical symptoms include profound fatigue worsened by exercise or exertion, headache, abdominal pain, muscle and joint pain and difficulty concentrating. A physical exam also often reveals low-grade fever, sore throat, tender lymph nodes and certain abnormalities of the immune system. Unfortunately, since there's still no agreement about what causes CFS, no definitive treatments exist.

But that's probably not what your problem is anyway. And we'd like to suggest a simple test to find out for sure: Just take your sweetie on vacation, get plenty of rest and if your love life revives, you're golden.

GUILT
When Religion and Sex Clash

Sexual guilt is when a voice inside your head insists you are doing—or even just thinking—something you shouldn't. In small doses guilt can be a good thing, keeping us gentlemanly and under control. But at its worst, guilt can scare you away from passion or sexual pleasure and inappropriately turn sex into an evil.

Guilt is not a natural thing; somewhere, somehow, you were programmed to think that certain aspects of sexuality are bad. It could come from your parents or what you perceive as societal rules or expectations. But most often, particularly for those with damaging levels of guilt, it's religion that does the negative programming.

"It's amazing to me how many people I see suffering from a lack of sexual desire who blame their dysfunction on their religious upbringings," says William R. Stayton, Th.D., a Baptist minister who is also a sex therapist in Philadelphia.

Although religious faith can infuse sexuality with rich meaning far beyond the flesh, it can also inspire sexual guilt that throws a wet sheet over your entire love life. In fact, William H. Masters, M.D., and Virginia E. Johnson, of the former Masters and Johnson Institute in St. Louis, reported that "religious orthodoxy is a major contributor to all the sexual dysfunctions."

One study of religious faith and sexual dysfunction, conducted in Australia, concluded that "Christian belief was positively correlated with sex guilt; and . . . members of conservative Christian churches consistently indicated higher levels of sexual dysfunction."

Whether the source of one's guilty feelings about sex come from church or somewhere else, they seem to be widespread. The University of Chicago researchers who conducted the 1994 *Sex in America* survey found that about half the men and women who masturbated said they felt at least a little guilty about it. And in our mail survey of *Men's*

Health readers, when we asked, "Do you ever feel guilty or ashamed about sex?" nearly one in four respondents said yes.

Which is not too surprising considering the weird, sex-obsessed, sex-negative nature of our culture and the complex impact of religion. But what really surprised us, in a kind of happy way, was that these numbers steadily declined with age—from 32 percent among guys under 25 to 12 percent among guys over 55. Apparently, sexual guilt is one of those hurts that time eventually heals.

It's Not All Bad

Of course, a little bit of sexual guilt is not all bad—in fact, a twinge or two can be downright fun. Many therapists have noticed that there's something about busting up a polite social taboo—like having wild oral sex, for instance—that can be a huge turn-on for lots of people. The physician/psychiatrist team who conducted the *Janus Report on Sexual Behavior*, a nationwide survey, noted that "interestingly, many individuals we interviewed felt that without at least a bit of guilt, sex loses some of its appeal; for some, the defiance of authority was a turn-on."

Sexual guilt also serves the useful purpose of keeping our wolfish desires in line. In a study of 143 male college students, researchers found that guys who had the lowest levels of sexual guilt also tended to be the most sexually aggressive and used the greatest level of physical force to get what they wanted from women. Guys who were smothering in guilt inside may not have been entirely happy, but at least they were more inclined to be gentlemen.

On a more sinister note, in another study 61 male sex offenders (mostly child molesters) answered questionnaires to determine their levels of sexual guilt. Then they were shown a series of erotic slides, including portrayals of fairly deviant acts, while strapped to a device that measured their erections. The study showed that the men's feelings of guilt about sex did not affect in the slightest their sexual arousal when shown the slides. But when compared to what these

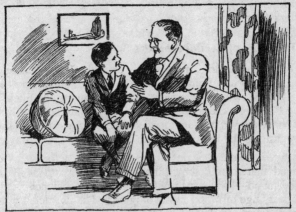

The NEW WAY

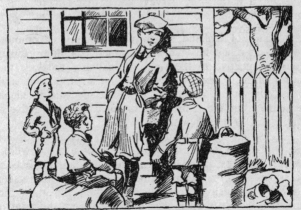

The OLD WAY

—From *Safe Counsel* by B. G. Jefferis, M.D., and J. L. Nichols, 39th edition, Intext Press

sweaty-palmed underachievers had actually done, the researchers found that "the number of paraphilic (deviant) acts attempted or completed . . . tended to increase as sex guilt decreased."

A Theology of Sexual Pleasure

There are, of course, many passages in the Bible that celebrate the glories of physical love ("Your two breasts are like two fawns, twins of a gazelle, that feed among the lilies."). But it's mainly the scowling, sex-negative parts of the Bible that have carried over into modern religious instruction, laying guilt on the multitudes with a heavy hand, Dr. Stayton says.

"Whenever you separate sexuality from spirituality—saying, in effect, that the body is bad and the soul is good—you're setting yourself up for problems. People who want to be good wind up having a very hard time integrating those two aspects of their lives. But this is one of the primary tasks of being human: to integrate the spiritual and the sexual," says Dr. Stayton.

This kind of dualistic, sex-negative teaching is commonplace in churches, he says. For instance, "an almost unanimous perspective in the field of sexuality today is that masturbation is healthy, desirable and an important adult sexual adjustment. Yet almost all Christian sexuality education curriculum either presents masturbation as negative or ignores it as if it did not exist."

It's easy enough to read the Bible in such a way that it does not seem to present any clear picture of whole, healthy sexuality. In the Garden of Eden Adam and Eve ate the apple—and for the first time realized they were naked (and, by extension, sexual). Only then did they feel ashamed. Christ himself was distanced from the taint of carnal desire by being born of a virgin. And St. Paul, when he wrote that "it is better to marry than to burn (with desire)," seemed to suggest only rather grudgingly that sex within marriage was allowable, though spiritually less blameless than celibacy.

But read a different way, the Bible "is basically a very sex-positive book," Dr. Stayton says. What's needed is a "theology of sexual pleasure" that affirms the God-given joy of human sexuality for its own sake and not just as a dutiful way of making babies. After all, he points out, "it could be said that the Creator intends sexual pleasure for the human creature. For example, females have an organ, the clitoris, that has no other function than sexual pleasure."

And if sex is only for making babies, why are we capable of having sexual pleasure long before we're fertile—in fact, even before we're born? Obstetrician/gynecologists, peering at the sonogram of an unborn male baby, sometimes observe that the little guy already has an erection.

Helping people to overcome crippling religious guilt in therapy is inclined to be a long, slow process, Dr. Stayton says. But the first step is to change their thinking about religion and sex. "If they believe that God created them and that God created them sexual, then their sexuality is a gift. And what good is the gift if we don't use it?" One of the main elements of sex therapy is simply giving people permission to express their sexuality, he explains. A second element is providing accurate information about sexuality—something guilt-stifled people are often short of if they've grown up in strict, religious homes where even talking about sex is taboo.

Sex As Spiritual Liberation

It's not hard to imagine a very different world where physical joy and spiritual faith are on friendlier terms—like the Tantric and Taoist traditions of Asia. These ancient traditions, so different from our own, "celebrate the naturalness of sexual pleasure and the spiritual potential of sexual relations," according to Robert T. Francoeur, Ph.D., professor of embryology and sexuality at Fairleigh Dickinson University in Rutherford, New Jersey. "Tantric and Taoist sexual union is viewed as a way to spiritual liberation, a consciousness of and identification with the Divine."

Anyone who has made passionate love to someone they

love knows what that ancient writer was talking about. And it isn't that far away from something blessedly spiritual.

It's almost, though not quite, like being in church.

ILLNESS AND SEX
Don't Let Disease Stop You

Sex and health are inseparable, as you can see in great detail should you choose to cruise through part three of this book. The opposite is also true—sex and sickness don't mix well. When you're sick, your immune system's responses dampen your sex drive and reduce your levels of circulating sex hormones. Any surgery throws the body into a tizzy and can produce feelings of vulnerability or even self-disgust that outlast the physical recovery period. Chronic diseases result in pain and fatigue and take their psychological toll both on the patient and the partner. When chronic illness strikes, especially in midlife and beyond, it is tempting to "throw in the towel" on sexuality and tell yourself you've had your fun.

It would be silly for anyone to proclaim that sickness doesn't matter or to promise no end of former pleasures. What your sex life does *not* need is one more unrealistic standard to meet. But by the same token, there's no cause to be despondent when you have sexual feelings while ill. In fact, if you and your partner are willing to make changes to keep physical affection in your lives, that shows a positive outlook. And it's probably good medicine, too. "Love heals in so many ways," says Reed C. Moskowitz, M.D., director of Stress Disorders Medical Services at New York University Medical Center in New York City, in his book *Your Healing Mind*.

Some diseases clearly do more sexual damage than others. We've provided specific advice about five of the leading disablers. Keep in mind, though, that you should ask your doctor for advice on this matter. Unfortunately, doctors sometimes live down to their reputation as body mechanics and ignore this subject. If they cannot answer your questions, at least they should be able to point you to support groups that can.

If you're about to have surgery, the *Kinsey Institute New Report on Sex* contains some strongly worded advice: "Insist on being told exactly what to expect in terms of future sexual functioning. You have a right to this information, especially since there appears to be a direct relationship between not getting the information and later problems with sexual response."

Consider it part of a broader right: While we're alive, we all have a right to the happiness of pursuit. In spite of our diseases and disabilities, we are sexual beings, always.

Alcoholism

Alcohol is man's ancient friend and enemy. In moderation it gets us in the mood and loosens the buttons of inhibition. After two or three drinks, however, it starts to dampen arousal and interfere with erectile function. And as for the long-term effects of heavy drinking, they are flat-out disastrous. One researcher has estimated that 70 to 80 percent of male alcoholics have decreased sexual desire or potency or both.

Persistent alcohol abuse decreases testosterone while at the same time increases estrogen levels. The resulting symptoms include loss of body hair and muscle mass, damaged fertility, swelling of the breasts and, ultimately, alcoholic hypogonadism—shrinkage of the testicles. Yes, alcohol abuse is a masculine rite. And yet in the end, it can literally de-sex us.

So unlike the diseases that follow, the answer here isn't to find ways to have sex while remaining an alcoholic. For you and all around you, get off the drink. Consider the return of sexuality one of the many rewards.

Arthritis

About half of the 36 million Americans who suffer from arthritis say it interferes with their sex lives. There's the pain, of course. But there's also insecurity, often manifested by interpreting a partner's honest concern as thinly veiled distaste for a body she once considered attractive.

The disease doesn't impair sexual response directly, but the pain, the fatigue and the general feeling that you're just not very sexy anymore take a toll on the libido. So it's important to make lovemaking as easy as possible, each and every time. The standard advice: Limber up your limbs, warm up with a bath and/or massage and experiment with time of day, or timing the pain medication, to create a better time for sex. Experiment, as well, with new positions: The "spoon position" (woman on side, knees drawn up, man behind her, fitting his body to hers), for example, may be most comfortable for women with hip pain. For men with hip pain, try on your side, facing each other. The Arthritis Foundation puts out a booklet, *Living and Loving*, with these and other tips; call 1-800-283-7800.

If you follow all the advice, you just might find an additional benefit. Arousal and climax can boost the levels of endorphins, the body's natural painkillers, and corticosteroids, which can reduce pain and inflammation in the joints. Some arthritis sufferers report being pain-free for more than six hours after having sex.

Cancer

With cancer, as with any chronic debility, it's time to let go of old beliefs, like the one that says sex should happen spontaneously. You have to schedule it for times when you're not fatigued or uncomfortable.

The particular devastations of this disease depend on the sites of metastasis, but cancers of the sex organs, of course, have the most direct impact on our sexual function and our sexual identity. Wives need special attention from their husbands after mastectomies; men need the same kind of loving support from their wives while recovering from prostate or testicular cancer.

Cancer patients should discuss sexual capacities with their doctors. Each case calls for different parameters.

Diabetes

Half of men over the age of 50 who have diabetes are impotent. That's a commonly recited fact, but it's only partly explained by the medical fact that the disease will, in time, damage the tiny nerves in the body's far-flung regions. The other culprit in diabetic impotence is the depression and psychological stress of coping with a chronic disease.

Whether it's congenital or adult-onset, diabetes can impair male sexual performance. Heavy alcohol use and poor blood sugar control make the problem worse. There's some evidence that the patient's acceptance of his condition makes things better. If you're in the process of coping with adult-onset diabetes or know someone who is, you may not want to leave its sexual aspects to your primary physician. See a urologist who specializes in male sexual dysfunctions.

Heart Disease

After the heart attack comes fear of sex. Most heart attack survivors say a sense of their own fragility now holds them back, spoiling what was just about the only moment of abandon left in life. And the fearful image of having cardiac arrest again, right then and there during sex, makes some couples put off their love lives indefinitely. Wives fear this as much as husbands.

The happy truth is that having another heart attack during sex is highly unlikely. Assuming you're resuming relations with a spouse of many years, your heart rate won't climb past 120 beats per minute, tops. We all know of someone who died in the saddle—Nelson Rockefeller will be remembered for it long after his tenure as vice-president is completely forgotten. But let us tell you about a little study the Japanese did. Of 5,550 men who died suddenly, it turns out that only 34 of them died during sex (18 of heart attacks). The key fact here is that 30 of those 34 were *not* having sex with their wives! They were having sex with someone much, much younger, and they all had been drinking. The Lord works in nonmysterious ways.

Anyway, about 80 percent of cardiac patients can safely resume reasonable, relaxed sexual activity. You should resume sex only after discussing it with your doctor, and you may have to bring it up. Some cardiologists are just as blushing about sex as anyone else.

There's a high incidence of both premature ejaculation and erectile failure in the year after a heart attack, even among those men who aren't on any medications. The cause is psychological rather than organic—the guy is nervous about his heart rate and is trying to detect chest pain, rather than responding to the pleasures of the moment. He's suffering from a type of performance anxiety.

Finally, don't shirk your physical conditioning. Like exercise for anyone else, it can improve your sexual activity.

LOW SEX DRIVE
When Stress Steals Your Thunder

Guys are supposed to be ripe and ready, anywhere and anytime, at even the most distant sighting of a panty line.

And that's part of the problem.

Because what if you really aren't aroused very much or very often?

There's no popular role model of the male who just isn't that interested in sex—even Woody Allen, that famous wimp, seems absolutely obsessed with it. A man who feels about as sexy as a mailbox most of the time begins to feel lonely, alienated from the great Brotherhood of Guys, and worried that there must be something seriously wrong with him.

The irony is that these guys have so much company. Millions of American men and women have such low levels of sexual desire that it's become a great concern to them. In fact, studies show that low sexual desire is the main complaint of up to 55 percent of couples who show up at sex therapy clinics, making it the most common sexual complaint of all. And over the past 20 years, especially

A FEW KEY QUESTIONS TO ASK YOURSELF

To help identify the source of your low sex drive, therapists suggest you ask yourself a few penetrating questions (and answer them honestly).

- Is this problem truly a sexual disorder, or is the sex problem really a consequence of other issues in my relationship?
- Is it mainly a problem of differences in desire between my partner and me?
- Are either of us taking some medication that might be to blame?
- Is the decreased desire actually secondary to some other sexual disorder (for instance, erection problems or pain during intercourse)?
- Is it she who doesn't turn me on, or do I have trouble getting aroused by anyone? (If it's only her, you're likely to have relationship problems.)
- If I increased my interest in sex, what bad things might happen?

There may be some hidden advantages in displaying little interest in sex, explain Jennifer Knopf, Ph.D., and Michael Seiler, Ph.D., in their book *Inhibited Sexual Desire*. For instance, maybe you're afraid of letting your partner get closer to you. Maybe you're afraid of being able to perform sexually. And if you are often pushed around by a domineering partner and you give in to all her requests for sex, "What will you have left to help you even the score or reassure yourself that you have some power in the relationship?"

the last decade, the incidence has dramatically increased, researchers say.

One other interesting development is that, though historically it's been mostly women who complained of this problem, in recent years many more men have been showing up at sex therapy clinics complaining of a limp-noodle libido. Why? Sexologists are full of theories, but nobody really knows. Some studies from the 1970s and 1980s suggested that women's newfound aggressiveness was a huge turn-off to many men; when they found themselves in bed with a jackbooted feminist, they just wilted. Others have suggested that our whole sex-saturated culture, filled with pubescent girls oozing out of their Calvins, seems to suggest that everybody should be having sex, sex, sex—as wild as possible, as often as possible. There's so much implied societal pressure to be a sexual superstar that when people (especially men) just don't feel like it, they tend to define it as a problem.

It's easy to forget that until fairly recently in history, low sexual desire (especially in women) was considered a virtue. As recently as the early 1900s, John Harvey Kellogg peddled cornflakes as an (unsuccessful) treatment for dampening carnal desire, not inflaming it.

How to Define It

Low sexual desire (we'll resist the urge to start calling it LSD) is also sometimes called decreased libido or hypoactive sexual desire disorder. Whatever you call it, its official clinical definition is this: having sexual urges, fantasies or activity less than twice a month.

The most relevant definition, though, is the definition offered by the person who complains about it, says Beth Alexander, M.D., associate professor in the Department of Family Practice at Michigan State University College of Human Medicine in East Lansing. In general, she says, that means "a level of sexual desire that either causes difficulty in a relationship or causes individual concern on the part of the patient."

It's important to remember that nobody defines a "normal" sex life the same way, and that differences in desire are another common source of sexual conflict in relationships. (Remember the scene in the movie *Annie Hall* in which

Woody Allen tells his shrink: "We hardly ever have sex—maybe three times a week." And then Diane Keaton tells her shrink: "We have sex constantly—three times a week.") That's why very often it's not the person with low desire who's in real distress—it's that person's partner.

Also, adds Dr. Alexander, "because of the wide variability in what constitutes 'normal' sexual drive, it is usually a change in libido that prompts concern."

A Tough Nut to Crack

"Although hypoactive sexual desire may be the most common complaint among couples who seek treatment for sexual problems, it may also be the most difficult sexual dysfunction to treat," according to David Farley Hurlbert, clinical director of Marriage and Sex Therapy at Darnall Army Community Hospital in Belton, Texas.

That's partly because there are so many different things that can cause it—and often more than one thing is involved. There may be relationship problems, like unresolved conflict or fear of intimacy. There may be psychological problems, like depression, stress, anxiety or guilt. It's possible the problem is secondary to some other problem, like the inability to get or maintain an erection. There may be physical problems, like hormonal abnormalities, medication side effects or illness. Or all of the above.

And, of course, at the heart of it all is the ephemeral nature of desire itself. In her groundbreaking work *Disorders of Sexual Desire and Other New Concepts and Techniques in Sex Therapy*, the late Helen Singer Kaplan, M.D., Ph.D., found that unlike sexual arousal—the ability to get an erection—sexual desire exists primarily in the mind. It's not so much a lack of ability to perform as a lack of motivation to do so.

And frequently, if you're not motivated to make love to her, that means there's some other problem in your relationship. In fact, observes Dr. Alexander, "Most patients who complain of decreased sexual desire have a relationship problem, not a true sexual problem."

One study conducted by Dr. Kaplan and her colleagues found that the most common cause of depressed libido was unresolved anger or conflict in the relationship. This only stands to reason. After all, if your relationship is livid with anger and conflict, avoiding sex is a completely normal response—your "problem" is not a problem at all, but a healthy reaction to an unhealthy situation.

Is It Physical?

In some ways it would be a whole lot simpler if the problem turned out to be purely physical—a thyroid disorder, say. And therapists say that many people really would prefer taking a pill or having an operation rather than having to deal with the complex, tentacle-like entanglements of an unhappy relationship.

But the truth is that if you're under age 50 and otherwise healthy, it's really unlikely that your flagging sex drive can be blamed on a physical problem, Dr. Alexander says. Nevertheless, if you do seek professional help, your doctor may ask that you get a complete physical and a few lab tests to rule out that possibility.

Here are some physical problems that might lower sex drive.

Low Testosterone

It's known that testosterone is a sort of natural aphrodisiac for both men and women. It triggers sexual desire in the brain with the help of chemicals, like dopamine, that act as messengers between nerve cells and the brain. Women who've passed menopause, and men diagnosed as having low testosterone, are sometimes treated with low-dose testosterone to put a little zing back in their sex lives.

Evidence suggests that in men between their late forties and early seventies, testosterone levels may sometimes drop by up to 40 percent, often from medication. In a few of these men (10 to 15 percent), levels may dip sufficiently to dampen their sexual desire. "I see a lot of older men who have decreased testosterone levels, often as a result of med-

ications they're taking," says Andre T. Guay, M.D., director
of endocrinology at the Lahey Clinic in Burlington, Massachusetts. If you have reason to believe your medication may
be involved, ask your doctor if you can have a blood test to
see if you're a candidate for testosterone replacement therapy.

In the old days guys with a demonstrable testosterone
deficiency had to get a shot twice a week, which can produce mood swings after the shot and lulls in energy and
libido after it begins to wear off. Now there's a testosterone
patch, like the nicotine patches would-be ex-smokers wear,
that delivers a small but steady supply of testosterone to the
bloodstream. In clinical trials, five weeks of treatment with
the Testoderm Testosterone Transdermal System produced
significant improvements in mood and sexual function in 63
percent of patients. The men reported having at least three
times more erections and orgasms than they had before
wearing the patches.

Medication Side Effects

Many high blood pressure drugs are known to have adverse
effects on erectile function, but some researchers also
believe that lowered sex drive is a much more common side
effect than is generally acknowledged. "Even antihypertensive drugs that aren't supposed to cause problems, like the
calcium channel blockers, often do," says James Goldberg,
Ph.D., a research pharmacologist in California. He says the
blood pressure medicine Captain may be the least likely to
affect sex drive.

Secondary Causes

It's also possible that your low sexual desire is actually secondary to some other sex problem. In men, studies have
shown, by far the most common problem is trouble getting
or maintaining an erection; in women it's inability to have
an orgasm.

In one study of 47 men with low sexual desire at the Sex
and Marital Therapy Program of the University of Chicago
Medical Center, researchers sketched a portrait of the "typi-

cal man" who has the problem. Usually, they say, he's in his late forties to early fifties and he almost always has some other sexual problem (generally an erectile problem). Therapists trying to help these guys should first figure out if there is a physiological problem like this and focus on treating that first, they say.

Try Sweat Equity

If you're reluctant to darken the door of a sex therapist's office, or if things aren't really that bad, there's at least one thing you can do to help yourself: Start working out regularly, if you don't already. A fairly impressive body of research suggests that exercise can enhance a flagging sex drive.

In one study, men who got an hour of aerobic exercise three times a week had sex more, masturbated more and had more frequent orgasms than their couch potato counterparts. Researchers speculate that exercise affects sex drive by boosting circulating levels of testosterone; in another study testosterone rose significantly after men ran on a treadmill for 30 minutes.

Just remember to take a shower before you ask her to dance.

MALE MENOPAUSE
What's Real and What Isn't

"As I write this, I am 62 years of age," one of the respondents to our *Men's Health* magazine survey noted, "and my desire has diminished just in the past couple years."

He may feel all alone, but he's not. As many men enter old age, their sexuality starts to go AWOL. Call it a mental impotence—their machinery may be in good working condition, but their sex drive sputters. The libido goes limp. That most basic of male needs, the one that has shaped their waking and sleeping habits since puberty, has departed, and has taken a big chunk of their gender identities with it. This is not accepted calmly by some men. "You might as well be dead," says another survey respondent of the loss of sexual appetite.

A dearth of desire could be caused by several factors: individual psychology and attitude, loss of interest in your partner, stress, the side effects of medication or the onset of depression. But a number of cases can be blamed on a hormonal problem: The testicles are not making enough testosterone.

Testosterone performs many bodily wonders. So even if you think you can live without your sex drive, this is not something you want to ignore.

When most men reach 50 years of age, testosterone levels begin to slump. By the time we're in our seventies, our total testosterone levels are 10 to 20 percent below what they were when we were age 30, and our levels of so-called free testosterone—what's actually available for metabolic use— are perhaps one-third to one-half what they were in our prime. Along the way, our muscles and bones get weaker; we lose both muscle mass and bone density, which provides us with skeletal strength. And our sex drive ebbs.

Does that mean most elderly men are suffering from a testosterone deficiency? Probably not. The drop-off leaves most men within the limits of what science still assumes to be normal. But some men drop far below normal. How many men? Nobody knows. But Adrian Dobs, M.D., professor of medicine at Johns Hopkins University in Baltimore and a leading testosterone researcher, will tell you one thing for sure: "I think it's underdiagnosed."

Let's Call It Something Else

The term male menopause is catchy because we instantly understand its point: Men can go through hormonal changes, just as women do. But it's also misleading, and not just because men don't have a monthly period that pauses. In women the ovaries close up shop. Estrogen production drops almost to zero. They become infertile. They have a much greater problem with bone loss and the suddenness of the hormonal change brings on hot flashes.

In men, by contrast, the production of testosterone falls gradually, the levels don't drop nearly as far and sperm production continues. Maybe we should imitate the Europeans and call it andropause. Because it's nothing like menopause.

But we're stuck with that name, at least for the present, chiefly because of the flurry of publicity that followed an article by Gail Sheehy in the April 1993 issue of *Vanity Fair*. In "Is There a Male Menopause?" the author of the bestseller *Passages* answered her own question, not surprisingly, in the affirmative, calling this phenomenon "the unspeakable passage, fraught with secrecy, shame and denial." (Gosh, Gail, thanks for your support!)

Trouble was, the anonymous anecdotes that provided the emotional hooks for her story all revolved around tales of impotence. This is nonsense. First of all, the majority of elderly men do not become impotent, and second, not all cases of impotence can be blamed on a testosterone deficiency.

Yes, testosterone is believed to play a small role in potency (it's involved in the creation of an enzyme that helps blood flow into your penis). And most causes of impotence may be age related. But they relate to an increase in fatty deposits that impede penile blood flow or to an increase in prescription drug use. Further, Sheehy's anecdotes portrayed men in their fifties and sixties who were still trying to behave as if they were 25. With 25-year-old women, no less. These men weren't suffering from testosterone deficiency. They were suffering from performance anxiety.

"Gail Sheehy goes too far in assuming that a gradual ebbing is the same thing as the loss," says Richard Spark, M.D., a professor at Harvard Medical School who was quoted in her article. "True, men aren't as sexually vigorous in later life. But people learn to economize. You marshal your resources for what you need." The other important point to remember is that the phenomenon is not the same in all men, as it is in all women. "Aging is not an equal-opportunity affliction," says Dr. Spark.

Other researchers dismiss the whole notion. "It's absolute baloney," says John B. McKinlay, Ph.D., director of the New England Research Institute in Watertown, Massachusetts, which has conducted the largest study to date on sexual function in men ages 40 to 70, the Massachusetts Male Aging Study. "We've studied 1,700 men, and there's no endocrine change in the middle years that's noteworthy.

"But even though there's no epidemiological, physiological or clinical evidence for such a syndrome, I think by the turn of the century we will have TRT—testosterone replacement therapy. There is a medicalization of male aging going on here, and it's because there is strong interest in treating aging men for profit, just as there is for menopausal women. I'm not antitestosterone, I'm just saying we haven't studied it enough," Dr. McKinlay concludes.

He's right. No large clinical studies have been done. But at the University of Pennsylvania in Philadelphia, endocrinologist Peter Snyder, M.D., is conducting a study of 100 men over age 65, all of whom have testosterone levels in the normal range. For three years they'll have been sporting a small patch on their scrotums; half the patches will be dispensing testosterone, the other half will be dispensing a placebo. His study is designed to find out not only whether some of the debilities of age can be eased by TRT but whether TRT might present a new set of problems—namely, an increased risk of sleep apnea, strokes, enlarged prostate glands and prostate cancer. Because of the potential risks, he says, "even this initial study won't be enough. I think it will be quite a while before we have the answers."

Back to What We Know

All of that controversy should not obscure the fact that a man who suffers from testosterone deficiency can be helped. If Dr. Dobs is right—that, as a medical phenomenon, it's underdiagnosed—that's not because a testosterone deficiency is so difficult to determine. Just the opposite. It's easily diagnosed, and easily remedied.

If you suspect you have a problem and your family physician concurs, you'll be sent to an endocrinologist, who will measure the testosterone levels in your blood. You'll be tested several times because it can vary greatly, depending on the time of day, season of the year, recent illnesses, stress, amount of exercise, alcohol consumption and mental state. But if it's consistently below the generally accepted threshold of 300 nanograms per deciliter, you're a candidate for treatment. That, by the way, would be the threshold for treating a man of any age.

In fact, treatment results reveal the critical role that testosterone plays in a man's well-being. In one study conducted in the early 1990s, 13 elderly men with low testosterone levels were given 100 milligrams a week of synthetic testosterone for three months. They gained muscle mass and decreased the levels of "bad" cholesterol in their blood without changing "good" cholesterol levels. But the best part is, because they felt so good and so sexy, they knew whether they were receiving the drug or not—despite the double-blind nature of the study that is supposed to rule out any placebo effect.

The biggest glitch in the treatment process is you—you may have a hard time getting up the courage to see a physician. "Men don't easily come to doctors with this problem," says Dr. Spark. But the test results could make it all worthwhile.

MEDICATIONS
When Side Effects Are the Main Issue

Medications are one of the leading causes of male sexual dysfunction—if not the leading cause. In the Massachusetts Male Aging Study, a random sampling of 1,700 men ages 40 to 70 in the greater Boston area, those men being treated for heart disease also suffered from complete impotence at a rate nearly four times greater than the entire group. Even drugs used to treat relatively nonthreatening ailments, like stomach ulcers or allergies, can bring nasty surprises.

We don't mean to belabor the obvious, but this has a disastrous effect on a patient's quality of life. Sometimes the doctor involved doesn't think so—after all, he's done his job, which is to prescribe the right medication for a particular problem and see some results. But if *you* think so, how regularly will you take your medicine, and for how long? Fortunately, unwanted side effects of prescription drugs are often reversible. In many cases you and your doctor can switch medications or tailor the dosage to alleviate the problem.

Erectile failure is far from being the only sexual side effect. If your doctor is starting you on a brand new medication and is talking just a bit too politely about sexual dysfunction as a possible side effect, he also could be referring to:

- Decreased libido
- Delayed ejaculation
- Retrograde ejaculation (semen ends up in the bladder because the neck of the bladder does not contract)
- Priapism (a prolonged, painful erection)
- Anorgasmia (inability to achieve orgasm)

A medication tends to cause just one of these effects; rarely do several sexual side effects appear together.

Which drugs are worst for you? Blood pressure pills are most notable, but after that it's impossible to draft a definitive list. "Virtually any drug can have sexual side effects in a small percentage of cases," says Jay Hollander, M.D., associate director of the Center for Male Sexual Function at Beaumont Hospital in Royal Oak, Michigan. "The list is vast."

Consider, too, all the new drugs coming on the market. Their side effects may not be fully known until they've been in general use for a few years. A classic example of this, Dr. Hollander says, is Prozac. When it first came out, *Physician's Desk Reference* noted delayed ejaculation as a side effect in less than 2 percent of cases. But subsequent studies report that effect on up to half of male patients. (Not all those patients are grumbling. One of our *Men's Health* magazine survey respondents wrote, "Since I began taking Prozac over two years ago, I am able to maintain an erection for a much longer time. It may not be as hard, but it is certainly more durable.")

The Blood Pressure Question

Drugs used to treat high blood pressure are called antihypertensives. We'll discuss them in particular because they provide a good illustration of how prescription drugs affect sex.

Millions of men have taken these drugs, and they have a long, sad history of causing impotence and/or other sexual dysfunctions. Yet the topic has been poorly studied. It seems men with high blood pressure who don't take any medication have more sexual dysfunction than men with normal blood pressure, proving that the disease itself is a spoiler.

But drugs definitely compound the problems. In one prominent study 75 men on antihypertensive drugs were asked about quality-of-life issues. Every one of the doctors involved thought their patients' quality of life had improved. But only 48 percent of the patients thought so. And 99 percent of their wives (or companions) thought they were worse off. If it were up to them, the pills would be dumped down the toilet.

The conventional advice is to avoid the notorious betablockers; switch to a calcium antagonist, like nifedipine (Procardia XL) instead. But Dr. Hollander believes that any high blood pressure medication has the potential to weaken erections, simply because the mechanics of erection depend on raising the blood pressure within the penis. "The effect of lowering blood pressure itself can have as much impact as the side effect," he says.

All of which becomes an eloquent argument for correcting high blood pressure via lifestyle changes rather than drugs, if possible. One study of 79 men with high blood pressure showed that those who made the right lifestyle changes—cutting down on fat, salt and alcohol, getting more exercise and using relaxation techniques to tackle stress—not only lowered their blood pressures but also improved their sex lives. And it wasn't just the effect of going off the drug propranolol that mattered. Those who were given a placebo without making lifestyle changes reported lower sexual satisfaction than those who got back in shape. The lesson: Anytime the pharmacy can be avoided, it should be avoided.

Rx for Men on Pills

Large scientific studies of hundreds of men often obscure as much as they reveal. It can be difficult to tease apart a medication's side effects from the tangle of other changes, emotional and physical, that are happening around the same time. Sometimes it takes a while for the drug to announce itself. "Coming off the drug won't instantly change things, necessarily—and it won't instantly cause change in the first place," says Dr. Hollander. But his bottom line is, "If you notice a difference in your erections, you should discuss this with your doctor."

And, we would add, if your doctor can't or won't answer your questions, find one who will. Don't solve this on your own.

PENIS ENLARGEMENT
Bigger Means Costlier, Not Better

Perhaps you've seen the ads. PENILE ENLARGEMENT says the big, block letters. PENILE LENGTHENING. Then it mentions the name of a doctor, the fact that he's performed over 3,000 surgeries and 100 percent financing is available (translation: No way is your health plan picking up this one, pal). It ends with a local phone number for a "free 30-minute consultation."

The surgeons who run ads like this one made a presentation to their fellow doctors at the 1994 national convention

of the American Urological Association. *Men's Health*
senior writer Greg Gutfeld was on hand to see the slide
shows. Although the doctors talked about what a marvelous
feeling it was being able to bring joy to the lives of so many
men, the images on the screen overpowered their words. It
wasn't a pretty sight: The "enhanced" penises didn't look
enhanced at all. They looked like soggy loaves of sour-
dough bread. Or worse. "For one moment," recalls Gutfeld,
"I mistook a slide for the weathered face of Jack Palance."
The urologists in the room weren't amused. They didn't see
the humor in it at all.

Exactly what made these male members look so miserable? The procedure used to "lengthen" the penis simply
involves cutting the main suspensory ligaments that anchor
the penis to your pubic bone. This allows a portion of the
penis that is normally inside the body (we're talking about
an inch here) to hang outside. Problems: Your erections will
point straight out rather than up, and you'll have pubic hair
on the base of your newly exposed penis. This is usually performed in tandem with another procedure, "enlargement,"
that adds fat to the penis. It's a reverse liposuction of sorts.
Problems: After a few months your body reabsorbs the fat.
What isn't reabsorbed may become lumpy and bumpy.

So you're left with an all-terrain penis that you need to
shave.

Most urologists are dead-set against doing this surgery.
The Society for the Study of Impotence issued a statement
warning that the procedures haven't been proven to be either
safe or effective and "should be regarded as experimental
surgery." A member of the society, San Francisco urologist
Thomas Lue, M.D., was quoted in a medical trade publication saying, "I can save these patients a lot of money. I'll put
their penis on a desk and whack it with a hammer. It will
swell up for about six months and then go down. They'll get
the same results as the fat injections."

The thousands of men who've sought out this surgery are,
for the most part, anatomically correct. "They truly have a
problem," says Kenneth Goldberg, M.D., founder and director of the Male Health Center in Dallas, "and it's in their

GET LEAN AND MEAN, GET A BIGGER WEEN'

Want to gain an inch in length without spending thousands of dollars to let someone attack your penis with a scalpel? John Mulcahy, M.D., professor of urology at Indiana University Medical Center in Indianapolis, has a better idea: lose 35 pounds.

"You don't see a lot of naked men, but doctors do," he says. "And I'll tell you this: We never see a fat man with a big penis, and we never see an emaciated man with a small penis." Yet, in fact, they may be fishing with the same size poles. What happens is, as a man gains weight, his *prepubic panniculus*, a pad or fold of fat surrounding the base of the penis, gains in girth, too. "And that encroaches on the shaft of the penis," says Dr. Mulcahy. "When we get a 300-pounder, all we see is the head."

Dr. Mulcahy says that for every 35 pounds you gain, you effectively lose an inch of batting swing. Losing that 35 pounds might not reveal that full inch exactly. "The change is not as dramatic as when you're gaining weight," he says. But it's an excellent reason to stay away from candy bars.

minds. I mean, to go through what they go through and then to boast about gaining an inch in length. . . . "

At a cost of $4,000 to $7,000, that's quite an inch. It's just too bad nobody performs *confidence* enlargement surgery.

A Measure of Respectability

But that's precisely what the men who undergo this work claim they've gotten. Into the breach comes E. Douglas Whitehead, M.D., associate clinical professor of urology at Mount Sinai School of Medicine of the City University of New York and co-director of the Association for Male Sexual Dysfunction, both in New York City. In the past, Dr. Whitehead has been a critic of penile augmentation. "More than 90 percent of the people who have this surgery are totally normal," he says. "It's a psychological problem." But patients do benefit psychologically from the procedure, he says—so why not try to perform it in a responsible manner? To that end, he is now conducting what he calls an investigational study. He'll operate on more than 100 men, working as a team with a plastic surgeon and a psychiatrist at Beth Israel Medical Center in New York City. The old, unreliable fat transfer procedure has been dumped in favor of something called a dermal graft technique, in which strips of fat are slipped under the skin on the penile shaft. "We expect it to last," Dr. Whitehead says. Each patient is being evaluated both before and after surgery, and results will be announced in 1997.

Maybe we'll wait.

PERFORMANCE ANXIETY
What to Do When Fear Attacks

"In the back of my mind I feel I have to perform," writes a 34-year-old waste water treatment plant operator. "I know I really don't have to. Simple moves are very satisfying to her."

We'd like to thank this man for his clear, simple definition of performance anxiety. He's nervous about performing. That's what it is. That little worry, in the back of your mind, that you won't.

We all get that from time to time. But for some men, that worry moves to the front of the mind, takes over and leads directly to failure. In these cases performance anxiety isn't just a small voice, it's a significant mental problem that can shut down a sex life.

Serious performance anxiety usually manifests itself physiologically in one of three ways: erectile failure, premature ejaculation or, very rarely, delayed ejaculation. Most often it's erectile failure—the inability to "get it up" or, just as commonly, the inability to keep it up.

The sex researchers William H. Masters, M.D., and Virginia E. Johnson, of the former Masters and Johnson Institute in St. Louis, considered it to be the key to most dysfunctions. "Fear of inadequacy" as they called it, "is the greatest known deterrent to effective sexual functioning," they wrote in their 1970 classic *Human Sexual Inadequacy*. Of course, the two missed the boat in some areas, claiming that most sexual dysfunction was mental. Now we know that it's a lot more complicated. Much erectile failure is rooted in physical causes, like cholesterol-clogged arteries or reactions to prescription drugs, and premature ejaculation may be a matter of youth and hypersensitivity.

But the mental anguish we call performance anxiety will always be with us—and Masters and Johnson deserve credit for pinpointing and treating the problem. They coined a phrase to describe exactly what a man does when performance anxiety takes over. They called it the spectator role, a term that sex therapists have since turned into a verb, spectatoring. In essence, you become a spectator to your own sexual event, evaluating and observing yourself rather than losing yourself in the experience. Thus, fear of a problem becomes the problem itself. How? Fearful thoughts about your sexual performance literally crowd out the sensual pleasures of the moment, and without any sense of sexual pleasure getting through, you wilt. Of course. Which makes you even more fearful the next time and, well, you can see how it could beget a vicious cycle.

Getting Back in Touch

Beginning in 1959, Masters and Johnson treated hundreds of people at their clinic at Washington University in St. Louis. Couples arrived from all over the United States for two-week sessions. Therapy always involved both partners, even though it might seem to be a "man's problem," because it really was the marriage's problem; Masters and Johnson liked to say that the marital unit was their patient. Take a couple being treated for impotence, for example. The therapists would start by explaining to the guy that they couldn't teach him how to have an erection. It's a natural bodily process, like breathing or digestion. But he can learn how to *let* himself have an erection.

And so this two-week session pursued a form of therapy called sensate focus. The couples were ordered to go off by themselves, get naked, take on the role of "giving" or "getting" partner and basically start all over. They would touch, explore, give and get pleasure—but under no circumstances were they allowed to touch the pelvic area. It was forbidden—until they gradually recaptured their capacity for sexual pleasure and lost the habitual panic over whether or not he could "do it." "Sensate focus, when explored without overt performance pressures, becomes something that marital partners can shape and structure as they mutually desire," according to the book. "Sensate focus then becomes theirs, not something that has been systematized for them."

Letting the Problem Grow

Alas, Masters and Johnson are divorced now, and their famed Masters and Johnson Institute in St. Louis closed at the end of 1994 after 40 years of operation. But their ideas still aid therapists today, as an article in an issue of the *Journal of Sex and Marital Therapy* illustrates.

Barry A. Bass, Ph.D., a clinical psychologist in private practice in Baltimore, tells in the article of a man who'd been happily married for 25 years. One night he received a particularly upsetting long-distance phone call from his son—he found out that the son had been seriously ill while out of the country. Later that same night, he and his wife made love. And he couldn't keep an erection. But instead of ignoring this isolated event, putting it in the context of an emotional day and the possibility of his child's death, he began worrying about it. And worrying some more. "Not surprisingly, during subsequent sexual encounters Mr. H. began 'spectatoring' during sex and found it increasingly more difficult to achieve or maintain an erection," writes Dr. Bass.

"By the time I saw him, almost one year from the date he first experienced what might very well have been only a transitory dysfunction . . . Mr. H. had seen his family physician before being seen by two urologists, the second at a 'regional impotence center.' The total cost of these medical evaluations was over $2,500."

Mr. H. finally balked when the urologist recommended penile injections.

Dr. Bass uses the anecdote to warn that the pendulum may have swung too far. If, in the 1970s, doctors thought all sexual dysfunction was mental, today too many doctors think the origins are purely physical. In many cases both mental and physical causes are responsible.

A point well taken. But Dr. Bass's anecdote leaves us with the uncomfortable feeling that sexual shutdown as a result of performance anxiety could happen to any guy, any time, anywhere. That just doesn't ring true either.

For one thing, just about every man experiences small bouts of performance anxiety throughout his life, without it becoming a big problem. A 25-year-old *Men's Health* magazine survey respondent complained about "the competitive nature of men—we feel we absolutely have to give a woman an orgasm to be considered a real man. When in bed we automatically feel we are competing with every other man the woman has gone to bed with." And virtually every man over age 40 has experienced at least one no-go episode. Once that happens, says Barry McCarthy, Ph.D., professor of psychology at American University in Washington, D.C., "the male will not return to unselfconscious erections."

Maybe deeper forces are at work in Dr. Bass's anecdote. Stephen B. Levine, M.D., director of the Center for Human Sexuality at the University Hospitals of Cleveland, in his book *Sexual Life: A Clinician's Guide*, makes the point that performance anxiety can serve as a distraction from a life crisis. "For some people, making love seems to create a confrontation with one's own psychic truths," he writes. "Performance anxiety, which usually begins after one or two erectile failures, helps the man to avoid thinking about these truths." In particular, it seems to arise during five major changes in life: relationship deterioration, divorce, death of a spouse, vocational failure and loss of your or your spouse's health.

The fact that the same crises affect men's sex lives differently suggests that performance anxiety levels are highly personal. Some men appear more prone to it than others. These guys might suffer from high anxiety, for example, or from broader social anxieties. Or, they might be mentally rigid, unable to cast off myths that he should be able to get an erection at all times, or that real men don't pay attention to feelings.

By the way, women are susceptible to performance anxiety, too. They worry about being able to achieve orgasms—because they know how much it pleases men. And the resulting anxiety explains a portion of all those faked orgasms out there.

Are You Overgeneralizing?

Sensate focus is not the only treatment for performance anxiety. Some men are badly misinformed about their own bodies and are helped by education about realistic expectations.

They can also be helped by a new branch of psychology called cognitive therapy, which maintains that people react badly because of mental hang-ups, like all-or-nothing thinking ("I don't have a 100 percent rigid erection, so I don't have any erection.") or overgeneralization ("I didn't get it up last night, so I'll never, ever get it up again.") Once people recognize that these are, indeed, the kinds of things they say to themselves, they're ready for cognitive therapy, which can equip them with more rational messages for critical moments.

Even if a man's impotence is rooted in a physical cause, performance anxiety often complicates the matter. It makes things worse and can hamper lovemaking long after the physical difficulty is treated. So it has to be treated along with the physical problem.

If you're nagged by worries but they're still in the back of your mind and not affecting your performance yet, Shirley Zussman, Ed.D., a certified sex therapist and co-director of the Association for Male Sexual Dysfunction in New York City, has an idea for you. "I suggest trying to get into a fantasy to distract the distraction." She also stresses being selfish. Yes, you heard right, selfish. If excessive worrying about your partner and her reactions is causing trouble, then concentrate on yourself. "You can be a good lover only if you're aroused," she says.

Will these therapies and suggestions cure you of performance anxiety? Not exactly. "Nothing's a cure," says Dr. Zussman. "But it can be very helpful in terms of undoing the damage."

Ten Powerful Ideas

In a scientific paper published in the *Journal of Sex Education and Therapy*, Stephen B. Levine, M.D., and Stanley E. Althof, Ph.D., both of the Center for Human Sexuality at the University Hospitals of Cleveland, suggested that many cases of erection shutdown are really what they call an adaptive defense. In other words, it's serving some hidden need, whether that be withdrawal from one's sexual partner or a distraction from major life changes of the moment.

"The patient thinks he wants to have intercourse and something within him does not allow it," they write. To get men thinking about what that "something" could be, Drs. Levine and Althof float these notions.

1. The penis is attached to the heart.
2. Trying to be a rooster in a henhouse, eh?
3. In some Polynesian languages there is no word for impotence. When a man cannot become erect, he concludes that he must not have felt like it after all.
4. I think your penis knows something you don't know.
5. This limp penis of yours is your friend; let's try to find out how it is protecting you.
6. More than 200 years ago, the medical recommendation to cure impotence was to go home and have six amatory experiences without coital connection. The language has changed a bit in two centuries, but the idea of mak-

ing love for a while without attempting intercourse has not. I'd like you to try this time-honored tradition.

7. The penis is the organ of emotional attachment.

8. Almost everyone finds that making love for the first time with a partner is like a two-horse race: Fear runs against Excitement.

9. I know you want to get better yesterday, but I worry when a man is too quickly cured. I'd much rather help you stay potent than help you to have intercourse a few times.

10. I think you will eventually be fine!

PEYRONIE'S DISEASE
A Turn for the Worse

This disorder afflicts at least 1 or 2 out of every 100 men, and we hope you're not one of them. Peyronie's disease is not life threatening, but it often takes you out of the game of love—you might be put on the inactive list for many, many months. And your sex life may never be quite the same again. A 46-year-old Arizona man who has suffered with Peyronie's for the last five years tells us, "It's more devastating than impotence."

A man will know when he has Peyronie's disease because one morning he'll wake up and his erection will be crooked. It can happen that suddenly. The penis may also be hard at the base but soft up top, or skinny in the middle as if there were an invisible band clamp cinched around it. Or just painful. But most often it takes a sharp bend. Right-angle sharp, even.

As you might guess, something has gone seriously wrong beneath the surface of the penis. Inside the penis are two cylinders called the corpora cavernosa. These chambers fill up with blood during an erection. But they don't expand forever, of course; they're encased in a jacket or sheath, the tunica albuginea, which gives an erection rigidity when inflated. The tunica is like the leather on a football—it defines and limits the shape.

The penis can handle some bending—there's a built-in safety factor of about 10 to 13 times the normal erect-state pressure, says Irwin Goldstein, M.D., professor of urology at Boston University School of Medicine. "But beyond that, you run the risk of fracturing the tunica."

In Peyronie's disease, that's exactly what happens. The sheath gets torn and your body, in the process of repairing it, lays on so much scar tissue that, well, things take a turn for the worse.

Urologists have a favorite analogy for illustrating the unfortunate result. Imagine a long balloon. Blow it up a little—enough to put a piece of tape on one side. That tape is the scar tissue. It's not elastic, like the rest of the sheath, er, balloon. Now blow it up some more. The balloon is bending around that piece of tape, isn't it?

The problem with Peyronie's isn't the fractured tunica. It's a sad but true fact that plenty of guys bust their buddies in the course of wild sex or walking in the dark; in most cases, however, it scars and heals relatively quickly. But in men with Peyronie's the scarring process goes haywire. Too much scar tissue is created and it doesn't restore the sheath to its former glory. It just sits there, a knotty lump beneath the surface that's easily detected by both touch and ultrasound.

Since there's no such thing as a perfectly straight penis, don't march yourself off to a urologist because of that lifelong swoop to the left. But do see a urologist if you're experiencing a sudden shift in direction, painful erections or pain during intercourse. (This may sound weird, but take along a photograph of your penis in the erect state, since it's unlikely that you'll be able to summon ardent desire with your bare derriere on those sheets of paper that cover the examination table.)

Don't be distraught when the urologist merely says, "Hmmm, this bears watching." That could be the right thing to say. You see, it could just go away with time. Hope for that. Pray for that. Because Peyronie's disease has no simple cure.

How to Be Defensive

Peyronie's disease has humbled men for centuries. (It's named after the physician to Louis XV of France and it's pronounced pay-rone-eez.) It tends to mostly affect men of middle age and beyond. It is distinguished from an affliction called chordee in that chordee forces the penis to curve downward; chordee is congenital and is usually diagnosed by childhood.

How long this abnormal scarring will give you the bends varies. About half the time, if left alone, the pain slowly fades and the penis gradually straightens out. This could take months or years.

Dozens of different treatments have been tried to soften or eradicate the scarring, from radiation to steroid injections to vitamin E. Some are noteworthy only to the degree that they are worse than others, and do more harm than good.

"Peyronie's is physically disabling and psychologically disturbing," says Laurence A. Levine, M.D., professor of urology and director of the Male Sexual Function and Fertility Program at Rush-Presbyterian-St. Luke's Medical Center in Chicago. "Very few who suffer from it will have intercourse in the ways they did before the disease."

Dr. Levine is hard at work on yet another treatment. Fortunately, this one shows more promise than the rest. In 1991 he came up with the idea of injecting the calcium channel blocker verapamil (a drug normally used to treat high blood pressure) directly into the troublesome scar tissue of his Peyronie's patients. Each patient received injections every two weeks for six months. By the spring of 1995 he'd treated 60 patients, and had some data to report.

- Ninety-three percent of the patients suffering from pain said the pain went away after the first few injections.
- Eighty-nine percent said their sexual performance had improved.
- Sixty-one percent had a measurable decrease in curvature. The decrease was anywhere from 10 to 40 degrees, with a mean of 22 degrees.
- Two patients got worse.

Those who got better tended to be men who'd had the disease for less than two years, whose scarring did not involve a lot of calcification, whose scar tissue was of moderate extent (less than five cubic centimeters) and who suffered the most initial pain. No side effects were reported.

In most men verapamil injections did not decrease the size of the scar tissue itself, which leads Dr. Levine to conclude that the drug works not by dissolving the scar tissue but by softening it enough to make it release its tapelike grip on the tunica, thereby easing the curvature.

Having investigated this disease for years now, he's developed his own ideas about the cause. "My theory is, there is a decreased elasticity within the tunica of men with Peyronie's. Because of that, they have a greater propensity to tear." And that weakness is, he believes, "a genetic predisposition." It's almost as if the penile sheath gets old before its time.

Not everyone agrees with Dr. Levine's explanation—Dr. Goldstein believes the disease is more the result of constant trauma to the sheath over a period of years, and likens it to arthritis. But both doctors offer the same preventive advice. Dr. Goldstein calls it defensive sex. You have to be careful not to stress or bend the penis during sex. The most dangerous position is with the woman on top, bending backward "rodeo sex," as Dr. Levine says. It's especially dangerous if she's not in control of herself. If she slips off you and tries to come back down onto you, she might miss and . . . you know.

All in all, creative sexual positions are, shall we say, zesty, but a few ought to come with warning labels. Also, be careful when changing from one position to the next. "Everyone smiles about this," says Dr. Goldstein, "but I see the same injures over and over and over again. This is not some elusive, mysterious problem from France."

Drastic Measures

Only 20 percent of Peyronie's patients who are brave enough to seek medical help in the first place will end up seeking surgery to resolve their problems, according to Dr. Levine. The three main surgical solutions are:

1. The Nesbit procedure, which removes a patch on the normal side of the penis and straightens you out—but leaves you a bit short. It's the least invasive, says Dr. Levine; it works best when the man still has good erections, the curvature is less than 60 degrees and the penis isn't narrowed at any point by the disease—that band-clamp effect he calls a bottleneck.
2. Cutting into the scar tissue that's causing the problem, then placing a graft of skin or other material to straighten and reconfigure the penis. It's the best choice for the bottleneck-type symptoms or when the curve is greater than 60 degrees.
3. For men whose erections are poor because of the disease or other complicating factors, a surgeon will recommend implanting a prosthesis and possibly releasing the scar tissue.

Surgery should not be considered unless a year has passed and the deformity still persists (or in some cases continues to get even worse). Like we said: Pray it goes away.

PREMATURE EJACULATION
Don't Hurry, Be Happy

"Did you ever see a chimpanzee have sex?"

The person asking the question is Richard Kavich-Sharon, Ph.D., a San Francisco sex therapist. He doesn't *really* want to know whether you've been hanging out at the zoo; the question is rhetorical. "They're in and out, just like that," he explains, snapping his fingers. And then he draws the parallel to the naked ape. "When it comes to coitus, we're just fancy chimpanzees. In nature coitus is more like a sneeze."

So when someone comes to him with the problem of premature ejaculation, Dr. Kavich-Sharon is likely to say, "Congratulations. You're a healthy male."

What a nice approach. In fact, we hate to put this problem in the dysfunction section of this book. It implies that premature ejaculation is abnormal. Au contraire: It's common. Among the young, it's virtually normal.

"I consider rapid ejaculation in the vagina to be a characteristic of the majority of men beginning their experiences with intercourse," writes Stephen B. Levine, M.D., director of the Center for Human Sexuality at the University Hospitals of Cleveland, in his book *Sexual Life: A Clinician's Guide*. Moreover, the fact that you see this as a problem says something rather nice about you. You're not the wham-bam-thank-you-ma'am type. You want to "make love" instead of mate. "Therapists are not sought out for assistance by men who do not care about their partners' enjoyment, who view intercourse as the male's prize for seduction or who have intercourse only with prostitutes," writes Dr. Levine. "Homosexual men almost never ask for help for premature ejaculation. It is . . . the sense of hopelessly failing to provide a partner with what she needs and deserves . . . that brings coupled men in for help."

Okay, enough with pats on the back. You know and we know it may be normal, but that doesn't mean it's fun. Not for her, not for you. The good news: If your premature ejaculation is simply because of youth and inexperience and possibly a physical hypersensitivity, there's a quick fix. You want control? You shall have it. That is, after all, the essence of what you're seeking, and it fits the simplest definition of the problem, which is: Ejaculation before you want it to occur.

There are two basic approaches.

The squeeze technique was developed by famed sex researchers William H. Masters, M.D., and Virginia E. Johnson, of the former Masters and Johnson Institute in St. Louis. In this technique the woman circles the tip of your penis with her hand. The thumb is placed on the frenulum, that piece of skin on the underside of the penis below the head, while the fingers are placed on either side of the coronal ridge. And then she begins to give you a hand job. When you feel like you're going to come, she squeezes for three to four seconds, then releases. The squeeze will probably make you partially lose your erection. After half a minute or so, when the feeling of impending *boom* has lifted, she begins stimulating you again. Do it three or four times until you can't stand it anymore. Then you can reach orgasm. (The technique can also be applied to the base of the penis, if that works better.)

Once you gain confidence and control with her manual stimulation, you can move on to oral stimulation, manual stimulation with a lubricant, intercourse with her on top, making slow movements and finally to a side-by-side position.

The stop-start technique was developed by Duke University Medical School urologist James Semans, M.D., (honest) in 1956—although the same approach has been taught in other cultures for thousands of years. Instead of squeezing, simply stop stimulating until the feeling of climax subsides. It can be done as often as once a day for 15 to 30 minutes for several days or weeks, just like the squeeze technique. Can you imagine a better homework assignment?

Controlling the Problem

Employing either technique, you'll hopefully notice an improvement in your relationship as well as your sex life. Doing this with your partner gives you a common goal, improves communication between both of you and gets you acting as a team to solve what is otherwise a frustrating and sometimes finger-pointing problem. Therapists say treatments are always most successful when the couple shares the problem and takes joint responsibility for the solution.

Both techniques work, argued the late Helen Singer Kaplan, M.D., Ph.D., former director of the human sexuality program at New York Hospital-Cornell Medical Center in New York City, because they give you more awareness of the sensations that precede orgasm—and in recognizing those sensations, the ability to slow down in time to control your arousal. Awareness is the key. Some men try to delay ejaculation by thinking about baseball or taxes, wearing two condoms or drinking two shots of whiskey. All are aimed at reducing pleasure. All are exactly wrong. They turn arousal itself into the problem. Arousal is not the problem. A rapid ejaculator needs to confront his arousal, not dodge it.

"Methods that distract the man from his penile sensations ultimately make the problem worse because they interfere with his sexual sensory awareness even further," Dr. Kaplan wrote in her book, *PE: How to Overcome Premature Ejaculation*. The book, in its zillionth printing by now, is considered the finest on this subject. It's out in paperback and is a quick, 118-page read, footnotes included. If you've read this far, go get the book.

Premature ejaculation is something you want to fix while you're young. You will be able to fully enjoy your peak sexual years, of course. Also, you don't want to live with your dysfunction, not at such an early stage in your sexual life, because it establishes a pattern. After years and years of letting it define your sexuality, your problem can lead to other problems, all of which will be increasingly resistant to therapy.

Are Some Men Just Born This Way?

Not everyone agrees with Dr. Kaplan's belief that anxiety is the problem and awareness is the solution. Donald S. Strassberg, Ph.D., a sex therapist and psychology professor at the University of Utah in Salt Lake City, has done some pioneering studies with premature ejaculators. His findings:

1. They know as well or better than normally ejaculating men how aroused they are at every level of the sexual response cycle. So there's no difference in awareness.
2. They aren't any more anxious about ejaculation than men who can hold off longer. In fact, if premature ejaculators can masturbate more quickly, how can performance anxiety be said to affect that? They were actually clocked in a laboratory reaching orgasm 30 to 40 percent more quickly than most men.

Dr. Strassberg concludes that some of us are just plain hypersensitive to sexual stimulation. These men don't show any more anxiety than "normal" ejaculators, so you can't say it's all in their heads. Rather, "It's a physiological fact of life," he says. "It may be constitutional, to use an old-fashioned term." Nonetheless, their hair-trigger responses *can* be changed by the two techniques described above—not because it increases awareness but because any bodily reflex can be brought under greater voluntary control by the process of frequently approaching its threshold without reaching it. "I think that raises the threshold with time and practice," he says.

> The natural man has only two primal passions—to get and beget.
>
> —William Osler

Medical Solutions

There are always a few men who don't respond to the usual therapies. If the ol' frenulum squeeze does nothing for you, don't start dumping on yourself. You may be helped by fluoxetine.

Fluoxetine (Prozac) or clomipramine (Anafranil) are used to treat depression and obsessive-compulsive disorders, respectively. They belong to a class of prescription drugs called SRIs—serotonergic reuptake inhibitors, which affect the neurotransmitters mediating messages between brain cells. Ongoing trials with these drugs show great promise that they or some yet-to-be-developed SRI can treat men who are plagued with especially stubborn ejaculation problems. In one study, for example, 23 guys who ejaculated either before or immediately upon vaginal penetration were given Prozac for four months. Six months later 18 of the men still had improved control, which leads us to hope that even the worst cases can be helped without long-term drug therapy. But drug treatment for premature ejaculation is quite new—you'll need a doctor to refer you to a specialist who's doing this therapy.

PROSTATE PROBLEMS
What to Do When the Gland Grows

For most of your life, you've been tooling along blissfully, unaware you even have a prostate gland. Then, once you hit middle age, you start having problems. Your friends start having problems. Your doctor wants to give you a digital rectal exam and something called a PSA test every year. How come nobody ever told you about this?

Because this is our sexual machinery falling apart. It's embarrassing.

Yet some sort of prostate trouble ends up afflicting more men than any other major medical problem. Prostate cancer is second only to lung cancer in the number of American men it kills. The operation to relieve the symptoms of an enlarged prostate is the second-most common surgical procedure among U.S. males. And yet most men cannot name one symptom of prostate disease.

The prostate is called a sex accessory gland. It's the factory for your seminal fluid—all that good stuff that surrounds the sperm cells in your ejaculate. And when something goes wrong down there, it can have a major impact upon your sex life, as you'll see.

In the Prostate chapter of Part 1 we give details about the prostate's role and the various risk factors, from ethnic background to daily diet, that increase or decrease your odds of developing a disease. But the biggest risk factor of all is, simply, your age. If you know of a way to prevent yourself from getting old, *you* should be writing a book.

Prostatitis

An inflammation of the prostate gland is called prostatitis. If you get acute prostatitis, you'll get a fever, chills, acute pain, a burning sensation when urinating, a frequent urge to urinate and possibly blood in the urine. Chronic prostatitis differs only in that you may not have a fever and the pain is not as acute. But you have a bacterial infection in either case, and the resolution for either is a course of antibiotics. Don't be surprised if your doctor tells you to stay on the antibiotic for many weeks; antibiotics don't penetrate the prostate very well.

You can get a prostate infection at any age. Be glad it's only that. If it's any consolation, the standard medical advice is to augment your medicine with more frequent ejaculations in order to flush out the bacteria.

Nonbacterial prostatitis is an inflammation of the prostate without the infection. The symptoms are similar, though there may be fewer urinating problems. It's far more common than the bacterial variety. Unfortunately, there is no known cause and no known cure. Doctors can offer nothing more than ibuprofen and warm baths.

Finally, prostatodynia hurts like hell down there, too. But it's believed to be caused by a muscle spasm, or possibly a pinched nerve. Remedies include warm baths and sometimes an alpha-blocker prescription drug to relax the spazzed-out muscle.

Enlarged Prostate

The technical name for an enlarged prostate is benign prostatic hyperplasia (BPH). You want to know why a dog is really a man's best friend? Because of all the world's mammals, only man and dog suffer from this. Maybe that's why your retriever has been giving you such a soulful look.

The prostate is the Gland That Ate Chicago. It starts growing when you're age 40 and doesn't stop until you're 80, ballooning as much as five times in size. There are theories why this happens, but nobody really knows for sure. Not yet. You will know if you have a problem because of the hallmark symptoms.

- Your urinary stream slows in force and volume, sometimes to a mere dribble of its former self.
- You have difficulty getting started or maintaining a urinary stream.

- You feel the urge to urinate more often.
- You wake up several times each night to go to the bathroom.
- Yet when it's over, you don't feel like it's over.

By the time you're 85, and may you live so long, chances of being all too familiar with these symptoms rises to 85 percent. In the days before modern treatment the condition progressed to the point that men could no longer urinate, and their kidneys failed. That's how Thomas Jefferson died.

You get these symptoms because the prostate surrounds the tube, the urethra, that leads from your bladder to and through your penis. And when it swells, it narrows that tube. Also, there's a sphincter muscle right there at your bladder's drain (called the bladder neck) that's actually part of the prostate. It's normally closed so you aren't dribbling in your boxers all day long. It has to relax so you can urinate. In men with BPH some of the symptoms occur because the sphincter is not relaxing properly.

If you go to a doctor about this, he'll probably have you fill out a standard "symptom scorecard" that gives him a clearer idea of the extent of your problem. He'll perform a digital rectal exam to feel your prostate's size. Then, in a sitdown chat, he'll determine how much it's bothering you. That will help the two of you choose one of three courses of treatment.

1. Watchful waiting
2. Medicine
3. Surgery

Watchful waiting is reserved for those patients whose symptoms aren't yet bothersome—the enlargement is discovered only because of a routine physical, for example. They're advised to avoid caffeine and spicy foods, which can irritate the bladder. Also recommended: drinking lots of water, urinating more often, ejaculating more often, relaxing and taking warm baths. If it can be ignored, that's perfectly okay, because BPH is not cancerous. Some of these men will eventually have surgery because their problems will worsen. But nothing is lost by delay.

Medical solutions include prescribing either an alpha-blocker (such as terazocin) to help relax that sphincter muscle, or the drug finasteride (Proscar) that shrinks the gland by up to 30 percent. Based on small studies to date, between a third and two-thirds of men find relief from their symptoms after using an alpha-blocker. The alpha-blockers' chief side effect: dizziness.

If that doesn't work, there's a standard surgical solution: a transurethral resection of the prostate. Urologists call it the Roto-Rooter operation because a small tube (called a resectoscope) is slid up through the urethra to the prostate. The tube comes equipped with a lens and a loop of wire. Electrical current is passed through the wire to cut the obstructing tissue. Most men who undergo this operation are satisfied with the results. Which is a good thing, because Medicare spends more than $1 billion on this operation every year.

Surgery becomes necessary when an enlarged prostate causes bleeding, recurrent infections, loss of kidney function or a complete inability to urinate. Disadvantages: Because the sphincter muscle is carved away, the patient will experience retrograde ejaculation—his semen goes up into his bladder during orgasm, and comes out in his urine later. As side effects go, it's basically harmless. The same

> Three times as many people get killed by prostate cancer as get killed by handguns in this country. Would you stand and watchfully wait while someone was holding a gun to your head? And could you go to sleep at night, and sleep restfully, knowing that gun was cocked at your head?
>
> —Donald S. Coffey, Ph.D., professor of urology, oncology, pharmacology and molecular science at Johns Hopkins University School of Medicine/Francis Scott Key Medical Center in Baltimore and former head of the National Prostate Cancer Project

cannot be said of impotence and incontinence, two conditions you hear a lot about, anecdotally, but that barely show up in controlled studies.

A warning is in order here: Just about *any* surgery can have negative consequences on sex life, especially in older men, and for reasons that are more psychological than physical. Having said that, you'll be reassured to know that a major multicenter Veterans Affairs study of 556 men that compared watchful waiting with surgery found no added sexual dysfunction after surgery. In fact, men who had surgery reported slightly improved sexual performance afterward, when compared with the watchful-waiting group.

There is a less invasive operation: a transurethral incision of the prostate. Instead of carving out a whole hunk of prostate, the doctor merely slices the gland to make it spread open and relieve pressure on the urethra. On mildly enlarged prostates it works nearly as well as a resection, but results in less retrograde ejaculation. As a form of treatment, it is probably underused.

Prostate Cancer

Every three minutes, a man is told he has prostate cancer. It will kill over 40,000 American men this year. And yet it's one of the most controversial cancers, and is poorly understood.

Doctors hope—though they don't know for sure—that early detection will increase your chance of survival. And so the American Cancer Society recommends yearly digital rectal exams starting at age 40 and a prostate specific antigen (PSA) test starting at age 50—or age 40 for African-American males and any man with a family history of the disease. Your family doctor can perform these tests—don't bother hunting down a specialist. The very good reason to have these tests annually is that when prostate cancer is most curable, it is also symptomless.

A digital rectal exam is exactly what you've always feared. A doctor snaps on a rubber glove and slips a lubricated finger up your anus; when he probes forward an inch and a half up there, he can feel the back of the prostate gland. He does this because he can feel the difference between a normal prostate (it feels like the soft muscle at the base of the thumb) and an enlarged prostate (it feels firm and rubbery, like the thumb muscle when you squeeze it against another finger). Prostate cancer feels like a knuckle—a hard nodule in there. A digital rectal exam also can discover rectal problems, hemorrhoidal problems and prostatitis, which is why it's part of a comprehensive physical.

> Sex lies at the root of life, and we can never learn to reverence life until we know how to understand sex.
>
> —Havelock Ellis, "Studies in the Psychology of Sex"

No, it's not fun. It's especially discomforting if you get an erection when the doctor touches the prostate. If that happens, it's simply because of all the nerves that pass right by the prostate on their way to the penis, and not because you secretly want to take a walk on the wild side.

The PSA test is quite new and a lot easier on you because it's performed on a blood sample. Formally approved by the Food and Drug Administration for prostate cancer screening in 1994, it correctly detects nine out of ten cancers, making it far more predictive than, say, a mammogram for women. But the problem is, it also finds "cancers" that are *not* there—the level can rise above the magic number of four if you have BPH or an undiagnosed prostate infection. This false positive problem scares a lot of men, who then go on to have biopsies that come back negative.

A biopsy, as well as an ultrasound, can further narrow the diagnosis. Only a few years ago a biopsy was almost as complicated as surgery, and required a stay in the hospital. Today it's done in a doctor's office—he goes up into your rectum with a little gun and fires a few needles into your prostate to gather the tissue specimens. If the biopsy is positive, you'll get a technical diagnosis that describes the extent and malignancy of the cancer.

Here's a seldom asked question: If most men start getting annual PSA screens when they're 50, is there a time when you should stop getting them? Some doctors say yes. "You do it only in men who are going to live ten years, at least," says E. David Crawford, M.D., chairman of the urology department at the University of Colorado School of Medicine in Denver. "What do you do if you find it?" The dilemma is whether men over the age of 70 should be treated. Why torment them with the knowledge that their bodies harbor slow-growing cancers? The unpleasant fact of life is that many elderly men will die of something else before prostate cancer gets them. Should they risk surgery and the potential unpleasant side effects in order to eek out a few extra days of life?

This argument may sound odd, since most cancers are jumped on as soon as they're detected. That's because most cancers respond to conventional treatments, like chemotherapy. Prostate cancer does not. There are three basic forms of treatment; they are enmeshed in scientific argument because no large-scale studies have determined which method saves the most lives at minimal cost to the quality of life.

All in all, prostate cancer is still mysterious. Autopsies indicate that four out of ten men over the age of 50 already have cancer cells in their prostates right now. One in five will develop into a life-threatening carcinoma—but there's no way to predict which ones. And once detected, "there is no way to tell whether a patient has an aggressive tumor or an indolent one," says Joseph E. Oesterling, M.D., professor and chairman of urology at the University of Michigan Medical School and director of the Michigan Prostate Institute, both in Ann Arbor.

So please be a patient patient if your doctor doesn't tell you what he's going to do, but instead lays out these three alternatives to mull over.

Watchful waiting: Simply, it's a gamble that prostate cancer won't kill you before something else does. You'll watch the progress of the disease and continue to get tested. That's a reasonable course because the disease is so often slow growing. Of course, you stand the small risk of letting the cancer advance too far to be treated. If your health otherwise proves sturdy, you'll deeply regret your decision of years past.

Radiation therapy: This is a good treatment option for elderly men who want to survive until something else takes them. When done well, it's safe and it avoids surgery's impairments of urinary and sexual functions (although patients do report more troubles with bowel function). The risk is that the radiation won't get it all. Up to one-half of all radiation patients experience a rise in their PSA levels five years later.

Radical prostatectomy: Removing the prostate gets all the cancer if the cancer is caught in time. We've seen large-scale studies that found 85 percent of patients to be cancer-free after ten years. The American Cancer Society says that if caught while the disease is still located within the prostate gland, the five-year relative survival rate is 92 percent.

The risk of erectile dysfunction is not nearly what it used to be. Nonetheless, because the nerves that control erections pass so close to the prostate, even so-called nerve-sparing surgery can result in anywhere from 15 to 65 percent of men being rendered permanently impotent. (And even the lucky ones will have slightly weaker erections.) Where you might fall within that huge range depends upon your age—the younger the better, the quality of your erections before the surgery, the size of the cancer and your surgeon's skill. The hospitals that perform hundreds of operations yearly have better track records. There is every reason to shop around for this surgery.

The surgery also results in temporary incontinence for virtually all men, and permanent incontinence for a few. You can prepare for surgery with Kegel exercises. For more information, see Kegels on page 171. Exercising your groin muscles will give you greater control of the voluntary sphincter and may shorten the period of postoperative incontinence. Better than 90 percent of men are "dry" a year and a half after the surgery.

If cancer has spread beyond the gland, treatment includes

radiation in combination with hormonal therapy—basically, "chemical castration" that shuts down the production of testosterone, which fuels the growth of the prostate.

In the Years to Come

Prostate disease may have been ignored in the past, but it's getting a tremendous amount of attention now. In the next several years researchers anticipate developments such as these.

• The National Cancer Institute is conducting a seven-year trial of the drug Proscar on 18,000 men across the United States to see whether the drug, now being used to treat BPH, may also prevent prostate cancer.

• Former junk bond king Michael Milken had surgery for prostate cancer after emerging from prison in the early 1990s, and thereupon donated $50 million to a Manhattan-Project-style assault on the disease in conjunction with Seattle scientist Leroy Hood. Hood hopes to apply genetic engineering to someday clone cells that would attack and destroy the cancer.

• Gene therapy is also underway at Johns Hopkins University in Baltimore, where researchers believe they have located a genetic defect responsible for prostate cancer. The defect, which seems to block the production of a protective enzyme, could be corrected by a yet-to-be-developed drug.

• Better, less invasive surgical methods for BPH are in the works, including laser surgery, ultrasound treatment and radio waves.

• Better PSA screens are in the works, too. Perhaps by the time you read this, a new PSA test will eliminate some of the false positive readings and better distinguish between a level raised by cancer or by BPH. Eventually, PSA tests may tell us the difference between cancer cells that are destined to spread quickly and those that are so slow-growing they pose no real threat to the elderly patient.

SEX ADDICTION
When Loving Is Loathing

Where do you draw the line between a fiercely healthy male sex drive and one that's slipped into something desperate, compulsive and out of control?

The truth is that it's virtually impossible to do with absolute certainty.

Some guys love to have lots of sex, and they're happy and well-adjusted. No problem. Yet, clearly, there are other men in our society whose sexuality has been taken over by the dark side of the force. The priest who preys on altar boys. The compulsive womanizer. The prominent investment banker who goes cruising for hookers in the seediest part of town, night after night. The happily married and devoted father of an 11-year-old daughter, who secretly pursues sex with 11-year-old girls even though he hates himself for it.

Out of the Shadows

It used to be said that a woman with a voracious sexual appetite was a nymphomaniac; a guy whose horniness never quit suffered from satyriasis. But in 1983, with the publication of a book called *Out of the Shadows: Understanding Sexual Addiction* by Minneapolis family therapist Patrick Carnes, Ph.D., the term sexual addiction came into increasingly widespread use. Dr. Carnes, who worked with alcoholics and drug addicts, noticed many similarities between them and people who had developed an unhealthy obsession with sex. As one scholarly writer put it, "uncontrolled sexuality is an addictive process in which anxiety, loneliness and pain are temporarily relieved through a sexual high not unlike that obtained from drugs or alcohol."

Dr. Carnes also noticed that many of these people had multiple addictions—in one anonymous survey of 75 sex addicts, 62 either were recovering from alcohol or drug addiction, gambled or shopped compulsively or had eating disorders. When it came to impulse control, they seemed to have no "off" button.

A slew of other books and articles quickly followed Dr. Carnes's book, along with self-help groups and professional treatment programs that purported to help sex addicts regain control of their lives.

Nay from the Naysayers

There has been a small backlash against the whole "sexual addiction" concept. Marty Klein, Ph.D., a licensed marriage counselor and sex therapist in Palo Alto, California, contends that sex addiction doesn't exist. Rather, he says, the term refers to a set of moral beliefs disguised as science; it's a new twist on an old theme—sex as sickness. Other reasons to be skeptical of the whole idea, Dr. Klein and others say:

• To say that somebody is addicted to sex means that you're implicitly comparing his behavior to "normal" behavior. But since the range of normal sexuality is so vast, calling a man an addict taints him with a "disease" for what is often reasonable sexual behavior, Dr. Klein says. Proponents, he says, are ignorant of the range of typical human sexuality.

BREAKING FREE

If you're concerned that your sexual behavior is unhealthy or out of control, you may want to contact a self-help group. (They are anonymous in the sense that whatever is said in the group stays in the group.)

Sexaholics Anonymous, Box 300, Simi Valley, CA 93062
Sex Addicts Anonymous, P.O. Box 3038, Minneapolis, MN 55403
Sex and Love Addicts Anonymous, P.O. Box 88, New Town Branch, Boston, MA 02258

• The growth in popularity of the sex addiction idea has paralleled the growth of narrow, restrictive, highly conservative attitudes about sex. Mental health professionals are simply being used by people with these conservative political views and have made people who do not fit into a narrow, traditional sexual lifestyle feel bad, immoral and, now, mentally ill, according to Eli Coleman, Ph.D., associate director of the human sexuality program at the University of Minnesota Medical School in Minneapolis.

• Recovering from a genuine addiction, like heroin or alcohol, means complete abstinence from your poison-of-choice. But nobody's asking sex addicts to give up sex completely; only to learn to express themselves sexually in a healthier way.

So by this definition, sex can't truly be an addiction or even a compulsion (compulsions are when a person is driven to do something even though it brings him no pleasure, but sex addicts take great pleasure from sex, if only fleeting).

• The whole idea of sex addiction has become popular partly because it's easier for people with problems to say they have a disease and therefore avoid taking responsibility for their own behavior. Sex addicts join self-help groups that provide a warm, phony cocoon but no real help, Dr. Klein argues. And a high percentage of sex addicts are recovering substance abusers who love being in recovery.

Ten Signs of Addiction

To define sex addiction precisely is difficult, admits Julius P. Lundy, Ph.D., a sex therapist in San Antonio, Texas. But to say that sex addiction doesn't exist is clearly wrong. Most experts concur that it is a legitimate, actual problem, and is at least similar to drug and alcohol addiction.

A person who likes to have a lot of sex generally has a feeling of well-being after sexual activity. But an addict feels despair, depression, shame. And addict is obsessed with a certain sexual behavior, gets anxious if he can't get it and can't stop doing it even if he wants to stop. He'll pursue sex in a desperate, out-of-control way, and he'll continue doing it despite all kinds of adverse consequences—loss of his job, his marriage, his freedom. He just can't stop. He's out of control.

In an effort to establish a clearer consensus about what sex addiction actually means, Dr. Lundy polled 93 other mental health professionals and sex therapist. Among these therapists there was the greatest agreement about the following ten statements.

• Many sex addicts feel ashamed to have anyone know about their sexual activities.
• Many sex addicts describe feelings of euphoria when engaged in their sexual activities.
• Some sex addicts live a fearful double life.
• Sex addicts, most generally, suffered physical abuse, sexual abuse or emotional abuse in their childhood.
• Because of their addictions, some sex addicts often violate ethical standards, principles and oaths of their professions (doctors, lawyers, ministers).
• As part of their addictive cycle, sex addicts' moods shift from euphoria to depression.
• Some sex addicts focus on their sexual activities in order to escape, deny or numb their negative feelings.
• Sex addicts' behaviors often interfere with their spiritual or religious lives and practices.
• Many sex addicts attempt ways to engage in their sexual activities with little regard for place or time.
• Some sex addicts jeopardize their own health or safety by not taking reasonable precautions to protect themselves during sex.

What Causes It?

A generally agreed upon definition of addiction is a behavior that produces pleasure and provides escape from internal discomfort, in addiction to the following two characteristics: The addict repeatedly fails to control the behavior, and the addict continues the behavior despite significant harmful consequences.

By definition then, when sexual behavior is compulsive and continued despite serious, adverse consequences, it is addiction, writes Jennifer P. Schneider, M.D., Ph.D., a specialist in addiction medicine at the University of Arizona College of Medicine in Tucson.

There's an emerging school of research that suggests that sex addiction may have the same biochemical basis as other addictions such as getting hooked on cocaine, amphetamines or compulsive gambling. The ultimate goal of all these addictions, this theory suggests, is a brain reward: Whether it's triggered by chemicals (like cocaine) or behaviors (like illicit sex), the big, addictive kick is the release of some monstrously pleasurable brain chemical that produces a feeling of euphoria. You come to crave this feeling and do whatever it takes to get it, even though it has destroyed your marriage, your kid's college fund and your own sense of self-worth.

Support for this idea comes from the fact that certain medications such as antidepressants have been found to help reduce the addictive cravings for various drugs and also certain sexual paraphilias (what used to be called perversions).

Psychologists suggest a different explanation. Sex addiction begins with some dysfunction in the family, whether it's sexual abuse, alcoholism or a rigid, emotionally detached family where sex is never discussed at all, suggests Dr. Coleman. The child comes to believe that sex is shameful, powerful and dangerous. If he was abused, he comes to believe that he was the cause of the abuse and develops feelings of unworthiness and low self-esteem. He begins searching for a fix to soothe this inner hurt. It may be alcohol, dope, food or compulsive sexual activity.

This provides temporary relief, a fleeting euphoria, but after it's over, the loneliness and shame return. There's an increasing need to cop a fix again, to relieve the hurt—at the same time the sex itself increases the sense of shame and worthlessness. The same cycle may occur in restrictive households where a child is punished for masturbation, can't stop and develops a shame-based personality, says Dr. Coleman.

Getting Help

Whatever the explanation—and whatever you wish to call it—if any of the foregoing sounds uncomfortably familiar, you may need to get help.

Psychotherapy, certain medications and self-help groups have all been shown to be helpful, Dr. Lundy says. Most self-help groups are based on the 12-step program pioneered by Alcoholics Anonymous (the first step is admitting that you're powerless over your addiction and you need help). Do these groups do any good? Sex addicts say they do, says Dr. Lundy. A lot of the power in this thing is in the secrecy, the shame, the guilt. Once people learn to open up about it, to share their secrets with other people who are having the same problem, the healing can start.

You have to remember, though, that you're not talking about a cure, you're talking about arresting the behavior, he says. And don't expect results to come too fast. Getting this way took a lifetime, and dealing with it is just the same.

Even so, if it restores joy and lightness to your sex life, it's worth it.

SEX THERAPY
When You're Ready to Make a Change

The very words "sex therapy" still make some people giggle. They might think it's euphemism for massage parlors or Freudian psychology gone nuts. What a pity. We'd argue that sex therapy is even more respectable than other forms of therapy, considering its success rate: Anywhere from one-half to two-thirds of its patients report improvement or cure.

It's successful precisely because it is *not* like classic psychoanalysis, where you spend years on the therapist's couch, endlessly pondering the possibility of Oedipal conflicts with your mother. Sex therapy since the 1960s has used behavior therapy and, more recently, added doses of an approach called cognitive therapy. Both treatment methods are understandable and action-oriented. Their common goal is to get you fixed. Or, more precisely, to help you fix yourself by giving you everything from new insights to interesting homework assignments. (Don't worry—you won't have to perform on some office couch.)

Indeed, sex therapy has been so successful that many sex therapists have written self-help books about their methods, enabling people to deal with sexual problems without the cost of formal counseling sessions. As a result, sex therapists often complain that they don't see any easy cases anymore. And maybe they don't: Studies have shown that up to half the people seeking sex therapy today have difficulties far beyond the bedroom. When deep-seated emotional problems are causing or compounding the sexual dysfunction, therapy will take longer and be more analytical.

Who Needs Help

For some people sex is blissfully simple. In other relationships it can become a weapon or a payoff. It gets entangled in anger, resentment, insecurity, isolation, manipulation, guilt and blame. Fortunately, sex therapy has been so well-accepted by the mental health professions that many good marriage counselors now incorporate sex therapy into their work.

Not all sexual problems are created equal. Some problems, like impotence and premature ejaculation, have the highest rates of cure among therapists. One of the hardest dysfunctions to cure is low sexual desire. Some sex therapists may specialize in these sub-categories. Sex therapists may treat something as obscure as frotteurism (the compulsion to touch people sexually), but more likely they deal with cases like your garden-variety sexual boredom or a couple's libido difference that has gotten intolerably unworkable.

Other cases may deal with those couples who are having trouble making the necessary changes in their sex lives as they age. Some men, for example, haven't faced the fact that, at age 55, they don't have the perfect penis they had at 25. They need to be stimulated physically to get an erection. They sometimes lose an erection. The old just-hop-on-board approach isn't working anymore. Now that their orgasms are no longer automatic upon first erection, they become demoralized. As therapists say, they need to re-write their "sexual script." They and their partners need to find new ways to arouse and stimulate each other if they're going to remain sexual friends.

A couple can make that happen by themselves, but some couples just don't. Our culture is open about sexual desire but closed-mouthed about sexual problems. No wonder people feel they need guidance or "permission" or the focus that a dozen sessions of therapy can bring.

There are probably fewer than 10,000 sex therapists practicing in America. They generally charge anywhere from $75 to $175 per hour. There is an accrediting organization: the American Association of Sex Educators, Counselors and Therapists (AASECT). It issues a national membership directory that also spells out certification procedures and contains the group's ethical code. Call AASECT's headquarters in Chicago at (312) 644-0828. Like any phone book, not everyone's number is listed—some highly competent sex therapists are nonjoiners.

Don't rely on AASECT's directory by itself; try to get personal referrals. If you think you have a mostly physical problem and want to get checked out by an expert on the male sex organs, you're probably looking for a urologist. Ask your family physician for a referral. If you believe you have more of a "couple" problem, ask your minister or ask around among marriage counselors or family therapists. Most will "refer out" if they think they can't handle your problem. But whatever it is, be specific about it. This is not the time to be coy.

Within the space of a five-or ten-minute phone call, you'll check out potential therapists and they'll check you out. Most therapists, for example, refuse to see couples if either partner is conducting an affair, especially if the affair is still a secret and the therapist is asked to become an accomplice to the deceit. The same rule applies to other secrets, like bisexuality.

While they're trying to find out exactly what's wrong with

you, try to find out what's wrong with them—why they might be wrong for you, at any rate. Ask specific questions about their training, qualifications and specialties. Some therapists might say they *can do* sex therapy, but look for someone who's trained in it, practices it and, hopefully, sees a lot of cases similar to yours. That's usually good— although sometimes that's bad, too, because the therapist may have a pet theory that he or she tries to apply to everyone. "Beware of rigidity," advises Oakland, California, sex therapist Bernie Zilbergeld, Ph.D., author of *The New Male Sexuality*. "A good therapist focuses on each patient's situation and needs and is flexible enough to come up with methods that suit the patient."

STRESS
The Need for Personal Control

Two facts to give pause:

• In the five top-rated soap operas, you'll see an average of 6.6 sexual incidents per hour.
• Three out of ten men ages 18 to 59 in the United States have either not had sex at all in the last year or only "a few times."

In America's public life there's Cindy Crawford, Claudia Schiffer, Whitney Houston, MTV, *Melrose Place*, slip dresses, couch dancing, the hot blondes in every beer commercial and the artist formerly known as Prince.

In Americans' private lives are 5:45 A.M. alarms, Pop-Tarts, beepers, lunch at the desk, laundry, the kids' soccer practice, groceries, unopened mail, unanswered voice mail and dinner at 10 P.M. out of a pizza box.

Sex is everywhere and nowhere. Some blame AIDS. We vote for stress.

When Harvard economist Juliet B. Schor came out with her book *The Overworked American*, it hit the best-seller lists because it confirmed what everyone instinctively knew—people are pushing (and being pushed) too hard. Yes. Americans are working more—the equivalent of a month more every year than the typical American worked in 1969, Schor estimates. Since 1972 our leisure time has dropped by 40 percent. We work a total of over two months more than our counterparts in Germany and France. Oh, we have plenty of *stuff*—twice what we would have had in 1948. But we're also working harder than people did in 1948. We're glutted with goods but suffer from something called time famine; working mothers, especially, talk about craving sleep the way a starving person talks about food.

Women are not the only ones working harder. Despite the complaints, men now do more at home *and* at work. (Beginning in the 1980s a historic change occurred. Single men now have fewer domestic demands than married men.)

The overload takes a disproportionate toll on couplehood, Schor argues. Two-earner couples have less time together, which researchers have found reduces the happiness and satisfaction of a marriage. These couples often just don't have enough time to talk to each other. . . . When job, children and marriage have to be attended to, it's often the marriage that is neglected.

Some dismiss this trend as a "yuppie sex" problem, but they must lead very insulated lives. Couples of all ages and incomes are exhausted by the so-called normal demands of modern life.

And nothing could be less conducive to the leisurely playfulness needed for romance—especially between two people who've celebrated a few anniversaries already.

Normal life is hectic enough. But when major change is added to the mix—a move, a new job, a new baby, the illness or death of a parent—your physical or emotional health can be affected in seemingly unrelated ways. Everyone reacts differently, of course, but men are famous for clamming up. Especially if they've always had trouble identifying and talking about their feelings, a period of great stress will cause them to withdraw into silence. "That turns women off," says Oakland, California, sex therapist Bernie Zilbergeld, Ph.D., author of *The New Male Sexuality*. "Women like to relate. They draw sexual energy from the communication and togetherness of the relationship. When men under stress pull away, women often suffer a loss of libido as well."

Physically, stress is every bit as damaging. Stanford biologist Robert M. Sapolsky wrote a lively book, *Why Zebras Don't Get Ulcers*, that explains what happens at the cellular level of stress. At its onset, says Sapolsky, the male brain slows its release of one hormone, which slows the production of two more hormone, which slows testosterone production in the testicles. But that's not all. "Decline in testosterone secretion is only half the story of what goes wrong with male reproduction during stress. The other half concerns the nervous system and erections. Getting an erection to work properly is so incredibly complicated physically that if men ever actually had to understand it, none of us would be here. Fortunately, it runs automatically. In order for a male to have an erection, his parasympathetic nervous system must be turned on."

Well, that system also runs the body's normal, noneventful activities like breathing and digestion. It's the opposite of the sympathetic nervous system, which kicks into action during emergencies. They are very much in opposition; when the sympathetic system is switched on, one of the things it does is suppress the parasympathetic. "It becomes difficult to establish parasympathetic activity if you are nervous or anxious," writes Sapolsky. "You have trouble having an erection." Among other things, the sympathetic nervous system constricts blood vessels—and blood flow to the pelvic region in particular.

His bottom line is that "stress will knock out male sexual responses quite readily." It's a nonsexist sex basher: Female libido is knocked out quite readily, too.

What to Do about Stress

A key principle of stress management is that you cannot eliminate stress from your life, but you can change the way you respond to stress.

The human response to stress is not terrifically subtle. You respond to psychological stress in pretty much the same way you respond to physical stress. The intricate biological reactions geared to escaping a hungry lion on the African savannah—constriction of blood vessels, for instance—do not do you a lick of good when you're sitting around worrying about the mortgage this month or smoldering over the recent coup pulled off by your worst enemy at the office.

To avoid the ravages of constant stress, you have to learn how to turn off your stress response. Lord knows, Americans have been trying; they have table-hopped among the various fashionable therapies of the last few decades: abdominal breathing, aromatherapy, biofeedback, jogging, meditation, massage, prayer, visualization, autogenic training, imagery, hypnosis, behavioral modification, emotional restructuring and cognitive-perceptual change . . . to name a few.

Table-hopping is actually okay. Because of the unique stressors in their lives, and their unique responses, everyone has to find their own relief from stress. That's why so much of the general advice about stress reduction sounds trite and lame—in being broad enough to cover everybody, it's not specific enough for anybody. But in risking another cliché, we'll tell you that your daily outlook is critical. (If you want to read more about specific strategies for coping with stress, here are some recommended titles: *Learned Optimism* by Martin Seligman; *The Success Syndrome* by Steven Berglas, Ph.D.; *Why Zebras Don't Get Ulcers* by Robert M. Sapolsky; and *Your Healing Mind* by Reed C. Moskowitz, M.D.)

Sapolsky summarizes the common themes of stress therapy in his final chapter: "This is the message that fills stress management seminars, therapy sessions and the many books on the topic. Uniformly, they emphasize finding means to gain at least some degree of control in difficult situations, viewing bad situations as discreet events rather than permanent or pervasive ones, finding appropriate outlets for frustration and means of social support and solace in difficult times."

Sapolsky zeroes in on four components of stress management that must be managed themselves—they're useful as long as you don't go overboard and embrace them as mantras.

Optimism. In the face of life's lesser problems, it's helpful to hope for improvement. As the old cliché goes, see the glass half-full, rather than half-empty. "But do not deny the possibility that things will not improve," he says. "Balance these two opposing trends carefully." Otherwise, your bubble will someday burst, and you'll be devastated. In effect: Hope for the best, prepare for the worst.

Control. "Those who cope with stress successfully tend to seek control in the face of stressors but do not try to control in the present things that have already come to pass. They do not try to control future events that are uncontrollable and do not try to fix things that are not broken or are broken beyond repair." It's like the old prayer: God grant me the courage to change the things I can, the serenity to accept the things I can't and the wisdom to tell the difference.

Information. Knowledge can relieve stress or be a source of stress. "Information is not useful if it comes too soon or too late, if it is unnecessary information, if there is so much information that it is stressful in and of itself or if the information is about news far worse than one wants to know."

Outlets. Find one you can use regularly. As Joseph Campbell, an author famed for exploring cultural myths, said: Follow your bliss. "Prayer, meditation, ballroom dancing, psychoanalysis, Bach, competitive sports—each may help some people but not others," says Sapolsky.

He forgets to mention one more outlet. It's a time-honored way to relax, rejuvenate yourself, brighten your mood and forget about your troubles.

Need a great stress-buster? We vote for sex.

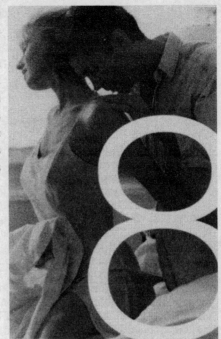

SEXUAL
DISEASES

AIDS
Glimmers of Hope

In the early days of the epidemic, before anyone had any idea what they were dealing with, it was known as gay cancer.

Homosexual and bisexual men, mainly on the coasts, began developing an odd array of symptoms: unexplained fatigue and weight loss, fever and chills, swollen lymph nodes and sometimes soft, ugly brown spots that first appeared on their feet and legs—sign of a rare cancer called Kaposi's sarcoma. Most puzzling of all, they often developed a deadly form of pneumonia that is extremely unusual in otherwise healthy young men.

Looking back, it's hard to believe it was only 1981 that these symptoms were first linked to acquired immune deficiency syndrome (AIDS), the scariest sexual scourge in history. It's hard to believe that HIV-1, one of two main strains of the virus that causes AIDS, was only identified in 1984.

It seems like AIDS has been with us forever. But in many important ways, the story of this terrifying disease has only just begun. A handful of tragic landmarks:

- By 1992 AIDS had become the leading cause of death among American men ages 25 to 44, according to the Centers for Disease Control and Prevention (CDC) in Atlanta. By 1995 it had become the leading cause of death among all Americans ages 25 to 44.
- By early 1995 more than 440,000 cases of AIDS had been reported to the CDC since the beginning of the epidemic (three-quarters of them among people ages 25 to 44).
- Worldwide, by 1995 there were about 20 million adults and children who were HIV positive, according to the World Health Organization (WHO) Global Program on AIDS. About 4.5 million of these people have full-blown AIDS.

- In 1994 alone, the WHO estimates, more than 13 million adults became infected with HIV. That's more than 35,000 new infections every day.

These numbers are all so big and so scary that they barely register. But the bottom line in all this is rather small and intimate: Since HIV is almost always transmitted by the exchange of body fluids during sex (mainly semen, vaginal secretions or blood), it all comes down to what you do or don't do in bed. And sure, maybe safer sex won't save the world—but it could save your world. For more on AIDS prevention and testing, see Safer Sex on page 513.

What It Is, How It Works

Normally, when your body is invaded by a microscopic intruder, your immune system mounts an awesomely complex counterattack. But what makes the HIV virus so ingenious, and so deadly, is that it invades the immune system itself. In particular, it penetrates and then begins multiplying inside a certain kind of white blood cell called CD4 T cells, which are key players in the body's immune response. As the disease progresses, a person's T4 cell counts steadily decline; people with full-blown AIDS often have counts one-twentieth of their normal value, doctors say.

HIV also attacks other immune system cells called macrophages, the Pac-Men of immunity, whose job it is to surround and engulf invading microorganisms. But once HIV has penetrated a macrophage, HIV remains undetected by the body's immune surveillance system and replicates freely . . . thus, the macrophage can serve as both a haven and a reservoir for HIV, explain Brian S. Koll, M.D., and Donald Armstrong, M.D., of Beth Israel Medical Center in New York City, in a medical research paper.

By crippling the body's ability to fight off microorganisms, HIV lays a person open to anything that happens to come drifting through the neighborhood—other viruses, foul bacteria, protozoa, fungi. A person whose immune system has been devastated by HIV is a sitting duck for all man-

COMMON SYMPTOMS OF HIV INFECTION

Unexplained weight loss

Unexplained fatigue

Swollen lymph nodes (typically in neck)

Loss of appetite

Chills and fever

Night sweats

Rashes, dark splotches or lesions on skin

Sore throat

Cough, shortness of breath

Abdominal pain, severe diarrhea

ner of opportunistic infections, and it's these secondary infections that are actually the major cause of sickness and death in people infected with HIV, doctors say.

Among the most common of these infections is *Pneumocystis carinii* pneumonia, which is found in about 65 percent of AIDS patients, according to Drs. Koll and Armstrong. It's also the leading cause of sickness in AIDS patients and the cause of death in about a quarter of cases. Certain kinds of cancers are also common, including Kaposi's sarcoma, Burkitt's lymphoma and non-Hodgkin's lymphoma. Then there's a whole range of bacterial infections that immuno-suppressed AIDS patients are prone to, including mycobacterium tuberculosis, which causes tuberculosis, and viral infections, like cytomegalovirus, a herpeslike virus that's found in nearly all gay men who are HIV positive.

Nevertheless, the disease can progress fairly slowly. The median time interval from HIV infection to onset of AIDS is around ten years, according to the CDC. That means that lots of people who are HIV positive do not yet know it—and are quite capable of passing along a death sentence to their sex partners between now and the time they begin to develop symptoms.

Many guys who are HIV positive feel perfectly fine and

aren't under any medical care at all, even though their blood and semen are deadly poison. The severity of symptoms, in those who develop them, range through a series of intermediate stages called AIDS-related complex to full-blown AIDS.

Since the beginning of the epidemic, the group most at risk for getting AIDS has been homosexual men. That's still the case, according to a CDC report in early 1995—44 percent of all AIDS cases in the United States were among men who have sex with men. Intravenous drug users, their sex partners and their children were the next most risk-prone group. And 18 percent of cases are now among women, who picked it up either through intravenous drug use or heterosexual sex with an HIV-infected man, the CDC reports.

Long-Term Nonprogressors

In the early 1980s, at the beginning of the epidemic, it appeared that the disease was inevitably fatal within a few years. But now there's evidence that a few people infected with the HIV virus—perhaps 5 to 10 percent—live for ten years or longer. The study of these long-term nonprogressors (meaning that the disease does not progress much beyond the initial infection) has become one of the most promising avenues of research by AIDS investigators in the 1990s.

One theory is that these people were simply lucky enough to pick up a mutant strain of HIV so weak it's virtually harmless. In 1994, Australian scientists reported a cluster of six people who became HIV-infected as long as 14 years ago, all through blood transfusions from the same donor. Yet all six of these people, plus the donor, are still alive and well—suggesting that they may have gotten a dummy strain of HIV. Oddly, though, in other cases of HIV infection through transfusions, some of the blood recipients died and others become long-term survivors.

Does it have to do with the fact that some people's immune systems are able to muster an extraordinarily powerful counterattack against HIV? This would be especially promising because if researchers could then figure out what it is about nonprogressors' immune responses that's different from those who have succumbed to the disease, perhaps a vaccine could be designed that would induce that response.

There's some reason to hope this may be happening. Researchers at Massachusetts Institute of Technology in Cambridge, for instance, have found that long-term survivors have more active CD8 cells, a class of cells that includes cytotoxic T cells, a kind of heat-seeking missile of the immune system that attacks and kills other cells infected with the HIV virus.

And researchers at the San Francisco Department of Public Health have found that about 1 in 12 men who have been infected more than ten years has counts of CD4 T cells that are still above half the average value—which is amazing, since T4 cell counts normally nosedive as the disease progresses.

But perhaps the most hopeful story of all was reported in mid-1995 when a five-year-old California boy, infected with HIV at birth, was found to be completely disease-free. Medical researchers say this is the first documented case in which anyone has ever fought off the disease entirely (provided that the boy is still HIV-free years from now). Tests had proven conclusively that he was HIV positive when the child was tested at 19 days and 51 days. But doctors reported that by the time he was a year old, the virus had vanished.

And perhaps, someday, it really will.

CHLAMYDIA
A Bacterial Infection That Tops the Charts

The most common of all sexually transmitted diseases (STD) very often produces no symptoms at all—until much later. Then things get serious.

Giving your girlfriend chlamydia is not exactly the same thing as giving her chrysanthemums. A chrysanthemum is a flower; chlamydia is a drag.

For males this sexually transmitted disease, caused by the

CHLAMYDIA: AT A GLANCE

Problem: A bacterial infection passed on most commonly during intercourse. It is the most common sexually transmitted disease, with roughly four million new cases each year.

Symptoms: Men usually experience mild pain during urination and/or a small amount of discharge from the penis. The discharge may be white or clear, thin or mucuslike. Symptoms generally show up one to three weeks after exposure. Ten to 20 percent of men have no symptoms at all.

Cure: In most cases antibiotics will knock this bug out in a week.

bacterium *Chlamydia trachomatis*, is usually no more than a minor irritation. But for women it can be genuinely devastating. If *C. trachomatis* spreads into the deeper regions of a woman's reproductive anatomy, it can cause pelvic inflammatory disease (PID), which may result in infertility or ectopic ("tubal") pregnancies. Experts estimate that up to half of the one million cases of PID reported every year in the United States are caused by chlamydial infections.

An STD for the Young

Although lots of people have still never even heard of it, chlamydia is the most common sexually transmitted disease in the United States. About four million people pick up the infection every year, according to the Centers for Disease Control and Prevention (CDC) in Atlanta. That makes chlamydia roughly twice as common as gonorrhea and 40 times as common as syphilis. In two military studies silent chlamydial infections of the urethra were found in about 10 percent of otherwise healthy young men.

It's especially common among sexually active men and women under age 25. Anybody who has had intercourse with a new partner in the past two months and doesn't use barrier contraceptives (like condoms or a diaphragm) is a likely candidate for chlamydial infection, experts say. (There's some evidence that barrier contraceptives can offer some protection against chlamydia, though how much is not clear. One analysis of 29 medical studies showed that women who used the Pill as their main form of contraception were roughly twice as likely to pick up a chlamydial infection, suggesting—though only indirectly—that barrier methods are protective.)

How do you know if you have it?

Well, that's part of *C. trachomatis's* secret plan for world domination. Chances are, you don't. Ten to 20 percent of men and up to 80 percent of women have no symptoms at all, at least not until more serious complications begin to develop. (Chlamydia is sometimes called the silent STD.) Which makes it all the easier for *C. trachomatis* to keep on stealthily spreading from person to person, San Diego to Austin to Indianapolis to your hometown.

If symptoms do appear, they usually show up one to three weeks after exposure. In men the symptoms generally look a lot like mild gonorrhea: pain and burning during urination, or a little bit of discharge from the penis. The discharge may be white or clear, thin, thick or puslike. (To put it bluntly, like nurses do on their coffee breaks, "All that drips is not the clap.")

You may also experience some pain or swelling of the scrotum. That's because chlamydial infections will sometimes spread from the urethra up into the epididymis, the tubes that carry sperm out of the testicles. The resulting infection, epididymitis, can be not only irritating but also may be linked to infertility. A study of 52 infertile couples concluded that "our results suggest an association between infection with *C. trachomatis* in men and unexplained infertility."

Occasionally, symptoms of chlamydia will turn up in more exotic places. Infections can cause proctitis (inflamed rectum) and conjunctivitis (inflammation of the lining of the eye). It's also been found in the throat (guess why).

In women the most common symptoms include vaginal discharge, pain during urination, stomach pain and vaginal bleeding after intercourse. Unfortunately, these are often signs that the infection is pretty far advanced.

Ditch the Dipstick

Because chlamydia can look so much like gonorrhea, especially in men, the only way to tell for sure is to get a lab test. (Just to make things more confusing: Studies have shown that about 20 percent of guys with chlamydia also turn out to have gonorrhea.)

Lab tests to detect *C. trachomatis* in men have not been terribly accurate and also were painful: The method of choice involved passing a swab up the urethra (yikes!) in order to obtain cell samples for culturing and analysis. Now a painless test called the PCR urine assay—which uses only a urine sample—has become available. In one study doctors tested 365 men who came into the STD clinic at Harborview Medical Center in Seattle using both the PCR urine assay and the urethral-swab method. The urine test proved almost equally accurate—and without the high-pitched screams. You get results in half an hour or so.

The Treatment of Choice

Despite all its dangers and discomforts, chlamydia is actually fairly easy to cure—more than 95 percent of infections are history after a week of antibiotics. The CDC recommends this easy plan for uncomplicated infections: 100 milligrams of doxycycline twice a day for a week or tetracycline four times a day for a week. (You can take both antibiotics in pill form.)

There's also an antibiotic called Azithromycin, introduced by Pfizer labs in 1992, which has two advantages: It's more powerful, and you only have to take a single, one-gram dose. Having to take a pill only once (or at most once a day) is an advantage if you have trouble remembering what you had for lunch yesterday. The disadvantage: That single dose costs around $32, compared to less than $10 for a week's worth of doxycycline.

Still, conclude researchers in a review of chlamydia treatments, "Azithromycin, doxycycline and tetracycline are virtually 100 percent effective against most *C. trachomatis* infections when the patient completes the regimen as directed."

Just to make sure the medicine did the trick, you should go back to the doctor or clinic a week after treatment for a follow-up visit. And one other thing you shouldn't forget: Your sex partner should also be treated, because doctors estimate that 50 to 60 percent of the partners of people with chlamydia infections are also infected. It doesn't do much good to get yourself treated if you return to a lover who is harboring a few million bacterial friends and relations of the bug that got you sick in the first place.

CRABS
How to Get Rid of Pubic Lice

Getting rid of crabs is fairly easy. It's getting over that creepy feeling, and patching things up with your lover, that's the hard part.

Strictly speaking, an infestation of crab lice is not a sexually transmitted disease at all, because they can be transmitted by all sorts of close physical contact other than sex. They can even be transmitted by inanimate objects (like towels, bedsheets or clothes) because the blood-sucking little buggers can live without a host for 24 hours, and their eggs can survive for several days. (Just because your girlfriend has crabs doesn't mean she's been unfaithful—and vice versa.) Crabs go for hair: They can get into your scalp, eyelashes, underarms or pubic hair (in which case they're called pubic lice; an infestation in that particular spot is called *pediculosis pubis*).

Generally, the first symptom is horrendous itchiness in places you'd rather not scratch in public. On closer examination you may also notice reddened, pimplelike bumps or a red rash (caused by scratching as much as anything else).

CRABS: AT A GLANCE

Problem: Crab Lice are tiny animals that infest pubic hair and feed on blood through the skin. Eggs get laid on the hair.

Symptoms: A terrible itchiness around the genitals. Sometimes you'll also notice red, pimplelike bumps or a red rash. The giveaway: Tiny white eggs attached to the pubic hair close to the skin.

Cure: Washing thoroughly with a shampoo made for lice and also cleaning sheets, towels and floors where they may be lingering, waiting for flesh (crab lice cannot survive long without a host).

The giveaway are the eggs: tiny white dots (called nits) attached to the shafts of pubic hair down close to the skin. The crabs themselves—horrible, grayish, lobsterlike things with jointed bodies and teensy claws for hanging onto your skin—are so small you probably won't be able to see them.

Death Shampoo

There are at least a half-dozen over-the-counter medications for crabs available in drugstores for $15 or less, including A-200 Pyrinate, Nix and RID. There's also a prescription medication called Kwell. Here's the drill: Use the medication to wet and shampoo your pubic hair (and whatever other hair seems to be infested), leaving the lather on for ten minutes. Rinse. Then carefully comb through your pubic hair with the fine-toothed "nit comb" that comes in the package, to remove dead lice and eggs.

Clothes and bedding should be washed on the hot cycle for at least 20 minutes or sprayed with a different formulation of the same medication. (Usually all this stuff comes packaged together.) Thoroughly vacuum the floor around your bed (or wherever else seems likely). Clothes that can't be washed can be dry-cleaned or sealed in a plastic bag for two weeks so the rascals will die a slow, humiliating death.

It's a good idea to reapply the medication a week to ten days later, just in case. Then send your lover flowers.

EPIDIDYMITIS
When the Plumbing Starts to Hurt

Chances are you didn't even know you had an epididymis, but when it gets infected, you'll definitely get a wake-up call. Generally, it's in the form of a painful, swollen scrotum, often accompanied by a lump on the back of your testicles that's tender and hot to the touch. You may also have trouble urinating, or you may notice a discharge from the penis.

Located on the back of the testicles, the epididymis is a packet of tightly coiled tubing through which sperm cells travel and gradually mature, between the time they're manufactured and their launch into the unknown.

Any acute or chronic inflammation of this ductwork, often caused by a bacterial infection that's ascended from the urinary tract, is called epididymitis. For adult males epididymitis is the most common cause of pain in the scrotum, says Bruce H. Blank, M.D., clinical associate professor of urology at Oregon Health Sciences University's School of Medicine in Portland.

Though gonorrhea or chlamydia, two common sexually transmitted diseases, are often to blame, sometimes doctors never do figure out what's causing it. They just give you antibiotics, and that generally knocks it out of your system.

Your doctor may also advise you to lay in bed with a pillow under your rear to raise the scrotum, or suggest wearing an athletic supporter. Ice compresses can help reduce the swelling and inflammation, Dr. Blank says. Or you can try a hot bath, which soothes the pain and stimulates blood flow.

Occasionally, a stubborn epididymal infection will just keep coming back, despite repeated attacks with antibiotics. "If it occurs only sporadically, antibiotic treatment is all you

---

EPIDIDYMITIS: AT A GLANCE

Problem: A bacterial infection of the sperm-carrying tubing in the scrotum.

Symptoms: Pain and swelling of the scrotum. You may also feel a lump on the backside of your testicles; the lump may be red and feel hot to the touch.

Cure: While doctors aren't always sure what type of bacterium is causing the infection, antibiotics almost always work to kill the beast.

---

need; but with recurrent bouts, it's worth having a look at the entire urinary tract to make sure that nothing else is going on," says Michael Nasuland, M.D., professor or urology at the University of Maryland School of Medicine in Baltimore.

"Ask your doctor about having an intravenous pyelogram to check for kidney problems and a cystoscopy to rule out a problem with your urethra," Dr. Nasuland suggests. The pyelogram is a kind of x-ray in which a fluid with a contrasting color is injected to help display the innards; a cystoscopy is a visual test of the urinary tract using a thin scope.

GENITAL WARTS
How to Not Do the Bump

Discovering a wart on your privates can be an unnerving experience—but at least you're not alone. In fact, genital warts account for a million (slightly sheepish) doctor visits a year in the United States.

Known to physicians as *condylomata acuminata*, genital warts typically show up as small, hard, painless bumps—one or many—on the tip or shaft of the penis, scrotum, anus or mouth. They often show up in places that get a lot of friction during sex. In uncircumcised men they may appear under the foreskin. And in women they're likely to turn up in places not visible to the eye—deep inside the vagina or on the cervix. Left untreated, they'll gradually develop a fleshy, cauliflower-like appearance.

Skin tags—tiny flaps or outgrowths of skin—may occasionally look like genital warts, but "skin tags are harmless and not related to genital warts in any way," says Carol J. Bennett, M.D., associate professor of urology at the University of Southern California School of Medicine in Los Angeles. Skin tags, unlike warts, don't show up suddenly; often you're born with them. If you're worried about them—or your girlfriend won't sleep with you because she thinks they're warts—a simple office procedure can remove them for good.

Genital warts are caused by a highly contagious, slow-growing group of viruses called human papillomaviruses, or HPVs, which typically show up six weeks to eight months after exposure. The great majority of people who pick up an HPV infection show no symptoms at all, though they go right on passing it along to sex partners. Because it's so stealthy, and so contagious—60 to 90 percent of the male sex partners of infected women also develop HPV infections—HPV has reached epidemic proportions. As many as 24 million Americans may already be infected, with 3 million new infections turning up every year, according to estimates by the National Institute of Allergy and Infectious Diseases in Bethesda, Maryland.

"In the college-age population it's one of the most common sexually transmitted diseases we see. And even though HPV used to be thought of as little more than a nuisance, we now know these infections need to be taken seriously," says Sandra Samuels, M.D., director of student health services at Rutgers University in New Brunswick, New Jersey.

There's growing evidence that in women, ugly-but-benign warts can sometimes transform into potentially cancerous growths called dysplasia. Roughly one in ten women with dysplasia will go on to develop cervical cancer, which can be deadly. In men HPV may be linked to rare but loathsome penile cancers.

Out, Out, Brief Wart

If you discover a wart down there (or your sex partner does), it's important to see a doctor, who can positively identify the bugger. In men genital warts are usually identified simply by visual examination. In women, who often develop warts in out-of-the-way places, identification is more difficult. The doctor may have to use a lighted magnifying instrument to examine the interior of the vagina and cervix. Or a Pap smear (a test for cancers of the cervix) may be used. In fact, HPV in women is often discovered only after abnormal results on a Pap smear.

Fortunately, getting rid of the warts themselves is not all that difficult. Smaller warts can be removed surgically, with lasers or by cryotherapy (freezing them off using liquid nitrogen or nitrous oxide gas). Sometimes they're burned off with topical medications, like podophyllin or trichloracetic acid, applied two to three times a week for four to six weeks. Experimental drugs, like interferon, have also been used with some success.

Unfortunately, getting rid of the blasted things for good is another matter. Since there is (at least for now) no way of

---

GENITAL WARTS: AT A GLANCE

Problem: The warts are caused by a highly contagious but slow-growing virus that is spread through touch, often during sex.

Symptoms: Genital warts typically show up as small, hard, painless bumps—one or many—on the penis, scrotum, anus or mouth. In uncircumcised men they may appear under the foreskin. Left untreated, they'll gradually develop a fleshy, cauliflower-like appearance.

Cure: There is no medicine yet available to kill the underlying virus. Rather, doctors treat warts by removing them (methods range from cutting them off with lasers to freezing them off with liquid gases).

treating the underlying virus, all treatments amount to simply destroying the warts. But the warts may reappear eventually.

Still, it's important to get the warts removed, not only because your lover may think you're turning into a toad but because they're contagious. You can get HPV simply by touching them. The wart removal process may involve several visits to the doctor, and "it's best to avoid sexual activity during therapy since, because of the nature of the treatment, it would only lead to delayed healing," advises Alan N. Gordon, a gynecologist in Austin, Texas. And if it's you who's being de-wartified, be sure that your sex partner also goes to see a doctor. "At least 60 percent of patients' partners harbor lesions, which, if untreated, may lead to reinfection of the patient," notes Dr. Gordon.

Avoiding an HPV infection in the first place (whether as infector or infectee) is more difficult. Physicians often recommend using condoms, which may help somewhat, depending on the location of the warts. Also, just watch your step: HPV infections are more common in people who have multiple, casual sex partners and don't regularly use contraception.

GONORRHEA
How to Tell If It's "the Clap"

The only good news about gonorrhea is this: It can generally be blasted out of your system with high-powered antibiotics in a couple of weeks or so.

The rest of the news ain't so great. Gonorrhea, if left untreated, can cause nasty infections of the John Robert (such as "urethral stricture," which makes it permanently painful to urinate). It may spread to your joints, heart or brain. It's worse for women: If an infection invades her reproductive system, it can cause pelvic inflammatory disease, which may result in sterility. And babies born to infected women can be blinded by it.

Despite its dangers, though, gonorrhea is still amazingly common, especially among sexually active people under age 25—about a million cases are reported in the United States every year, and at least a million or more go unreported. Though these numbers have dropped a bit since the 1980s, the clap, ancient scourge of sailors on shore leave, is still "a huge medical problem," according to H. Bradford Hawley, M.D., chief of the infectious diseases division at Wright State University School of Medicine in Dayton, Ohio.

To make matters worse, guys who pick up gonorrheal infections don't become immune to future infections (unlike some other diseases). If you don't change your ways, you can just keep on getting it. James Boswell, the celebrated eighteenth-century biographer of Samuel Johnson, was also famous for something else: The poor devil got gonorrhea 12 different times.

The Bug That Does It

The bug that's responsible for all this pain and humiliation is a bacterium called *Neisseria gonorrhoeae*, which has an unnatural fondness for warm, wet, dark places. It flourishes and multiplies in the vagina, cervix or the urinary tract. It can also spread to the throat during oral sex, resulting in an

---

GONORRHEA: AT A GLANCE

Problem: A bacterial infection passed on through sex that, if left untreated, can spread to the joints, heart or brain.

Symptoms: Two to ten days after infection, men often notice a tingling sensation in the penis, then pain and burning during urination. Finally, a greenish, grayish, creamyish discharge begins dripping from the tip of the penis. Twenty to 40 percent of men have no symptoms at all, however.

Cure: Probably a single shot of a new, more powerful antibiotic, plus another antibiotic in pill form for a week.

unpleasant variant of the disease called pharyngeal gonorrhea. Or it can spread to the rectum during certain more
exotic explorations.

To keep from having to learn any more about this miserable
subject, "always practice safe sex: Use condoms and/or spermicides when you have sex, and avoid prostitutes," says Irwin
Goldstein, M.D., professor of urology at Boston University
School of Medicine. Studies have shown that using condoms
during intercourse is a "very effective" way of protecting
yourself from gonorrhea, according to the National Institute
of Allergy and Infectious Diseases in Bethesda, Maryland.
There's also good evidence that using a diaphragm or spermicidal foams, creams and jellies that contain nonoxynol-9
(which is lethal to the bacteria) can also cut your risk of picking up an infection, perhaps by as much as half.

The Deadly Drip

If it's too late for that sort of advice and you've already
picked up gonorrhea from a sex partner, the symptoms will
generally show up two to ten days later. In men the symptoms usually start as a weird tingling sensation in the penis,
followed by pain and burning during urination. After that it
progresses to the "drip"—what Dr. Goldstein describes as "a
colorful discharge that finds its way from the tip of your
penis onto your underwear—it's sort of a greenish, grayish,
creamyish color, and it's often associated with a visit to a
prostitute when you didn't wear a condom." No, you're not
possessed by the devil; it's time to see the doctor. (The
second-century Greek physician Galen actually named the
disease gonorrhea, Latin for "flow of seed," because he
incorrectly thought this vile seepage was semen.)

The great majority of infected men have these symptoms.
They are fairly revolting but also useful: At least you know
you have it. But some men, and most women (80 percent, by
some estimates), will have no symptoms at all until they've
developed more serious complications. This is a good strate-
gic move on the part of *N. gonorrhoeae*, allowing the little
bugger to keep on spreading.

How to Find Out for Sure

If this sounds like what you have, you need to see a doctor right away. Two simple tests can provide a quick, almost-certain answer. The doctor will probably do a Gram's stain test, which involves putting a smear of the discharge on a slide that has been stained with dye, then examining it under a microscope for the presence of gonococcus. It's accurate more than 90 percent of the time in males with symptoms and 50 to 70 percent of the time in males without symptoms. It's also fast—you can usually get an answer before you leave the doctor's office.

Many physicians also like to do a culture test, in which a sample of the discharge is put on a culture plate and "incubated" for at least two days to see what grows. Doing both tests increases the accuracy of the results.

Treatment: An Antibiotic Double Whammy

From ancient times until the end of the eighteenth century, if you'd gone to the doctor for gonorrhea (or syphilis), you'd probably have gotten a good "urethral irrigation"—meaning that the doctor would stick a catheter up your penis and flush it out with bizarre liquids ranging from mild acid to brandy. Mercury, a deadly poison, was also a big favorite, though it tended to make your teeth fall out.

It wasn't until the 1940s, with the introduction of penicillin, that a really effective treatment for gonorrhea (and syphilis) was found. Penicillin and other antibiotics, like tetracycline, ampicillin and amoxicillin, became the mainstays of gonorrhea treatment and are still widely used today. That may be what the doctor gives you.

But chances are you'll be given one of the new, more powerful (and more expensive) antibiotics, like ceftriaxone or cefixime. The reason is that sly strains of gonococcus that have developed a resistance to old-fashioned antibiotics have been discovered around the world. In one study 6,204 gonococcus specimens were tested. Twenty-one percent were resistant to at least one of four kinds of antibiotics (including penicillin and tetracycline)—but all of them were killed by ceftriaxone.

At the moment, the Centers for Disease Control and Prevention in Atlanta recommends this treatment plan: One shot of ceftriaxone (unfortunately, it can only be administered as a shot) plus another broad-spectrum antibiotic, doxycycline, taken in pill form twice a day for a week. The doxycycline is mainly to knock out a different disease, chlamydia, which tends to hitchhike alongside gonococcus—about 45 percent of men who have gonorrhea also have chlamydia.

You should take the full course of antibiotics and go back to the doctor's office for a follow-up visit. And—here's the hardest part of all—you should also let all of your sex partners know about your big news, and they should go get themselves tested even if they have no symptoms at all.

Hey, nobody said life was going to be easy.

HERPES
Separating Hype from Truth

Before AIDS came along, genital herpes was the sexual plague that grabbed all the headlines. Think about it: A highly contagious, incurable, sexually transmitted virus that already infects roughly 30 million Americans and that claims an additional 200,000 hapless new victims every year, according to estimates from the Centers for Disease Control and Prevention (CDC) in Atlanta. That means roughly 16 percent of all U.S. citizens over the age of 15 are now infected.

Yikes!

But what all the scare talk didn't reveal was that for most herpes sufferers, the virus isn't that big of a deal, more of a nuisance than a serious medical problem.

In fact, a huge number of these people are completely

HERPES HOTLINE

The Herpes Resource Center publishes a newsletter full of helpful advice and information called *The Helper.* Contact the Herpes Resource Center, c/o American Social Health Association, P.O. Box 13827, Research Triangle Park, NC 27709; or call (919) 361–8400. They also run a Herpes Hotline at (919) 361–8488.

---

unaware that they're herpes carriers. Problem is, not knowing you have it means not knowing you might be spreading it. Some researchers believe up to 75 percent of new herpes infections are transmitted by people who don't know they're infected.

Think of it in terms of the rule of thirds, explains Charles Ebel, director of the Herpes Resource Center at the American Social Health Association and author of the book *Managing Herpes: How to Live and Love with a Chronic STD*. About a third of the people who have herpes know it. About a third of those who have it don't know it. The remaining third have very mild symptoms—they may think they just caught their penises in a zipper—and may or may not know they're infected. Research suggests that this third group may actually be the largest group of all.

Any way you cut it, if you're sexually active, you have a betting man's chances of tangling with herpes at some point in your career.

How the Virus Works

To clarify, there are actually two types of herpes virus. Type one causes cold sores around the mouth. Type two causes infections in the genital area and is the one usually passed along via sex. Those are not air-tight distinctions, though, because a type-one infection can migrate south to your privates during oral sex, and a type-two infection can migrate north the same way. (There's another kind of herpes, herpes zoster, that causes chicken pox and shingles—but that's a different story.)

Once herpes penetrates your body, it takes up permanent residence, hiding in nerve cells along the lower spinal cord in a place called the sacral ganglia. It can remain dormant for days, weeks, years—even forever. But usually it periodically reappears anywhere from a couple of times a year to once a month or more. Various things can trigger its reappearance—sunlight, fever, drugs, intercourse, even the flu. (Lots of people think stress also triggers herpes outbreaks, but this remains unproven.)

The first outbreak, usually about ten days after exposure, is generally the worst: You may experience flulike symptoms, fever, headache, muscle aches or fatigue. After that, recurrences are usually confined to genital lesions and they usually grow briefer and less severe over time, according to Peter J. Lynch, professor of dermatology at the University of Minnesota in Minneapolis.

HERPES: AT A GLANCE

Problem: A virus (herpes simplex) that takes up permanent residence in your body and causes periodic outbreaks of sores around the genitals. An estimated 30 million Americans have been infected with the herpes simplex virus. There are 200,000 new cases yearly.

Symptoms: The first outbreak is usually the worst. You could experience flulike symptoms, fever, headache, muscle aches or fatigue. After that, recurrences are usually confined to genital lesions, clusters of blisterlike eruptions that are often raw and painful but eventually scab up and heal, usually within ten days.

Cure: There is no known cure. The prescription drug acyclovir (Zovirax), however, greatly reduces the frequency and severity of outbreaks.

Usually, about 12 to 24 hours before a recurrence (the so-called prodrome phase) your body gives warning that the virus is burrowing its way up toward the surface of your skin. You may feel itching, tingling or numbness where the sore is about to appear. Or sometimes people will feel a pain in the leg or buttock, or get a headache or fever.

Then comes the active phase. Clusters of blisterlike eruptions appear on or around the genitals, buttocks or fingers. They're often raw, painful or itchy. It may hurt to urinate. Sometimes the lymph glands in the groin are tender and swollen. Eventually, the blisters burst, crust up and scab over. Then the scab falls off and the skin appears healthy again, at least until the next outbreak.

This whole unpleasant parade of symptoms usually lasts a week to ten days, from the first feeling of itchiness or burning to the disappearance of the sores, Dr. Lynch explains.

The Important Stuff

If you or your lover already have herpes, you're only too familiar with this whole depressing story. The main thing you care about is how to avoid getting infected or infecting your lover without giving up sex altogether.

HOW DO YOU SPELL RELIEF?

- If your herpes sores are painful to the touch, wear loose-fitting clothes and underwear. At home, take the opportunity to be a nudist whenever possible.
- If it hurts to urinate, drink lots of water—that will dilute the urine and make it less painful.
- Take a warm bath or shower three or four times a day.
- Use a blow-dryer, set on low, to dry your privates after a bath or shower.
- Avoid using creams or ointments that keep the area moist (except for herpes creams).

Here's the most important stuff to remember.

• The most common way that genital herpes claims a new victim is when active sores make direct contact with the tender membranes of the vulva, penis, anus or mouth. Not only is this skin particularly soft, but sexual sport opens tiny cuts and abrasions in it, opening a pathway to the bloodstream. So to avoid getting herpes from (or giving herpes to) a lover, avoid direct contact with the sores during an active outbreak. Many physicians recommend avoiding sex altogether during outbreaks. But if that's not possible, just think of creative ways to pleasure one another without touching the sores.

Also, adds Ebel, as far as prevention goes, barrier contraceptives, like condoms, are the best thing we have to offer right now. Again, that's because condoms block direct skin-to-skin contact—but only if the lesions are confined to the penis.

• Don't rely on spermicides. Lab studies have shown that nonoxynol-9, the active ingredient in most spermicides, can destroy the herpes virus by dissolving its protein envelope in the same way it destroys sperm cells. Still, a rough-and-tumble human sexual encounter is much different (and much more interesting) than a lab experiment in a petri dish. There are really no good clinical studies to show that spermicides decrease the rate of infection, says Ebel. So use a spermicide, sure—but always use a condom as well.

• Don't forget that, like any other sexually transmitted disease that causes breaks in the skin, herpes increases your risk of HIV infection. One study of 471 heterosexual men and women, conducted by researchers at the National Institute of Allergy and Infectious Diseases in Bethesda, Maryland, found that those with genital herpes had twice the risk of picking up an HIV infection as those who were not infected.

• Don't forget that herpes can be transmitted even during periods when there are no visible sores at all or symptoms are so mild they're all but unnoticeable. You're not as contagious during these periods of asymptomatic viral shedding, but you're contagious nonetheless.

• During active outbreaks avoid touching the affected area, because you can transmit the virus on your fingers. Wash with soap and water to cleanse skin that's accidentally touched a contagious area.

• Avoid sharing towels or clothes during active outbreaks. It's remotely possible that you could pass the virus on this way.

Estimating the Risk

If you're seriously involved with somebody who has herpes—or you have herpes and are worried about giving your lover an obnoxious, lifetime gift—consider the following study (widely considered one of the best studies on herpes transmission rates to date). For about a year researchers monitored 144 heterosexual, monogamous, mostly white couples in which one partner had herpes and one did not. These were well-informed, conscientious people who took pains to avoid skin-to-skin contact with lesions and did everything else they were supposed to do. Even so, by the end of the study period 14 people were newly infected— roughly a 10 percent annualized risk. In 11 of the 14 cases it was a man who passed it on to a woman, which squares with findings from other studies: Women are roughly three times more likely to get herpes than men.

And in 9 of the 14 couples the uninfected partner got herpes after having sex when the infected partner had no visible sores at all.

The study also showed that condoms really do help—but that they're not perfect. Couples who used barrier contraceptives, like condoms or diaphragms, were less than half as likely to get infected. Still, 1 of the 14 unlucky couples who reported a new herpes infection during the study period also said they faithfully used condoms every time they had sex.

Acyclovir: The Closest Thing to a Cure

Though nobody's come up with a cure for herpes yet, the closest thing so far is the prescription drug acyclovir (Zovirax). It's the only drug approved by the Food and and Drug Administration for the management of herpes and is usually only prescribed to people with frequent outbreaks (usually eight or more a year). For them, though, it can be a godsend by dramatically reducing the frequency and severity of the outbreaks to the point where some guys actually get their sex lives back.

Acyclovir is not cheap. Suppressive therapy (two to four pills a day) can cost up to $100 a month. And though it reduces outbreaks, you'll still be contagious. On the other hand, according to the CDC, daily suppressive therapy reduces the frequency of herpes simplex virus by at least 75 percent among patients with frequent recurrences. It also seems to have very few unwanted side effects.

Which, for lots of guys, is close enough to a cure to declare victory.

SAFER SEX
How to Avoid the AIDS-Causing Virus

Fear of AIDS has transformed sex more completely than Woodstock ever did. Now almost everybody knows somebody who's HIV positive (meaning the person is infected with the virus that leads to AIDS) or has already died from AIDS. And "casual sex"—if there ever really was such a thing—has turned into a potential death sentence, a luscious apple shot through with poison.

The sheer speed of the epidemic's spread has been breathtaking. The first AIDS cases in the United States were only diagnosed in 1981, yet by 1994 over a million Americans were HIV positive and over 220,000 had died of the disease—more than four times the number of Americans killed in Vietnam, according to numbers compiled by the Centers for Disease Control and Prevention (CDC) in Atlanta.

So why does the epidemic continue to spread despite the fact that condoms are handed out on the streets of San Francisco and in the subways of New York City, and "safer sex" is even taught in schools? Because people still aren't listening. Because they're still not using condoms every time. Because sex is a primal force millions of years older than civilization and in the heat of the moment people—even you—may do things you later can't believe you did.

Can You Really Know Your Partner?

Even people who are taking every reasonable precaution may be at risk. Take the advice, routinely handed out by AIDS educators, to "know the people you're sleeping with." Well, at least in theory, that's a good idea. The trouble is that no area of human life is more rife with secrets—and lies—than a person's sexual past.

"When you ask people what they're doing to reduce their risks of getting AIDS, they often say, 'I'm being more careful about who I have sex with.' But this is really very little help because you simply can't tell by looking at someone if they're infected," says Robert Kohmescher, deputy chief of mass media communication development at the CDC's National AIDS Information Program. "After all, how do you think people are getting infected? They're getting infected by having sex with people they think are not infected."

And as time goes by, the chances of meeting somebody nice who's also an HIV carrier get greater: Already, 1 out of every 100 American men and 1 out of every 800 American women is HIV positive, according to the U.S. surgeon general.

In the age of AIDS, unfortunately, suspicion has become a virtue.

A Disease of Conscious Action

But despite all those uncertainties, perhaps the single most important thing to remember is this: AIDS is almost entirely a disease of conscious action. Almost everybody who gets infected does so by means of things they consciously did or did not do. HIV is not wildly contagious, like the flu; you can't get it through casual contact or a mosquito bite. Outside the human body, in fact, the HIV virus dies very quickly. The only way you can get it is through intimate (usually sexual) contact with infected body fluids. Which means that, for the most part, your fate—and your HIV status—is in your own hands. There are really only three ways to get infected with the HIV virus.

Sexual contact involving an exchange of bodily fluids (mainly semen, vaginal secretions or blood). This can be homosexual or heterosexual, vaginal, oral, anal or otherwise. Sexual contact is by far the most common route of transmission—so far over 65 percent of AIDS cases in the United States have been spread this way, according to the CDC.

Birth. Babies born to HIV-infected mothers may become infected before or during birth or through breastfeeding after birth.

Exposure to infected blood. Between 1978 and 1985, when blood screening for HIV was developed, up to 15,000 people got AIDS from transfusions of blood or blood products, according to CDC estimates. Today, though, all donated blood is screened for HIV and other viruses (seven tests are conducted on each sample), and the risk of getting infected this way is extremely low. (There's no risk of getting infected with HIV by giving blood because a new, sterile needle is used for each blood donation.)

Sharing needles or syringes with someone who is HIV positive is a much more effective way to get AIDS because a little bit of infected blood remains on the needle and is passed directly into your bloodstream when you use it. So far about 90,000 Americans have gotten AIDS this way. And don't forget that it's not only junkies who are at risk—any needle you stick in your skin could be dangerous.

"There have been cases of HIV infection by athletes injecting steroids, and we believe it's possible—though there have been no reported cases—of becoming infected via tattooing, acupuncture or ear piercing," says Peter Drotman, M.D., assistant director of the CDC's Public Health Division of HIV/AIDS.

The Riskiest Sex Practices

More specifically, here are the sex practices that are known to increase your risk of getting AIDS, in descending order of risk. (This list is adapted from a list compiled by Robert A. Hatcher, M.D., director of the Emory University Family Planning Program at Emory University School of Medicine in Atlanta, and the other physician-authors of *Contraceptive Technology,* the bible of contraceptive and sexually transmitted diseases (STDs).

• Any "unprotected" sex—meaning sex without a latex condom. Anal sex is especially risky because unlike the vagina, the rectum isn't naturally lubricated, so sexual sport using the anus as a receptacle often causes abrasions that open a doorway directly into the bloodstream.

"Studies provide compelling evidence that latex condoms are highly effective in protecting against HIV infection

---

WOULD I LIE?

If you have any doubt that people will lie like dogs in order to have sex, consider one study of 665 college students conducted by researchers from California State University and the University of California. A third of the guys (34 percent) admitted that at some time in their steamy pasts they had told a lie in order to have sex, and 20 percent said they would lie about HIV tests results in order to get somebody between the sheets. (Women were considerably more likely to be truthful—or so they said.)

"One can probably assume that (these) reports of (the students') own dishonesty underestimate rather than over-estimate the problem," the researchers wrote.

when used properly for every act of intercourse," according to a report from the CDC.

The most impressive evidence comes from studies of couples in which one partner is HIV positive and the other is not. In a European study of 123 such couples who also reported consistent condom use, not one of the uninfected partners became infected. By contrast, among 122 couples who used condoms inconsistently, 12 members became infected.

Remember to use latex condoms (not natural skin condoms, which can be penetrated by HIV) and plenty of lubrication to reduce the chance of breakage. Use only water-based lubricants (like K-Y Jelly; spermicidal creams; lubricants, like Astroglide and Lubafax; or good old saliva). Oil-based lubricants (like petroleum jelly, cold cream, hand lotion, baby oil or vaginal creams, like Monistat or Vagisil) turn latex to goo at an alarming rate. Also remember that other kinds of birth control methods (like the Pill, foams, sponges, IUDs, diaphragms and being sterilized) don't protect you. Only latex condoms help. For more information, see Condoms on page 358.

• Oral sex on a woman when you're not using a dental dam. This is especially risky if she's menstruating or has a vaginal infection with discharge. For protection use a dental dam (a sheet of latex used by dentists for oral surgery) laid over her vagina. Dams are available without a prescription in drugstores and are often displayed near condoms. Some people complain, however, that most of them transmit sensation about as well as an old magazine, so you might want to try an Australian model made specifically for oral sex rather than dental surgery. It's called the Kia-Ora Lollyes dam (Lollyes is an acronym meaning "latex on lips . . . yes") and is available through the Blowfish Catalog. For more information on ordering this catalog, see page 339.

Some people also use clear cellophane food wraps. "Food wraps that are labeled microwavable or microwave-safe should offer some protection against the HIV virus—but they've never been tested in a sexual context, so it's not clear how safe they are," warns Dr. Drotman.

• Oral sex on a man without a latex condom. HIV has been found in high concentrations in semen, and if you have sores or cuts in your mouth, your risk is greatly increased, according to the U.S. surgeon general.

• Semen in the mouth.

• Oral-anal contact.

• Sharing sex toys or douching equipment.

• Any kind of blood contact. That includes contact with menstrual blood, sharing needles or anything that causes tissue damage or bleeding.

• Having an STD that creates sores on your skin, like her-

SHOULD YOU GET TESTED?

If you answer yes to any of the following questions, you could be HIV positive, according to the U.S. surgeon general. Have the guts to get tested.

1. Have you ever had unprotected sex (vaginal, anal or oral) with a man or woman who:
   • You knew was infected with HIV?
   • Injects or has injected drugs?
   • Shared needles with someone who was infected?
   • Had sex with someone who shared needles?
   • Had multiple sex partners?
   • You normally wouldn't have sex with?

2. Have you used needles or syringes that were used by anybody else before you?

3. Have you ever exchanged sex for drugs or money?

4. Did you or any of your sex partners:
   • Receive treatment for hemophilia between 1978 and 1985?
   • Have a blood transfusion or organ transplant between 1978 and 1985?

pes or gonorrhea, also increases your risk of getting HIV because it opens a pathway into your bloodstream.

• Having unprotected sex with multiple partners, especially prostitutes or drug users, because it increases your risk by simple mathematics.

• Being uncircumcised. There's fairly convincing medical evidence that sexually active gay men who are not circumcised are more likely to pick up the AIDS virus—though it's not clear why. Keeping one's foreskin clean may be of some benefit, but the main thing, says Dr. Drotman, "is to use condoms every time you have sex," same as everybody else.

• Wet kissing. HIV has been found in tiny amounts in saliva, so there's at least a theoretical risk of getting infected through open-mouth, French kissing. Because of this possibility, the CDC recommends against it. There's never been a confirmed case, however, of HIV infection contracted this way.

• Vaginal or anal intercourse using a latex condom. Using a spermicide in conjunction with a condom reduces your risk even more. Spermicides have been shown to kill HIV, at least in lab tests. Still, since it's not clear how much protection spermicides actually offer, never use them without a condom as well.

• Oral sex on a man using a latex condom.

• Sports. You can't get HIV through sweat. You can get it through blood, though—so if somebody starts bleeding during a rough scrimmage, get him bandaged and avoid the blood.

Things That Are Safe

• Abstinence. The safest way to avoid getting AIDS is to avoid having sex altogether. (Then again, the best way to avoid death is not to live at all.) The next best thing is to have sex only with one steady, uninfected partner. (Of course, not all of us are so lucky.)

• Casual, nonsexual contact. In 11 studies that investigated more than 700 people who shared a household with

HIV-positive people, no evidence emerged that the virus could be transmitted by casual contact—shaking hands, hugging, dry kissing, sneezing or coughing, swimming together, sharing eating or drinking utensils, eating food handled or prepared by someone who is HIV positive or sharing toilets, bathrooms or kitchens.

Inside the body HIV is savagely virulent; outside the body it quickly dies. CDC studies have shown that 90 to 99 percent of HIV in a solution will die in a couple of hours if allowed to dry out. Also, since it's unable to reproduce outside its living host (unlike many bacteria or fungi), it can't spread or remain infectious outside the body.

• Sexual contact limited to massage, hugging, body rubbing, dry kissing, mutual masturbation or lusting in your heart. Intact skin provides a wonderful barrier between you and the outside world.

If you have close, repeated contact with somebody who is HIV positive, however, be careful. The CDC has reported two cases of apparent HIV transmission through skin or mucous membranes after repeated exposure to infected blood or other body fluids. In one case an HIV-infected mother with extensive and sometimes bleeding skin lesions apparently infected her child. In another an elderly woman apparently became infected while providing daily nursing care (including skin contact with body fluids) for a son with AIDS.

• Contact with saliva, tears or sweat. This has never been shown to result in transmission of HIV, according to the CDC. HIV has never been found in the sweat of HIV-infected people and though it's been found in tiny amounts in both tears and saliva, that doesn't mean it can be transmitted that way.

• Mosquitoes and other insects. This has always been a concern—but after extensive investigation researchers have never been able to show any evidence of transmission by insects. There are a couple of reasons for this. For one thing, when an insect bites a person, it doesn't inject its own or a previous victim's blood into you. Instead, it injects its own saliva, which is not HIV-infected. (Yellow fever and malaria are transmitted through the saliva of certain kinds of mosquitoes; HIV is not.) Second, HIV lives for only a short time inside the insect, so the insect doesn't become infected and transmit the virus to the next human it bites.

THE ANNALS OF IGNORANCE: 1888

Top ten warning signs of excessive masturbation:

1. General feebleness. Emaciation, paleness, colorless lips and gums.

2. Consumption (tuberculosis). Coughing, sore lungs, shortness of breath.

3. Defective development. The "self-abuser" remains physically and mentally small.

4. Sudden change in disposition. When a cheerful, pleasant boy suddenly becomes morose and peevish, it's a dead giveaway that "solitary indulgence" is the cause.

5. Lethargy. Weariness, indifference, dullness and vacantness in the eyes.

6. Insomnia.

7. Stupidity.

8. Fickleness.

9. Untrustworthiness. "A child previously honest will soon become an inveterate liar under its baneful influence."

10. Love of solitude. Very suspicious sign. "The barn, the garret, the water closet and sometimes secluded places in the woods are favorite resorts of masturbators."

—From "Plain Facts for Old and Young" by John Harvey Kellogg, developer of Kellogg's cornflakes, which were originally marketed as antimasturbation food

Getting the Test

If you have any reason to wonder about your HIV status, you really should get the test—for yourself and for everybody else you may want to wake up beside. HIV testing is widely available at community health clinics, doctors' offices and elsewhere. Most publicly funded testing sites are free or charge only a small fee; your doctor may charge up to $200.

Make sure that you understand the confidentiality policies of the center where you get tested. Most centers follow one of two policies: Confidential testing means the center will record your name with the test result. Your name will be kept secret from everybody except medical personnel or in some states the state health department. You should ask who will know the result and how it will be stored.

Anonymous testing (which is not available in all states) is where no one asks your name and you are the only one who can tell anyone else your test result.

If you've had a blood test for a routine physical, a marriage license or insurance—that's not good enough. You need to get a test specifically for HIV infection. Two main tests are used (the enzyme-linked immunosorbent assay (ELISA) and Western blot tests) and taken together; they're extremely accurate—the results are correct more than 99.9 percent of the time, according to the U.S. surgeon general. The tests themselves simply involve drawing a little blood from your arm to be taken to a lab for testing. The results can take anywhere from a few days to a few (very nervous) weeks.

The ELISA test can be performed quickly and easily. If it's positive, the doctor will repeat the test just to make sure. If you get two positives, you'll get a third test, the Western blot, which takes a little longer but is even more specific, to triple-check the first two results.

These tests measure AIDS infection indirectly by detecting antibodies that your body manufactures in response to the HIV virus. It's important to remember, though, that almost everybody develops HIV antibodies within 2 to 12 weeks after infection, but it can take as long as six months. That's why if you did something stupid less than six months before you got tested, there's an off chance you may be infected even though the test result was negative. To be positive, you need to get tested at least six months after doing something you know to be sexually risky.

Belgian researchers reported that they've developed an improved AIDS test that detects the HIV virus itself, not just antibodies to HIV—and provides results in a matter of days, not months. This test might be available to you soon, depending on further testing.

If your test result is negative—hey, go out and tank a cold one. But don't forget that coming up negative on your test doesn't mean that you're immune. Nobody is immune to HIV.

If you have a more specific question that's not answered here or want to find a place near you for confidential HIV testing or counseling, call the CDC National AIDS Hotline at 1-800-342-AIDS. For Spanish speakers call 1-800-344-7432. For the deaf (using TTY/TDD technology) call 1-800-243-7889. For written information contact the CDC National AIDS Clearinghouse, P.O. Box 6003, Rockville, MD 20849.

SYPHILIS
The Ancient Scourge Is Coming Back

Syphilis—a truly odious disease that's haunted the human race since at least 2000 B.C.—has made an amazing comeback. According to the National Institutes of Health in Bethesda, Maryland, about 40,000 cases of early-stage syphilis are reported in the United States every year and at least 50,000 more go unreported. Those are the biggest numbers since 1950.

These numbers are worrisome because syphilis can be a devastating disease all by itself and because there's reason to

SYPHILIS: AT A GLANCE

Problem: A bacterial infection passed on through sex that causes hard-to-diagnose sores and rashes and, if left untreated, can cause serious long-term problems.

Symptoms: Untreated syphilis passes through four stages.

1. *Primary—A hard, red, usually painless pimple, or chancre, appears at the site of exposure, usually on the genitals or around the rectum. The chancre generally has a moist, clear center surrounded by hard, raised edges.*
2. *Secondary—A measleslike rash appears on the palms, soles of the feet, genitals, underarms or elsewhere. Also, flulike symptoms appear.*
3. *Latent—All symptoms vanish, sometimes for decades.*
4. *Late—Severe numbness, loss of bladder control, blindness or death.*

Cure: *Treated with antibiotics, most likely penicillin. Early detection means easy cure.*

believe that people with syphilis are also more likely to pick up the HIV virus. Syphilis causes open sores, or lesions, on the skin, and it's well-known that any break in the skin opens the pathway for the HIV virus to enter your body. Several studies in Africa and the United States suggest that having syphilis makes you more prone to HIV infection. The Centers for Disease Control and Prevention in Atlanta recommends that people with newly diagnosed syphilis also have an HIV test.

Still, there are several reasons to be optimistic about this rather dismal-sounding story. First, even with the increase, syphilis is really not all that common. It's far less common than gonorrhea (possibly two million cases a year) or chlamydia, the most common sexually transmitted disease (four million cases or more a year).

Second, if it's diagnosed and treated early, a couple of shots of benzathine penicillin will generally blast syphilis out of your system. (If you're allergic to penicillin, other antibiotics, like tetracycline or doxycycline, will usually do the trick.)

And third, it's not all that difficult to avoid getting the disease in the first place. Avoid cozying up to anybody who has sores on or around their genitals, because that's the way syphilis is usually spread. Limit your sex partners and use condoms and spermicides, which can reduce your chances of picking it up. It's hard to get syphilis in any way except through sex. Outside the body the bacterium that causes the disease is very fragile, so it's nearly impossible to pick it up by contact with toilet seats, towels or other inanimate objects, according to the National Institute of Allergy and Infectious Diseases in Bethesda, Maryland.

A Quick-Moving Bacteria

Syphilis is caused by a corkscrew-shaped bacterium called *Treponema pallidum*. These insidious little buggers generally find their way into a new host when a person makes direct contact with the open lesions of an infected sex partner. Once *T. pallidum* gains entry to your bloodstream, it spreads throughout your body in a matter of hours.

After that, if the disease is not treated, it typically passes through four predictable stages.

Primary: The first symptom is a dull red spot that turns into a hard, red pimple, or chancre. It's usually painless and generally shows up ten days to three months after your first exposure to *T. pallidum.* Because the disease is generally transmitted through a romp in the hay, the chancre is most often found on the genitals or around the rectum. It can also appear on the lips, tongue or tonsils, the eyelids or the fingers. Gradually, the chancre turns into a clear pustule (which may exude highly infectious fluid) surrounded by hard, raised edges. Your lymph glands may also become swollen. (You can tell the difference between syphilis sores and those caused by herpes—which are far more common—by three signs: Herpes sores are usually painful, they come in clusters rather than singly and they look like little fluid-filled blisters rather than pimples.)

Secondary: The chance usually goes away in three to six weeks. But it's not gone. Anywhere from two weeks to three months later you'll develop a highly infectious skin rash. Sometimes it covers the whole body, but usually it's confined to the palms, soles of the feet or warm, moist places, like the genitals or underarms. You may also develop flulike symptoms—fever, fatigue, headache, sore throat, nausea, weight loss. All this stuff looks like any number of other things (the flu, an allergic reaction, measles, even sunburn), which is why syphilis is sometimes called the great imitator. These symptoms can last up to two years.

15 FAMOUS MEN WHO HAD SYPHILIS

1. Al Capone, gangster
2. Woodrow Wilson, U.S. president
3. Adolf Hitler, German leader
4. Vincent van Gogh, Dutch painter
5. Ludwig van Beethoven, German composer
6. Christopher Columbus, Italian explorer
7. George Armstrong Custer, U.S. Army officer
8. Henry VIII, King of England
9. Benito Mussolini, Italian leader
10. John Donne, English poet
11. Napoleon, French emperor
12. Paul Gauguin, French artist
13. "Wild Bill" Hickok, U.S. lawman
14. Charles Baudelaire, French poet
15. Ferdinand Magellan, Portuguese explorer

During these first two stages you can continue to infect other people.

Latent: The symptoms disappear completely. But once again, the disease is still there. People can walk around with latent syphilis for as long as 40 years with no apparent ill effects. Which wouldn't be a problem except that for about one-third of these people the disease will progress to its final, most malicious stage.

Late: When people talk about "the wages of sin," this must be it. In tertiary or late-stage syphilis the bacteria can attack any organ, including the heart, brain, central nervous system, bones, joints or liver. The results of this internal devastation may range from severe numbness to loss of bladder control, blindness, insanity or death.

One additional danger: If a pregnant woman gets infected with *T. pallidum,* she can transmit the disease to her fetus. The toll of this "congenital syphilis" is terrible: Forty percent of these babies die.

Diagnosis: Two Simple Tests

Any time you develop a suspicious rash or sore around the genitals, you should see a doctor. But sometimes even doctors have trouble identifying syphilis, partly because it's still relatively uncommon (many doctors have never seen it) and partly because there are other, more likely explanations for a genital sore (like herpes). In one study in Detroit, in fact, physicians failed to correctly identify primary syphilis lesions in 22 percent of cases.

This is why it's important to get a lab test to positively identify the enemy. Two tests are commonly used for syphilis—the Venereal Disease Research Laboratory (VDRL) test and the rapid plasma reagin test. Both of these tests detect antibodies (*T. pallidum*-fighting proteins) in the blood. Neither one is perfect but they're both fairly reliable. According to one study, the VDRL test is almost 100 percent accurate if given during secondary-stage syphilis (though less accurate during primary, latent or late stages).

The Beauty of Penicillin

In the early stages of syphilis infection one shot of benzathine penicillin will usually cure you. If you've been infected a year or more, a couple of shots spread out over three weeks is usually enough to do it. If you're allergic to penicillin, other antibiotics, like tetracycline or doxycycline, are next best and almost equally effective. Again, the length of treatment depends on how long you've been infected—if less than a year, you may have to take doxycycline for 15 days; otherwise, 30 days, according to *Contraceptive Technology,* the bible of sexual diseases and contraception.

It's important to remember that syphilis is quite treatable in the early stages, but once it has progressed to the late-stage disease, it's too late to reverse much of the damage. So don't wait around; if you have a suspicious genital sore, have it looked at right away.

If it is syphilis, all you have to suffer through is a shot or two. If you'd gotten syphilis back in 1892, you'd probably have been treated with mercury or arsenic, both of which are deadly poisons. Or consider this fiendish treatment, which

---

THE ANNALS OF IGNORANCE: 1925

Personally, although I do not believe in frightening anybody over sex matters, I feel it permissible to show photographs of the hideous condition of rottenness into which the victims of venereal disease descend. Show them pictures of people with heads half eaten away with sores and germs, and bodies crumbling away with syphilis. It will make them feel ill and sick for a day or two, but they will never forget the danger, and they will steer as clear of it as they can.

—From *A Complete Book of Sex Knowledge* by Bernard Bernard, D.Sc., editor, author, philosopher, scientist, idealist and champion athlete

actually worked (sort of) and won its inventor a Nobel prize in 1927: Infect the patient with malaria so that they develop a fever that remains greater than 101°F for 60 to 70 hours, and 104° to 106° for 70 percent of that time. If the malaria "burns out" too soon, reintroduce the fever with an intravenous of undiluted typhoid. A few guys were actually cured of syphilis this way, though about 13 percent died of malaria.

URETHRITIS
When Something Gets in the Plumbing

The urethra is the dark, narrow pipeline through which urine and semen exit the tip of your penis. Because it's warm, moist and cozy, and during intercourse opens directly into one of life's most interesting places, it's also the place where most genital infections get started in a guy, according to William R. Bowie, M.D., of the Division of Infectious Diseases, Department of Medicine, at the University of British Columbia in Vancouver.

Any infection and/or inflammation of the urethra is called urethritis. If the doctor is able to rule out gonorrhea, one of the most common causes of urethritis, it's known as nongonococcal urethritis, or NGU. If the doctor hasn't the foggiest idea what's causing it, but still needs a fancy name to describe it, he will call it nonspecific urethritis.

The good part: "Today, nonspecific urethritis is really quite treatable," says Irwin Goldstein, M.D., professor of urology at Boston University School of Medicine.

Whatever the cause, typical symptoms of urethritis include:

- Puslike discharge. Sometimes this pus isn't visible at all until the penis is "milked" (in a motion similar to masturbation). Or it may range from a slight drip noticeable only in the morning to a truly revolting, copious yellow or green ooze. "The more pronounced the discharge and the more acute the symptoms, the greater the likelihood of gonorrhea," notes Dr. Bowie. (One other clue is that if it's gonorrhea, it will usually produce symptoms within a week after your roll in the hay with an infected sex partner. NGU usually doesn't show up for two to three weeks afterward or sometimes much longer.)

- A burning sensation during urination.
- Itching in the urethra at other times.
- No symptoms at all. A fair number of men may be completely asymptomatic. In that case the infection is detectable only through lab tests—yet you can still infect your sex partner, who may develop nasty symptoms.

Which Bugs to Blame

If you notice any of these symptoms, it's time to go see a doctor. The physician will take a sample of the discharge (sometimes, unfortunately, by slipping a tiny swab up into your urethra, which may briefly turn you into a soprano). Then the discharge is either stained and examined under a

---

URETHRITIS: AT A GLANCE

Problem: A bacterial infection of the tube in your penis through which semen and urine leave the body. Any number of bacterial types could be the culprit.

Symptoms: Puslike discharge, pain during urination or an itch in the penis. Symptoms that are not typical of urethritis and may indicate something else (like epididymitis or prostatitis) include blood in the urine, chills or fever, an altered pattern of urine (increased frequency or urgency or urination during the night), altered urine stream or changed color of ejaculate.

Cure: Treatment with antibiotics works in most cases, though occasionally men suffer from longer-term infections that are harder to kill.

microscope (the Gram stain test) or allowed to grow for a few days in a lab dish (culturing).

In men the two most common bacteria responsible for urethritis are *Neisseria gonorrhoeae* (which causes gonorrhea) and *Chlamydia trachomatis* (which causes chlamydia). Very often, a guy who is carrying one of these infections will also be carrying the other—in one study 15 to 25 percent of heterosexual men with gonorrhea also had chlamydia. Because of this, the Centers for Disease Control and Prevention (CDC) in Atlanta now recommend a treatment plan that will knock out both of these buggers. A single shot of the high-powered antibiotic ceftriaxone, for instance, will often do the trick. For more information, see Chlamydia on page 493 and Gonorrhea on page 503.

Urethritis caused by something other than gonorrhea is actually far more common than gonorrhea urethritis, according to Dr. Bowie. *Ureaplasma urealyticum,* another common sexually transmitted microorganism, turns out to be responsible in 40 to 50 percent of men with NGU. Less commonly, the bugger will turn out to be *Trichomonas vaginalis,* a protozoan that causes foul-smelling vaginal infections. Sometimes herpes simplex is to blame. But all too frequently the culprit is never identified.

The Ones That Won't Go Away

The bottom line is that urethritis is a pain but it's usually not that serious. And it's usually not all that hard to wipe out with a week's worth of antibiotics, like erythromycin, tetracycline or doxycycline.

New, turbocharged antibiotics may also work—with only a single dose. In one Norwegian study of 130 men with chlamydial urethritis, one 1,000-milligram dose of the new antibiotic azithromycin proved to be just as effective as taking doxycycline twice a day for a week.

If your doctor identifies gonorrhea or chlamydia as the cause of your urethritis and you take your antibiotics like you're supposed to and refrain from sex until the treatment is over, it's extremely unlikely that you won't be cured. (The

CDC also suggests that you have your sex partner checked out if you noticed symptoms within 30 days after your last sexual contact. You should also abstain from intercourse at least until your partner has been treated.)

If it's NGU you have, 95 percent of men show partial or complete improvement after treatment. Unfortunately, up to 40 percent of these guys will start having symptoms again within six weeks.

"Sometimes these infections will retreat into the epididymis or the prostate or glands inside the urethra and they're a little difficult to get to—we may have to recommend a several-month course of antibiotics in stubborn cases," Dr. Goldstein says.

This second, longer course of treatment generally knocks out the infection in all but around 25 percent of men. For the small, hassled, hard-core group of guys who can't seem to get any relief, there's at least some comforting news, Dr. Bowie says. Though in the great majority of these cases the culprit is never identified, these mysterious infections will eventually just fade away by themselves (though there's no telling how soon). It's extremely unlikely that there will be any long-term damage (like infertility).

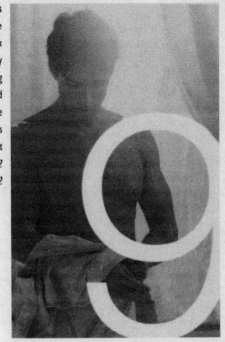

ARE WE REALLY
THAT BAD?

AFFAIRS
Why We Do It, Why We Shouldn't

Men cheat on their spouses more frequently than women, have more extramarital partners than women and do it earlier in their marriages. Men are also more likely than women to believe that extramarital sex is justified and report less guilt about it. That's what the vast sociological literature on the subject shows. You may assume it's true.

Sure, the numbers vary. A 1993 study conducted by the National Opinion Research Center showed that 21 percent of men and 13 percent of women had had an affair; another survey conducted by *Psychology Today* reported that 40 percent of married men and 31 percent of married women had been unfaithful. Other studies have come up with higher (or lower) numbers.

Well, whatever the exact figures are, one thing is clear: Adultery happens. In her book *Anatomy of Love*, Helen Fisher, Ph.D., an anthropologist at the American Museum of Natural History in New York City, writes of reading about 42 societal groupings from all over the world, and adultery occurred in every one. Some of these people were rich, some poor; some espoused Christianity, others worshiped the rocks and trees; some farmed rice, some took the Metroliner to work. But regardless of their traditions of marriage, despite their customs of divorce, irrespective of any of their cultural mores about sex, they all exhibited adulterous behavior—even where adultery was punished by death.

Even disapproving of affairs is no great help, it seems. One study found that although 75 to 90 percent of people surveyed thought extramarital relationships were wrong, 30 to 60 percent of the men and 20 to 50 percent of the women had had one anyhow.

So . . . what does that mean?

That people—especially men—are born to be wild?

The Selfish Gene

Well, yes—at least men are. That's the basic answer the late Dr. Alfred C. Kinsey came up with after surveying thousands of men and women back in the 1940s and 1950s: "There seems to be no question but that the human male would be promiscuous in his choice of sexual partners throughout the whole of his life if there were no social restrictions. . . . The human female is much less interested in a variety of partners."

That's also the answer you tend to get from evolutionary psychology, a relatively new field that looks for clues to our innate sexual nature by studying how our physical bodies and our mating behavior have been shaped by evolution over the past few million years.

For instance, consider the big balls theory. In his book *The Evolution of Desire*, evolutionary psychologist David M. Buss, a psychology professor at the University of Michigan in Ann Arbor, makes a case for the idea that man's polygamous nature is built right into our bodies—in the form of our testicles.

Among primates, he explains, testicles increase in size as a result of intense sperm competition, where sperm from two or more males may occupy the reproductive tract of a female at the same time. If you have bigger testicles than the guy who slept with her yesterday, you produce more ejaculate and thus your sperm is more likely to win out, fertilize her egg and ensure that your genes are passed on to the next generation. Chimpanzees, who are extremely promiscuous, have a three times higher testes-to-body-weight ratio than humans. But humans have much larger testicles (relative to body weight) than gorillas and orangutans. Hence, men's relatively large testicles provide one solid

> When two people make love, there are at least four people present—the two who are actually there and the two they are thinking about.
>
> —Sigmund Freud

piece of evidence that women in human evolutionary history sometimes had sex with more than one man within a time span of a few days. (The expression big balls, a reference to male strength and dominance common in many cultures, may refer to this, Buss says.)

More fundamentally, these thinkers argue, the central Darwinian goal of all organisms is to disperse their genes to the next generation and to do so as widely as possible. For a woman to pass her genes on by having a child involves an enormous parental investment of time and energy: nine months of pregnancy, perhaps years of breastfeeding, then decades of dirty socks and school lunches. So women's best "mating strategy" is to find a mate who will stick around long enough to ensure that the children who bear her genes will survive to adulthood. Hence her concern about commitment and relative lack of interest in short-term affairs.

A man, by contrast, requires a far lower investment in order to pass on his genes—possibly as little as a ten-minute roll in the hay. So the best way for a man to bequeath his genetic legacy to the next generation is to mate with as many women as possible and spend as little time with each as possible. Male promiscuity, they argue, is simply a primal instinct that reflects nature's attempt to maximize reproduction. And that's why, in virtually every culture ever studied, guys tend to fool around more than women do. For more information, see Evolution of Sex on page 29.

Why It's a Bad Idea Anyhow

Of course, we're not just gene-making machines at the mercy of biology. The evolutionary-psychology argument is just the latest take on what makes men and women so different, based on physiological developments that occurred long before mankind was civilized.

In practice, having an affair turns out to be a genuinely lousy idea most of the time. Why? Simple: It'll screw up your marriage and screw up your children, says Frank Pittman, M.D., an Atlanta psychiatrist and author of *Private Lies*, a book about affairs. "In the last 30 years of treating troubled marriages, I've only seen a handful of divorces that occurred when no one had been screwing around. This is important: The likelihood of an established first marriage ending in divorce is minimal unless someone has had an affair."

Here are a couple of other reasons why it's a bad idea.

Sex wrecks friendships. In an examination of 100 of his clients who'd had affairs (60 men, 40 women), Dr. Pittman found that only 10 were in sexually dead marriages, but 30 of them complained that they felt little or no intimacy with their spouses. Affairs were thus three times more likely to be the pursuit of a buddy than the pursuit of a better orgasm, he says. What is so sad, and seems so foolish about affairs, is that many of them might have been wonderful, utterly unthreatening friendships had they not been so naively sexualized.

> The possession of many wives does not always prevent their entertaining desires for the wives of others. It is with lust as with avarice, whose thirst increases by the acquisition of treasures.
>
> —Montesquieu

The sex is no better. One amazing thing he's noticed, Dr. Pittman says, is that even though it's usually assumed that affairs are about sex and that the affairee is irresistible in bed, "It is about as common for the infidel to acknowledge that the sex was better at home." And though you'd think that guys betray their marriages only for babes who look like Julia Roberts, "I have certainly not found a pattern of affair partners being better-looking than marriage partners," he says. "The main thing is that the affair partner is just different than the spouse."

It won't fix your marriage. Some guys believe that an affair is a good way to revive a dull marriage or to fix some problem in it. But "to have an affair in order to trigger a crisis from which the marriage might eventually benefit is truly a screwball, convoluted approach to problem solving," says Dr. Pittman. "Sometimes a guy will have an affair to avoid a divorce—his sexual needs are not being met, but he thinks it would be bad for the kids for him to split up with his wife. So he goes on the hunt. But an affair won't help a shaky marriage—it almost always makes it worse."

It's expensive. Since most of the time it's the guy who pays for the dates, dinners and hotel rooms, affairs can wind up being amazingly expensive, says Alvin Baraff, Ph.D., founder of MenCenter, a psychotherapy practice in Washington, D.C. That's one thing that surprised him when he began counseling philandering men. The other surprising thing is how quickly affairs lose their glitter and fun and how soon the men wanted to get out of them. "I've heard lots of horror stories about men trying to break off affairs."

Uh, like, death. Besides being the most universally accepted justification for divorce, infidelity "is even a legally accepted justification for murder in some states and many societies," Dr. Pittman points out helpfully.

If you're worried about what you've gotten yourself into—or might get yourself into—it's important to find the right person to talk to, Dr. Pittman says. If you value your marriage, see a marriage counselor or a couples therapist (a psychotherapist may be more inclined to encourage you to leave the relationship for your own personal betterment). For a list of marriage therapists in your area, write to the American Association for Marriage and Family Therapy, 1133 15th St. NW, Suite 300, Washington, D.C. 20005.

To get better, you'll have to work. You may also have to give up your secrets. Therapists differ on whether or not long-dead affairs need to be admitted to and re-examined, but there's no question that current ones will need to be revealed—and the affair will have to end—before the magic of couples therapy can work.

DATE RAPE
Some Real-World Guidelines

Does "no" always mean "no"? If it does, there are an awful lot of confused men out there.

One of our *Men's Health* surveys asked the question, "When a woman says no to a sexual advance, do you think she always means it?" Our respondents split right down the middle. Half of them said yes, *of course* she means it. The other half said of course she *doesn't* always mean it.

Please do not assume that half of our respondents are serial rapists. They all know—at least they profess to know—when she really means it. Everyone seems to agree that, as one guy said, "It depends on how she says no." It also very much depends upon who's asking. As another respondent put it, "For the two-drinks-and-let's-do-it guy, no doesn't mean no."

But when men try to explain why a woman would say no but mean yes, they sound like a bunch of physicists theorizing about subatomic particles. Apparently, there are a great many schools of thought on the matter. Like:

The who's-in-charge-here school—"She wants to let you know that she is in control."

The this-is-only-a-test school—"Some women want to see what type of person you are."

"It may be a test to determine a person's character."

The slow-down-pal school—"Women want to be courted."

"They want us to charm and caress them."

"Haven't you ever heard of foreplay?"

The coy-mistress school—"She wants to be pursued."

"Sometimes they like to play hard-to-get."

"Their upbringing—they were taught to say no."

"They don't want to appear 'easy and sleazy.' "

The bang-up-and-try-again-in-five-minutes school—"Her emotions are not ready to say yes yet."

"She may just want you to try to turn her on."

"She's just making the sexual contact more intense."

The hang-up-and-she'll-call-you school—"There have been many times I have backed off because of the word 'no' and five minutes later she is undressing me."

"I have had a woman say no, then yes ten minutes later."

The bitter-resentful-rhymes-with-witch school—"Most women like to tease men."

"They just like to jerk you around."

"If she doesn't mean it, then she's playing a game—and if I play, I could go to jail."

Finally, here's one fellow's rather original axiom for navigating this very, very slippery terrain: "One no means nothing, but two means stop immediately."

When No Means Yes, and Why

"No Means No" has been a key slogan of rape awareness advocates and campus Take Back the Night marches. But as anything more than a rallying cry, it does a disservice to men and women. First of all, many women admit to saying no when they mean yes. Second of all, there's no such thing as date rape—only rape. Rape requires force. And despite the long, sad history of misunderstanding between the sexes at critical moments, rape is not simply a failure to communicate. It's a criminal combination of sex and violence, arousal and hostility, that is egged on by peers, pigheaded clichés and alcohol.

These are some of the conclusions reached by Lance Shotland, Ph.D., professor of psychology at Pennsylvania State University in University Park, who has been studying courtship behaviors for 20 years and has done some of the pivotal work in the field.

Dr. Shotland theorizes that once a couple is alone and nuzzling, either partner can make a variety of responses to the mate's advances: token resistance (saying no but meaning yes), uncertainty (saying no but meaning maybe), compliance (saying yes but not really wanting to) and resistance (saying no and meaning exactly that).

In his latest work he polled 378 women taking an introductory psychology course at Pennsylvania State University. They filled out a 128-item questionnaire. Early on, they were posed this scenario and asked how many times they'd been there: "You were with a guy who wanted to engage in intercourse, and you wanted to also, but for some reason you indicated that you didn't want to, although you had every intention to and were willing to engage in sexual intercourse. In other words, you indicated no and meant yes."

About 37 percent of the women said they've been there, done that. That figure is highly consistent with what other researchers have found—among college underclassmen, mind you, most of whom are just embarking on the prerogatives of adulthood. One might venture to say that the majority of women have been ambivalent at some point in their love lives.

But it must be emphasized that women don't make a habit of this. So let's not start making dark generalizations, okay? The vast majority recalled one to five incidents, at most. Moreover, token resistance doesn't just occur "out of the blue," but for a very plausible reason at a very particular time in the relationship. Every one of these 141 women didn't engage in token resistance until on or after the 11th date with the guy. Furthermore, 70 percent of them had not yet had intercourse with their dates. The scene that emerges is this: A woman has been dating the same guy for months, they're messing around one day, some of her clothing is off and she's sexually aroused. She says no but means yes because she's in the process of changing her mind. She's getting to yes.

Men engage in token resistance, too. Several surveys—including ours—show that men say no but mean yes at least as often as women. Or say yes and mean no. And the surveys also show that some women don't take no for an answer. In studies of long-term relationships both men and women take turns at being reluctant, compliant and successful in finally arousing their partners. Gender differences all but disappear in this regard. Both sexes comply with a partner's greater arousal simply because they are eager to maintain the relationship. Psychologists say that people view an exclusive romantic relationship of any duration as an implicit deal: Fidelity is exchanged for availability. One of our survey respondents said, "It took a long time to recover from all the times my ex-wife said no. After remarrying, I wouldn't dream of saying no to my wife. No is very painful."

The 378 Penn State women told Dr. Shotland and his colleagues that they were saying no for three sorts of reasons—

they were manipulating the situation, they were worried about practical repercussions ("I might get pregnant.") or they were inhibited for moral or personal reasons. At the moment they were saying no, they meant no, says Dr. Shotland—but later on they agreed to sex, and only because of a process called memory consolidation do they recall saying no but meaning yes. The much smaller group of women who did it to manipulate were engaging in true token resistance—saying no and meaning yes at the same moment. They were much more likely to have

> If our elaborate and dominating bodies are given to be denied at every turn, if our nature is always wrong and wicked, how ineffectual we are—like fishes not meant to swim.
>
> —Cyril Connolly,
> "The Unquiet Grave"

begun a full sexual relationship with the guy already and were saying no for sexual reasons. Their biggest reason, by far, for token resistance: "I wanted to be in control—the one to say when." Other reasons: "I wanted to get him more aroused," "I was angry with him," "I wanted him to beg."

Maybe our survey respondents aren't so clueless after all.

The Truth about Rape

Of the 378 Penn State women, 87.3 percent said they'd said no and meant no at least once in their young lives, meaning that virtually all of them had experience in parrying an unwanted advance. Unfortunately, experience doesn't always count. How many college women are date-rape victims? Many figures are bandied about. "Right now the best answer we have is 15 percent," says Dr. Shotland.

If you're like us, you say to yourself, I don't do this. The guys I know wouldn't do this. Who's doing this? Research is helping to answer that question. Rape isn't purely random; not all men are potential rapists. "To some degree, rapists are a different breed," says Dr. Shotland. They are highly promiscuous and highly hostile. His latest work finds

TO BE A HARVARD MAN

The Faculty of Arts and Sciences will not tolerate sexual misconduct, including rape and sexual assault, whether affecting a man or a woman, perpetrated by an acquaintance or a stranger, by someone of the same sex or someone of the opposite sex.

Rape includes any act of sexual intercourse that takes place against a person's will or that is accompanied by physical coercion or the threat of bodily injury. Unwillingness may be expressed verbally or physically. Rape may also include intercourse with a person who is incapable of expressing unwillingness or is prevented from resisting as a result of conditions including, but not limited to, those caused by the intake of alcohol or drugs.

Being intoxicated does not diminish a student's responsibility in perpetrating rape, sexual assault or other sexual misconduct.

Harvard University Policy Statement on Rape

May 1993

---

that roughly 60 percent of date rapes occur within the first two or three dates. Dr. Shotland has a theory about the rapists in these cases. They are basically young sociopaths, with histories of antisocial and misogynist actions and attitudes. They may actually think that any woman who agrees to a date is automatically agreeing to have sex, or they may think that "all's fair," and they can employ any combination of sneakiness and/or force to achieve that end. They might even be capable of raping total strangers but hide behind the guise of a date, like a wolf in sheep's clothing.

In sum, this guy isn't misunderstanding women. He has no intention of understanding women. His sexual aggression knows no bounds.

The Gray Area between True and False

The legal definitions of rape vary slightly from state to state, but they all turn on the issue of force and nonconsent. Legally, men are expected to take no for an answer. Even the lack of a yes can mean no. A woman does not have to resist to be raped if the prosecution can show she was sufficiently threatened by force into not resisting. A New Jersey Supreme Court ruling went so far as to maintain that there was "no burden on the alleged victim to

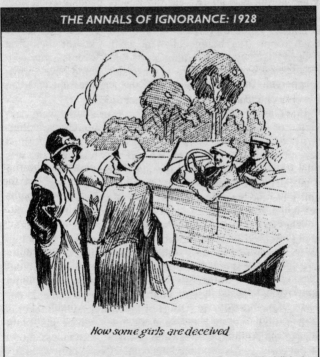

THE ANNALS OF IGNORANCE: 1928

How some girls are deceived

—From *Safe Counsel* by B. G. Jefferis, M.D., and J. L. Nichols, 39th edition, Intext Press

have expressed nonconsent or to have denied permission."

Then what is date rape? Date rape is the gray area, the big, fuzzy zone in which juries fear to tread. When two people know each other, and she says she was forced but he says she agreed, it's just her word against his. He said, she said. That makes it difficult for a jury to decide who's telling the truth.

A Florida jury, for instance, decided to believe William Kennedy Smith when he was charged with raping Patricia Bowman after meeting her in a bar one night. But an Indiana jury did not believe Mike Tyson. His accuser, Desiree Washington, was an 18-year-old beauty pageant contestant and Sunday school teacher less than half his size. Tyson's defenders noted that Washington willingly went up to his hotel room after being called at 1:30 A.M. for their first "date." His lawyers also maintained that Tyson is a guy who paws every woman he sees—and so she should have known better. But does all that mean she wasn't raped? Even Tyson's chauffeur that night took her side.

In a Glen Ridge, New Jersey, case four youths were convicted of raping a 17-year-old girl, even though she voluntarily accompanied them to a basement and performed several sexual acts. You see, the girl was retarded; she was functionally an 8-year-old. So, in addition to being guilty of a morally repugnant deed, a jury found these four fellows guilty of rape because she was incapable of valid consent. A yes under those circumstances clearly does not count.

Whether or not you get hauled into court on charges, being accused of date rape can jeopardize your academic career if you're a college student. Most colleges have date-rape policies that call for suspension or expulsion regardless of legal action. (Some colleges have been sued for pursuing these cases because they inevitably fail to protect the defendant's rights as fully as a court of law.) In academia there is such a thing as date rape—and the rules can be just plain bizarre. At Antioch College the political-correctness mood of the early 1990s produced a sexual-offense policy requiring that men ask women for explicit consent every step of the way. "May I undo your bra?" "May I kiss your breast?" "May I touch you there?" How silly. How sad.

Can't We All Get Along?

You don't have to attend Antioch to fear that a yes the night before will somehow become a no the morning after. Despite what feminists would have you believe, false rape allegations are not uncommon. One study of all rape charges reported in a Midwestern city of 70,000 during a nine-year period found that 41 percent of them turned out to be false!

This unnamed city was no crime mecca, so the police department had the ability to thoroughly investigate all such charges. Furthermore, a rape charge could be deemed false only if the complainant recanted—that is, if she herself said she'd made it all up. Which is what 41 percent of them actually did after undergoing both a hospital exam and a polygraph (lie detector) test. Many of the women lied to get an alibi because they worried about being pregnant—and not by their husbands. Others did it to gain revenge—they were spurned by a man or found out that he'd bragged about their little tryst. But despite the male myth, nobody cried "rape" to extort money.

Subsequent studies of police records of all rape complaints brought during the preceding three years at two Midwestern state universities found exactly half were later recanted. The author of the studies, Eugene Kanin, Ph.D., is professor emeritus of sociology at Purdue University in West Lafayette, Indiana. He told us his paper presenting this research was so controversial that it had been turned down at two scholarly journals before being accepted by the *Archives of Sexual Behavior*.

There's really nothing you can do to protect yourself against false charges, says Dr. Kanin, "except, don't be a dope." And keep your pants up. These are big risks for men who take the Playboy philosophy a tad too far. Casual sex is dangerous. A century ago you would have worried about being tracked down by a furious brother. Today you have to worry about being tracked down by a furious lawyer.

In a way, this is the same message Camille Paglia delivers to women. Paglia, the author of *Sexual Personae*, has criticized academic feminists for misleading a generation of young women about the inherently problematic nature of sex. "Feminism keeps saying the sexes are the same," she has written. "It keeps telling women they can do anything, go anywhere, say anything, wear anything. No, they can't. Women will always be in sexual danger. . . . There never was and never will be sexual harmony."

Other cultures at other times have dealt with sexual dangers by imposing veils, chaperones or curfews. Only in America in the 1990s would a young woman wander into a fraternity party by herself, get drunk, go upstairs with a guy and then be shocked by a cruel turn of events. Such a young woman, says Paglia, "is an idiot. Feminists call this perspective 'blaming the victim.' I call it common sense."

Even the incorrigible womanizer Sam Malone, Ted Danson's character on *Cheers*, was scripted not to take on a drunken Kirstie Alley after pursuing her so ardently for so many episodes. Let's pride ourselves on being gentlemen, not predators. Let's incorporate into who we are, sexually, the quality of our amorousness, not the quantity of our encounters. And let's be proud of our values so that we don't inadvertently contribute to any pigheaded notions about women deserving what they get.

Then we'll have nothing to worry about.

Likewise, the women we date.

LOVE AND SEX
Men Separate the Two . . . or Do They?

It's hardly news, but we'll mention it again: There's a whole lot of confusion between men and women about whether sex and love are the same or different, or sometimes the same and sometimes different—or something else entirely. A thousand movies, ten thousand novels and millions of really screwed-up relationships have struggled with this bedeviling question.

The usual rap against men, of course, is that we separate love from sex. That we are capable of having sex with somebody we barely know, just so long as she has terrific, er, legs. Women, by contrast, are said to need some kind of emotional connection with a man before they're willing to connect in the flesh. In barroom discussions of these great issues, this perception is generally reduced to: Women give sex to get love; men give love to get sex.

But, of course, nothing's ever quite that simple.

"My wife does not understand why every tender moment with me leads to sex, nor does she understand why I am lustful when making love—to her it seems that I am very selfish," a 40-year-old medical transcriber wrote us as part of our *Men's Health* magazine survey. "She makes me crazy when we are in bed or elsewhere—she has a knockout rear end and I want to have her when I want to have her, but it is because I love her that I want her so badly sometimes. Maybe I do get lustful, but no other woman does that to me and this is after 16 years of marriage.

> There can be no solution to any of the world's problems without a wholesome approach to love and sex. Nearly all destruction or self-destruction, almost all hatred and sorrow, almost all greed and possessiveness, spring from starvation of love and sex.
>
> —Jolan Chang in *The Tao of Love and Sex*

"I have tried to explain to her that my lust for her and my love for her are inseparable and that I don't think either would be as strong without the other, but my lust is directed at no other woman and neither is my love. I think sometimes she wants me to separate the sex part from the love part so she can be sure I love her and not her body. I don't separate the two because her body is part of what she is."

In this case, it seems, it's not the guy who is separating love and sex—it's his wife. And that's not so awfully uncommon: Women do tend to be suspicious of men's sexual interest in them, often seeking some confirmation that our attraction is deeper, more personal or more emotional than mere carnal desire. Yet lots of men don't make a distinction—and don't want to.

Researchers from Bowling Green State University in Bowling Green, Ohio, ran a survey in which a group of college students (149 women and 48 men) responded to the question "What is a romantic act?" Of the top ten most frequently mentioned things (taking walks, giving or receiving flowers, kissing, candlelight dinners), seven were mentioned by both men and women. (One thing lots of women mentioned—hearing the words "I love you"—men hardly ever mentioned.) But perhaps the most unusual finding, the researchers reported, "is that whereas men mentioned making love as an act of romance, women did not."

It's almost as if, for men, actions—whether it's having sex or washing her car—are love; to women, it's feelings that count.

Romantic Foreplay

"Women do tend to be less willing to be sexual if the emotion is not there—they have a greater need for a kind of romantic foreplay before sex than men do," says certified sex therapist Shirley Zussman, Ed.D., co-director of the Association for Male Sexual Dysfunction in New York City. "They need touching, talking, caressing, reassurance, some sense of personal connection before having sex."

One of our survey respondents, a chiropractor, made a similar observation: "I feel that many women don't realize that men use lovemaking to gain intimacy, whereas women need intimacy prior to lovemaking."

Then again, there are plenty of men who think of love and sex as two entirely separate things, and make no bones about it. This came through clearly in the voices of men who answered our survey, including one guy who said he was a former NFL defensive back: "Probably the most misunderstood fact of men's sexuality is the detachment men can make between sex and feelings."

Another said: "Women don't understand that sex, for a

man, is a bodily function that needs to happen on a regular basis. Romance (love) and sex are not the same thing; it's great when they happen simultaneously, but they are independent in my mind. Love is a blessing. Sexual relief is a necessity."

"Women don't seem to understand that men are for the most part driven by pleasure," added another guy. "We are hungry wolves seeking to satisfy a deep appetite. . . . This is not to say that we are uncaring or savages, but only that we see the difference between a physical act and an emotional feeling. For men, lovemaking is the emotional feelings that arise after the physical act takes place. Women, for the most part, intertwine the two.

"But women should heed this advice: You know when a man has made love to you when he holds you, kisses you, cuddles with you and whispers sweet compliments to you long after the physical act is over. If he simply gets up, wipes himself off, says 'Thanks—you were great, babe!' and gets dressed, it was only sex."

The Reasons They Gave

A study by two psychologists from Catholic University of America in Washington, D.C., gives a little more insight into the love/sex divide between men and women.

The researchers surveyed 303 white, married men and women to find out which of 17 reasons would cause them to feel justified in having an extramarital affair. Twenty percent of the men and 30 percent of the women said nothing would justify an affair. But among the rest, 77 percent of the women, versus only 43 percent of the men, said that falling in love would be reason enough to have a fling. By contrast, 75 percent of the men, versus 53 percent of the women, said that sexual excitement would be a good enough reason. Guys were after sex; gals were after love. No wonder we can't get along.

The data supported the observation that men separate sex and love, the researchers added. "Women appear to believe that love and sex go together and that falling in love justified sexual involvement."

"But just because men tend to separate love and sex doesn't mean they're all cold, carnal wolves. I think men are also seeking the kind of closeness and intimacy through sex that women seek—but they're usually unwilling to admit it, even to themselves," Dr. Zussman says.

Besides, there are some genuine advantages in keeping love and sex separate. Because in a very practical way, they are different. A University of Pittsburgh study found that over half the women who said they were happily married also admitted they had trouble reaching orgasm or becoming aroused. Emotional fulfillment and sexual technique are two entirely different things, and confusing them can be dangerous, Dr. Zussman says. "After all, as you get older or if you get sick, you're likely to have sex less often—but that doesn't mean you love each other any less. If love is sex, then the longer most people are married, the less they love each other."

And for many long-lived, happily married couples, whose affection for each other has only deepened with the years, quite the opposite is the case.

MONOGAMY
Why the Pair-Bond Endures

The old dark male idea that marriage is actually a female plot to enslave men economically in exchange for sex will probably never die. We wonder whether monogamy is not just some social invention for somebody else's benefit. Whether it's even really natural (at least for men). And in a society where the divorce rate and the marriage rate are always teetering in rough balance, it's easy to be skeptical of the notion that marriage works at all.

Not so long ago, the word we got from anthropologists and zoologists was that monogamous pair-bonds were common among animals, especially birds, like geese and swans, suggesting that it was also natural for us. Zoologist Desmond Morris argued in his 1967 book *The Naked Ape* that the whole point of human sexuality was "to strengthen the pair-bond and maintain the family unit."

But more recently, reports from the scientific front haven't been quite so encouraging. It turns out that lots of birds fool around (at least 40 percent of indigo buntings get a little on the side, researchers report). And anthropologists have found that nearly 1,000 of the 1,154 past and present human societies ever studied have allowed men to have more than one wife. (Societies where women are allowed more than one husband—polyandry—are extremely rare.) In Western cultures, where having more than one wife at the same time is generally illegal, many men practice serial monogamy: having more than one wife, one after the other. This isn't entirely unrelated to polygamy.

Ward and June Were Right

Even so, some form of monogamous bond between a man and a woman is still the norm all over the world—imperfect as that bond often is. This is true even in societies where polygamy is allowed. University of Michigan researchers found that although in 83 percent of all tribal societies men are permitted to take multiple wives, only 20 percent of the men actually do so. And in a review of all American sex surveys during a recent two-year period, two Columbia University psychiatrists found that among adults 25 to 59 years old, relative monogamy appears to the norm: Eighty percent of heterosexually active men and 90 percent of heterosexually active women in this age group report having had only one sex partner in the preceding year.

No matter what a society permits or encourages or requires, most people seek out for themselves some form of monogamy, says Frank Pittman, M.D., an Atlanta psychiatrist and family therapist.

And what's so bad about that?

There's a fair amount of evidence that men actually get a better deal out of marriage than women do (to put it rather coldly). Marriage protects men from depression and makes women more vulnerable to it—twice as many married women are depressed as married men, according to Neil Jacobson, Ph.D., a psychologist at the University of Washington in Seattle who has done groundbreaking work with women, depression and marital therapy. It's the best evidence that marriage is an institution that primarily benefits men, he maintains.

Other studies have shown that at all ages, husbands report higher levels of marital satisfaction than do wives. Single women report more life satisfaction than married women; the opposite is true of men. And husbands who lose their wives have lower survival rates than still-married men. Widowhood, by contrast, seems to have no effect on women's health.

And the University of Chicago researchers who conducted the 1994 *Sex in America* survey were surprised to find that their data supported "an extraordinarily conventional view of love, sex and marriage." Of the 3,432 people they interviewed,

> In any relationship in which two people become one, the end result is two half-people.
>
> —Wayne Dyer, American psychologist

those who were happiest with their sex lives (both physically and emotionally) were married people. About 88 percent of married people said they received great physical pleasure from their sexual lives and about 85 percent said they received great emotional satisfaction, they reported. By contrast, the least satisfied were those who were not married, not living with anyone and who had at least two sex partners.

That's not to suggest that you have to be married or otherwise committed to be happy. Lots of people have worked out different kinds of arrangements that seem to suit them just fine. Even so, observes Helen Fisher, Ph.D., an anthropologist at the American Museum of Natural History in New York City, in her book *Anatomy of Love*: "Human beings almost never have to be cajoled into pairing. Instead, we do this naturally. We fall in love. We marry. And the vast majority of us marry only one person at a time. Pair-bonding is a trademark of the human animal."

Fidelity Is a Decision

Here are a few suggestions for making your pair-bond work.

Don't marry people who don't like you. "I don't mean to denigrate love in choosing a partner, but the most important element is whether the two of you like each other," Dr. Pittman says. "Friendship is an infinitely more stabilizing basis for marriage than romance. Also, don't marry a woman who doesn't like men but considers you different from all other men—because she'll eventually discover that you have indeed absorbed many of the hated characteristics of your sex.

"Another important point is to consider the degree of friendship your prospective mate has with her parents, because the best indicator of how someone is going to be in a family is how that person has been in a family before."

Don't mistake your mate's gender for her self. Sure, your mate is a female, but that doesn't necessarily mean she likes to cook, sew and hang little ruffled things all over the house. Seems obvious, but couples frequently get so hung up in the gender dance, thinking of their partner as a man or a woman rather than a fellow human being, Dr. Pittman says. "Everything you need to know about the experience of your partner's gender can and must be learned from your partner."

Be honest. Sometimes guys will convince themselves that they're doing themselves a favor by hiding things from their spouses, that telling them a lie is better than fessing up. But there is no truth that is as destructive as any lie.

Decide on fidelity. When it comes right down to it, Dr. Pittman says, fidelity is a decision. It's not a feeling or an inclination. It's about what you decided to do or not to do. And basically, despite it all, compared to flitting from partner to partner like a pollen-dazed bee, monogamy is much more likely to make you happy for a lifetime.

OGLING
The Science of the Gaze

"It is better to be looked over than overlooked," Mae West once said.

If Mae West were alive today and attending college, she'd be accused of "positioning herself within the dominant patriarchal discourse."

With the coming of the gender wars, something has happened to ogling. Among some women it is no longer perceived as merely oafish. It is called unwanted sexual attention, and it is a high crime. It is felt to be a form of sexual bullying, a standard behavior of the domineering male who wants to make women into objects instead of people.

Ardent academic feminists have lifted the term "the Male Gaze" from feminist art and film criticism and have turned it into the operative metaphor for the oppression of women. According to them, all sexual attention is unwanted, offensive and demeaning. Ogling is the height of political incorrectness. It is denounced as sexism, heterosexism, lookism.

Few women would go *that* far; most women don't officially hate sex. Rather, most actually like it. But values have shifted dramatically on this issue. It wasn't so long ago that men would stand around unabashedly engaged in a pastime called girl watching. They would draw hourglass shapes in the air with their hands and say things like "Va-va-VOOM!" At worst, these men were perceived to be unsophisticated.

Now, like everything else since the 1950s, ogling strikes people as a lot less harmless. And yet, isn't it odd? As ogling has become less acceptable between two people, the mass media's use of female beauty to attract our attention has risen in direct proportion. Today it is forbidden to openly ogle the girls—but assumed that we will gaze at the girls in beer commercials, and that we can't get enough of Sharon Stone.

In Praise of the Copulatory Gaze

Ogling may be on the outs as a human mating strategy, but for our primate cousins it still works pretty well. In nature fixed-eye contact elicits one of two basic responses—retreat or approach. Among those who study the genetic aspects of behavior, the intent stare at a potential mate is called the cop-
ulatory gaze, says Helen Fisher, Ph.D., an anthropologist at the American Museum of Natural History in New York City, in her book *Anatomy of Love*. She describes it as a two-to-three-second look—and an abrupt look away while you stick your toe in the dirt or

> The truly erotic sensibility, in evoking the image of woman, never omits to clothe it. The robing and disrobing:
> That is the true traffic of love.
>
> —Antonio Machado, Spanish poet

something once you're caught. A male and female baboon will trade these exchanges until they finally are comfortable enough to look deeply into each other's eyes simultaneously. Then a courtship is born. "This look," says Dr. Fisher, "may well be embedded in our evolutionary psyche."

Sure feels that way, doesn't it? Most men would swear they're hardwired to ogle. "But honey, a guy just can't help it!" is the oft-heard plea when his wife or girlfriend tells him to put his eyes back in his head and his tongue back in his mouth. Hey, we're only being attuned to reproductive potential, for which a woman's face and form were the original advertisement. Does sex sell? Of course—and the very first thing it sold was the propagation of the species. It's nice to know the mechanism still works, even though sex has less and less to do with reproduction, and just as the disembodied sex that's everywhere in our advertising has little to do with the product at hand.

Here's the surest sign that our culture casts a cold eye on the practice: There is no nice word for it. Ogling, leering, checkin' out the babes—all have negative connotations. And yet it does fulfill a need. "If no one was ever allowed to risk offering unsolicited sexual attention, we would all be solitary creatures," writes Katie Roiphe in her book *The Morning After: Sex, Fear and Feminism on Campus.*

It also fulfills our needs as men. The trite-but-true fact of life is that men are more aroused than women by visual stimulation—we're the ones who buy most of the pornography and pin-up calendars. Ogling not only reflects the degree of our sexual interest generally, but probably serves to maintain it, too.

So it all comes down to this: Every man has a choice to make. You can be discreet or blatant. You can be admiring or threatening. "It can be flattering to women," says Maureen O'Sullivan, Ph.D., professor of psychology at the University of California at San Francisco. "It's all in the style and manner and context in which it is done."

There are guys who do it in an assertive, aggressive way, who seem to be getting off on their own power to intimidate, who leave women thinking that he undressed them with his eyes. There are times it's inappropriate; when a women is merely trying to do her job, an ogle seems like a mean-spirited attempt to undermine her professionalism. There are potentially dangerous contexts; when it comes from a stranger on a gritty street or in a deserted parking garage, it is especially aggressive and threatening. Ogling can feel like the prelude to a crime, not a kiss.

But there are plenty of guys who look at women in an admiring way, says Dr. O'Sullivan. The right kind of look can make the right woman feel good. Or feel bad when it's *not* given. "Middle-age women," she says, "complain because they are invisible when they walk down the street."

Can men ever win on this? It's tough. But we'll keep trying.

ONE-NIGHT STAND
It's Best Left As a Fantasy

They were both starved for love. When he pulled into her driveway that day to ask directions, she just happened to be sitting on the front porch drinking iced tea. Her husband and kids were away at the state fair for a week. By that evening they were drinking brandy together, and a part of her wanted to "be taken, carried away and peeled back by a force she could sense but never articulate, even dimly within her mind."

Which is exactly what happened the next night. As they danced cheek-to-cheek in the kitchen, he told her he wasn't like other men. He was an artist. A poet. A free spirit. A vegetarian. So she led him up to her bedroom and they made love until dawn, as she found out just how strong this hard-bodied guy really was: "She, who had ceased having orgasms years ago, had them in long sequences now with a half-man, half-something-else creature."

The one night stretched to three. Then she went back to her responsibilities, and the half-something-else creature left town. In the end they loved each other enough to set each other free.

As a fantasy of casual sex, this one's hard to beat. Fabulous sex, no slip-ups, and they never see each other again. They hardly know each other, but they really love each other. He loves her intelligence. She loves his manliness. It only *seemed* casual, this fling. Actually, it was fated. It was out of their control. They'd been moving toward each other, not just their entire lives, but for several lifetimes. Top that.

The Bridges of Madison County was such a runaway bestseller that it was promptly turned into a movie starring Meryl Streep and Clint Eastwood. Alas, Robert Kincaid and Francesca Johnson never fall out of love with each other, and *Bridges* becomes a story of opportunity missed and love lost. In death they are reunited as their ashes are scattered at Roseman Bridge. Yes, there's only one thing worse than an empty, meaningless one-night stand: A one-night stand that makes the rest of your life empty and meaningless.

But What about Reality?

Bridges is a lovely story—which is to say, it's anything but your average assignation. Robert and Francesca were chaste.

The one-night stand is the province of the promiscuous. The definitive 1994 *Sex in America* survey conducted by University of Chicago researchers found that about a quarter of people with two partners in the last year also had a one-night stand—but nearly two-thirds of people with three or more partners in the last year had a one-night stand during that time. They were also more likely to have been "strongly affected" by drugs or alcohol the last time they had sex.

So, although you can count on Hollywood to pretty things a bit, the one-night stand is largely the domain of the frequent-flier crowd, if you catch our drift.

It's also a lopsidedly male fantasy. There are all kinds of physical and behavioral signs that indicate men's long history of greater interest in casual sex. Let's mull over just one: Worldwide, the average male would prefer to have 18 sex partners in his lifetime; the average woman would prefer 4 or 5.

Eons ago, the guys who had more than 18 sex partners had more offspring, who often tended to inherit the desire to have more than 18 partners and . . . you can see where this is headed. Men have an "evolved desire" to fool around, say evolutionary psychologists. Genetically, it's been in the works for a few million years. Empires and civilizations have risen and fallen, Puritans and their scarlet letters have come and gone and new and deadlier diseases keep on coming. None of this lays a glove on the instinct to stray. It will always be with us. When you think about it, the attitude reflected in a *Redbook* headline—A Married Man? A One-Night Stand? In 1994?—is rather touching in its naivete.

We love short-term encounters so much our standards basically sink like a stone at the prospect of having one. The sexes couldn't be farther apart on this one: Women's standards for a one-nighter dip only slightly in comparison with their eligibility criteria for a more permanent mate. Not guys. We don't care if she's dull, poor, witless, sneaky, stingy or half-nuts. We care only that she's not coyote ugly—and that she won't start calling us every day for weeks. No fatal attractions, please!

Men's standards may go down—but our arousal skyrockets. Sex with the same old partner can go flat because of something scientists call habituation. The sexual high brought on by "fresh flesh" can become an end in itself, especially among middle-age men. The exhilaration is compounded by the thrill of the chase, the big ego boost when the chase succeeds or the feeling that it is a man's reward for success and achievement.

The ego boost is a reason why women indulge in one-night stands, as well. They are just as susceptible to its promise of joy and positive regard, however fleeting. They want to know how marketable they are, too. Women, like men, use casual sex to evaluate potential partners—who paradoxically must shun casual sex. (The appearance of promiscuity on Kincaid's part would have been a turn-off.) If they already have a partner, they can use it to keep those options open. But more women than men tend to use the one-night stand as a ticket out of a current relationship.

In a sense, it's a wonder that women wander at all. They have so much more to lose. Because of contraception, they don't have to fear unwanted pregnancy but more than ever they need to fear the chilling possibility of violence and disease. It takes a particular kind of person to defy those odds—or, indeed, to enjoy defying the odds. Experts say that women who seek out one-night stands on a regular basis are either the newly divorced, who are making up for lost time, or they're inveterate thrill-seekers. Helen Fisher, Ph.D., an anthropologist at the American Museum of Natural History in New York City, says in her book *Anatomy of Love* that there may be a "physiology of adultery." People respond differently to novelty. Some avoid it. Some seek it out. The latter are "sensation seekers," and they usually have low levels of monoamine oxidase, an enzyme in the brain. They are seemingly wired since birth to create a maximum of excitement in their lives.

Maybe that's why some men like their sauce on the side. Then again, some don't. "I'm not into casual sex," said one respondent to our *Men's Health* magazine survey. We asked men whether they'd ever said no to a woman, and plenty had. The number one reason: He was married. Number two

The Two Paths

AT 15
STUDY & CLEANLINESS

AT 15
CIGARETTES & SELF-ABUSE

What Will The Boy Become?

AT 25
PURITY & ECONOMY

AT 25
IMPURITY & DISSIPATION

AT 36
HONORABLE SUCCESS

AT 36
VICE & DEGENERACY

AT 60
VENERABLE OLD AGE

AT 48
MORAL-PHYSICAL WRECK

—From *Safe Counsel* by B. G. Jefferis, M.D., and J. L. Nichols, 39th edition, Intext Press

reason: She was married—usually to his best friend. Run-ner-up reasons: Because he didn't have the time, the energy or the inclination. Because she'd been drinking. Because he'd been drinking. Because it would be morally wrong. Because she's a stranger, and whatever she has, it might be contagious. Because their relationship was headed south and—dare we say it, guys? Women think they have a monopoly on this line, but sometimes sex without love is an empty experience. So, despite the studies that show men jumping at any opportunity for sex, some men look before they leap. As one respondent protested, "I do have some standards."

The man who does but somehow has found himself the next morning in a strange bed anyway—he's got problems. If he's married, the first problem is, does he kiss and tell? Therapists argue that both ways. The don't-tell argument: If it was just a horrible accident and you've resolved never to have it happen again, why compound the suffering by telling your spouse? (Francesca didn't exactly sit her hubby down for a chat when he got back from the state fair.) The do-tell argument: Your marriage will suffer because you'll be car-rying around a dirty little secret, which will strain the mar-riage and result in some loss of intimacy on your part. Take full responsibility for what you did, and hopefully, the emo-tional dust-up will eventually result in more intimacy and a stronger marriage.

The only way to avoid that decision is to avoid the encounter.

OPEN MARRIAGE
A History of the Impossible Dream

In some ways open marriage seems like every guy's dream of heaven. You have your main partner for love and support, but you also have the hat-check girl. And your boss's secre-tary. And the girl who sells you your Lotto ticket. Your wife understands. In fact, she feels free to have lovers, too. You have an arrangement. Nobody gets hurt. Everybody gets along fine—especially you.

So why doesn't this ever work?

Well, every once in a blue moon it does seem to work (we end this chapter with one such tale). But of all the marital arrangements that have been tried in cultures all over the world, group or open marriage (also called polygynandry) is one of the rarest birds of all, according to Helen Fisher, Ph.D., an anthropologist at the American Museum of Natural History in New York City. "You can count on the fingers of one hand the number of peoples who practice group marriage," Dr. Fisher writes in her book *Anatomy of Love*.

> Open marriage is nature's way of telling you you need a divorce.
>
> —Marshall Brickman

Though it's been defined differently at different times and places, we'll just say open marriage means some kind of stable relationship involving more than one man and more than one woman. It's different from swinging, which is more of a sexual free-for-all.

One culture that's tried such a set-up is the Pahari, a tribe in northern India. Among the Pahari, wives have to be bought from their fathers—but they're so expensive it sometimes takes two men, pooling all their dough, to come up with enough cash to buy a single wife. Then the three of them live together, with the two husbands sharing the wife. If the men get rich, they can buy a second bride—and then each man can make love to either woman.

Hmmm. Can't you just imagine what would happen? A hint creeps out of the 1875 autobiography of a Mormon woman, written during a period when polygamy (one husband, multiple wives) was widely practiced by members of the Mormon Church—and jealousy, gossip and backbiting among wives was common. "Each wife finds pleasure in telling all the little weaknesses of the other wives to her (friends) . . . (and) each notices every article of clothing that the others wear," she wrote.

The Oneida Community

Nevertheless, Americans have always had a fondness for tinkering with marriage, just as we love to tinker with everything from carburetors to corporations. In fact, during the latter half of the nineteenth century, a groundswell of sexual and marital experimentation swept across the northeastern United States. Bearded, long-haired radicals celebrated the joys of free love, proclaimed the equality of men and women, demanded the abolition of marriage (which they considered an enslavement of women) and set up communes in which they practiced what they preached.

> We sleep in separate rooms, we have dinner apart, we take separate vacations—we're doing everything we can to keep our marriage together.
>
> —Rodney Dangerfield

The most famous of these free-love communes was the Oneida Community, founded in 1848 in a small town in upstate New York and run by a religious zealot named John Humphrey Noyes. At its height, 500 men, women and children lived at the Oneida Community in one enormous building called Mansion House. Everybody had a private room in the mansion, not unlike a college dorm, but everything else—including clothes, children and sex partners—were shared. Noyes ran the place with a tyrannical hand, discouraging romance between individuals (he considered it selfish) but encouraging copulation between adult men and women. In theory every man in the place was a potential sex partner with every woman.

But this wasn't some nineteenth-century Woodstock; Noyes laid down strict rules about sex. If a man was attracted to a woman, he applied to a special committee. The committee approached the woman to see if she'd be willing, and if she agreed, the man would visit her room for a few hours in the evening—but strictly for sexual pleasure. There was no responsibility to develop a relationship if it was not wanted.

Also, Noyes decreed, no children were to be born. So in order to prevent conception, the men learned to practice a technique called coitus reservatus, in which you're able to orgasm repeatedly without ejaculating. Until they learned to control their ejaculations in this way, men were permitted to have sex only with older women who'd passed their childbearing years.

In 1868 Noyes lifted the ban on babymaking, and people started having kids. Unfortunately, Noyes also arranged to have the younger men make love only to the older women—while he kept the delectable young nymphets to himself. In 1879 the men revolted. Noyes was accused of raping a couple of women and he fled; within a few months the community fell apart.

The most interesting thing about the Oneida experiment, Dr. Fisher observes, was that despite his dictatorial regulations, Noyes was never able to keep men and women from falling in love and forming clandestine pair-bonds with one another. Attraction between people was more powerful than his decrees.

Or as Margaret Mead once observed: "No matter how many communes anybody invents, the family always creeps back."

Trying It Again

In 1972, with the publication of the best-seller *Open Marriage* by Nena O'Neill and George O'Neill, the whole idea got a new airing, but this time in a culture newly liberated by the sexual revolution, the Pill, encounter groups and all the rest of it. In their book the O'Neills defined open marriage (as opposed to old-fashioned closed marriage) as "an honest and open relationship between two people, based on the equal freedom and identity of both partners . . . in which there is no need for dominance and submission." Honesty, commitment and personal growth were supposed to come first, even before sexual fidelity, which they scorned as the false god of closed marriage. If either one of you wanted to take another lover, fine—just so long as you were honest about it. In fact, they wrote, "outside sexual experiences, when they are in the context of a meaningful relationship, may be rewarding and beneficial to an open marriage."

A fair number of people experimented with these looser marital arrangements in the 1970s and 1980s, but like the Oneida Community, the whole thing fairly quickly petered out. Fear of AIDS didn't

> I haven't known any open marriages, though quite a few have been ajar.
>
> —Bob Hope

help. But some of the underlying ideas also seemed faulty. For instance, the O'Neills claimed that jealousy is primarily a learned response, determined by cultural attitudes, and that by talking about it couples could overcome their sexual possessiveness. They pointed to other cultures (like the Eskimos) where they said jealousy "is almost completely absent." But when sociologists took a closer look at these other cultures, they found that jealousy, in fact, is as universal as sex. And one researcher who questioned 50 people in open marriages found that 89 percent of them said there was not any less jealousy than in any other kind of marriage.

A psychoanalyst who studied eight open marriages over a period of nine years found that often these ultraliberated folks were secretly fighting a powerful superego—that is, people who are engaged in open marriage are not infrequently in combat with strong sexual inhibitions, too. They went to such lengths to be open because they weren't really open at all.

And a sociologist who conducted extensive research on the open marriages of over 100 couples made one truly bizarre discovery: A statistically significant number of them wanted to enter the clergy or a convent, or were already in the clergy!

Go figure.

More recently, the University of Chicago researchers who conducted the 1994 *Sex in America* survey found that the people who were happiest with their sex lives (physically and emotionally) were those who were married the old-fashioned way. Over 85 percent of married men and women said they got tremendous emotional and physical pleasure from their sex lives. By contrast, the least satisfied were those who were not married, not living with anyone and who had at least two sex partners—the very people who are supposed to have the hottest sex lives, the researchers reported. "The human animal," Dr. Fisher observes, "seems to be psychologically built to form a pair-bond with a single mate."

One Guy's Story

And yet . . . in our heart of hearts, lots of guys still wish it could be true. And sometimes, despite it all, strange sexual arrangements—even something close to open marriage— actually does seem to work.

One of our survey respondents, a 52-year-old electrical construction manager who says he's been "an exercise nut since 1958 and still has an avid sexual appetite for his wife of 22 years," told us the following story.

Occasionally, he said, he and his wife would fantasize about a couple they'd met in 1974 who were eight or nine years younger than they were and with whom they'd become great friends. "In 1991, after 17 years of friendship with them, we finally got up enough nerve to ask them if they would be interested in swapping partners for an evening. They said that they had wanted to ask us, too, but were afraid of upsetting us. We both have had very good, prosperous marriages and didn't want to hurt anyone.

"At first we would go out dancing and light partying, then go back to one or the other's house and take the other's partner and be separate for about 1½ to 2 hours. That was taking place on a once-or twice-a-month basis. All four of us definitely enjoyed it, and it sure did spice up our sex lives. We have finally gotten to the point of all four of us in bed, which is a blast, and we have had three or four true orgies with them.

"We would never think of doing this with any other couple, and I know they feel the same. Once when my wife was in California visiting our daughter, this other couple called me and asked me to come up and spend the night with them. I called my wife and she said okay. Well, my friend and I made love to his wife for hours. We still are great friends with these people and probably will be for a long time. As long as we all love each other and help each other in times of need, we feel okay, but never would we betray our friends nor they us."

Who says it's not—sometimes—possible?

PROSTITUTES
You Won't Get Us to Cast the First Stone

"That's what I do," 31-year-old Rosemary Garcia was saying to the television cameras. "I'm a prostitute."

Hey, it's just a job! But on this day in 1991, she'd been riding around with televangelist Jimmy Swaggart. He picked her up at a truck stop, she said, and they were looking for a motel with porno flicks when he was stopped by police.

Swaggart had been caught with a prostitute before, outside a motel in New Orleans in 1988. He begged forgiveness, and his multitude of followers said, shucks, Jimmy, we're sinners all. But here he was, messing with prostitutes again. For a preacher man, that's a guaranteed career-ender.

Long before Mary Magdalene, women were accepting money from men in exchange for sex. They still do, despite the popular notion that the Pill and premarital sex ought to have put the world's oldest profession out of business by now. The definitive 1994 *Sex in America* survey conducted by University of Chicago researchers found that about 16 percent of men ages 18 to 59 had paid for services. Only one thing has changed in the last few decades: Fewer men now go to a prostitute to become "initiated." Of U.S. males who came of age in the 1950s, 7 percent lost their virginity to a hooker, compared with 1.5 percent of men coming of age in the late 1980s and early 1990s.

If sex is supposedly so available now, why do men still pay hard cash for it? All kinds of reasons. You've heard of the Madonna/whore dichotomy? Some men want to marry good girls and save the rollicking sex for bad girls. They'll never get over the notion that sex is dirty—so they want dirty sex. Other men aren't getting it at home. What they might be hearing from a partner is that sex is not okay anymore. Or they're happily married—but have a strong need for novelty. Still other men want a weird kind of lovin'. They need to be rocked like a baby, spanked like a child or boffed in a coffin on the living-room floor. And, you know, a lot of women just won't go along with that.

A prostitute takes all comers.

But mostly, men are willing to pay for oral sex. In fact, although nobody has done the definitive scientific study of what men ask prostitutes to do for their money, all signs indicate that fellatio, not intercourse, is the most popular item on the menu. Maybe it's because men love it so much. Maybe it's because prostitutes who are getting paid by the trick have found that it makes for quick, easy, surefire orgasms. It's been estimated that among New York City's streetwalking prostitutes, three-fourths of their contacts are limited to fellatio.

Who Are These People?

Despite popular images of prostitutes as man-hating lesbians or nymphomaniacs, all kinds of women get into this line of work. The profession ranges from the cocaine addict who gives quick fellatio and takes $5 to get her next vial of crack, all the way up to a Los Angeles MAW (model-actress-waitress) who gets $1,500 a night while she waits for her big break. In between are streetwalkers in several price ranges, illegal aliens who work in massage parlors run by gangs, teenage runaways, women who work in the so-called escort services that you can find listed in the phone book or the back of any urban weekly, part-timers who work in bars or strip clubs and call girls with their private clientele who call themselves sex workers and turn up their noses at the streetwalkers.

The streetwalkers are the ones you see. They're the ones

who cause traffic to slow, who run up to the rolled-down windows to negotiate, who drive the neighbors nuts, who get busted. They're estimated to comprise only about a third of the total scene.

Every once in a while, the curtain is pulled back and the public sees the upper end of the business, the part that is hidden most of the time. That happens when a Sydney Biddle Barrows ("The Mayflower Madam") or a Heidi Fleiss ("The Hollywood Madam") is arrested. It is said Fleiss charged a minimum of $1,500 a night and kept 40 percent for herself—the industry standard. One of her "girls" told all to *Cosmopolitan*; "I Was a Heidi Fleiss Girl" was filled with tales of being tied to the bed, smacked around or merely touched lightly all over in front of a mirror by a famous actor while he masturbated himself. And the story of her last job, the job that convinced her to quit: a "threesome." The guy put a leash around the other girl's neck and made her walk around his house on all fours, barking like a dog.

The Consequences of Paying

David M. Buss, a psychology professor at the University of Michigan at Ann Arbor, in his book *The Evolution of Desire*, tells us that prostitution "can be understood as a consequence of two factors operating simultaneously—men's desire for low-cost casual sex and women's either choosing or being forced by economic necessity to offer sexual services for material gain." Is it really that simple? A little low-cost casual sex? Well, it's casual. Nobody worries about a working girl calling your house the next day.

But it's not low-cost. Even if it's cheap. There is the danger of being set up for robbery. There is, in some states, the danger of being arrested for patronizing a prostitute and having your name publicized (some neighborhood groups send "letters of shame" to johns or place their names on public display in order to get the action out of their area). And there has always been the danger of catching a nasty disease. Many prostitutes have AIDS, and most of the drug-addicted women have the HIV virus by now. But, because of the lower transmission rates from women to men, prostitutes tend to get the disease rather than spread it. They have condoms for their protection, not yours.

It's these little details that get left out of movies like *Pretty Woman*.

Although some people think it will fade away, we doubt it. Especially after we learned that human males are not alone in this endeavor—pygmy chimps in Africa have been observed trading meat for sex. How fitting: When caught, most men feel like they've made monkeys of themselves.

SEXUAL HARASSMENT
The New Rules of Engagement

A lot of men are saying this is silly, this is getting out of hand. They're saying, "Everything I say or do can be characterized as sexual harassment."

And sometimes they're right.

Sexual harassment, at its simplest and worst, is a person using a position of power to obtain sex. Sleep with me, get a promotion. Refuse to sleep with me, you're out of here.

But sexual harassment has become something bigger, broader and more than a little vague. Corporations, fearing lawsuits that are increasing in number and jury awards, are now desperately trying to stamp out anything that could possibly be construed as creating a "hostile environment" for women. And some women, taking their personal gender war into the office, are finding hostility whenever and wherever they can.

Here are some egregious examples.

• A veteran columnist for the *Boston Globe* was fined $1,500 when he chided a male colleague for not planning to attend a staff basketball game, saying, "What are you, pussy-whipped?" The remark was *overheard* by a female staffer, who complained to the editor. The fine was withdrawn when the story received national attention.

• A male graduate student at the University of Nebraska was reprimanded for placing in his office a small photo of his wife in a bikini.

• A female attorney successfully sued the Securities and Exchange Commission for sexual harassment because a number of romantic relationships sprang up between staff attorneys and supervisors—and she was *left out*.

• A female professor at Pennsylvania State University claimed she was sexually harassed by a print of the Goya painting *The Naked Maja* that hung in her classroom.

Could it get any worse for men? It could, and it has. Some women in positions of power now think the rules of equality don't apply to them. Once they're the boss, suddenly sexual harassment charges are no longer a way to make everything fair but merely a weapon to be used only by women against men. So a woman manager will think nothing of posting a cartoon in her office that reads, "If you want a job done right, get a woman to do it," or asking a man to put a new jug, which she could very well lift herself, atop the water cooler. Or asking a male subordinate to shovel snow, empty the trash and fix her car, which are the kinds of things that men who worked in the Jenny Craig weight loss centers in the Boston area claim they were asked to do. Eight of these men have sued for sexual harassment, and their stories of being told by female bosses, "I dreamed of you naked" and "You're sensitive for a guy" received national publicity—simply because that's the same old stupid stuff that men used to do to women.

> If you don't like my sweet potato, what made you dig so deep, dig my potato field three, fo' times a week?
>
> —Blues lyric from "You'll Never Miss Your Jelly," recorded by Lil Johnson

Sex discrimination as a legal reality began in the late 1970s, about the time that a majority of women took on jobs outside the home. With the workplace now so thoroughly coed, most everyone agrees that the sexes simply have to learn to work together. Most everyone. Even though sexual harassment has been talked and talked about, some people still don't get it—or don't want to get it, says Stephen M. Paskoff, a lawyer and president of an Atlanta workplace legal training firm, Employment Learning Innovations. "Do some men not understand that their behavior can be offensive and demeaning? Yeah. In some cases it's expressed as anger. 'What's the big deal?' they say. 'People are too sensitive.' "

Maybe so, but the law by now is pretty clear-cut. Teresa Harris, a manager at Forklift Systems of Nashville, sued Charles Hardy, the president, because he'd say stuff like, "Let's go to the Holiday Inn to negotiate your raise." He'd ask her to reach into his pants pocket to retrieve change. A real fun guy, huh. Harris's case finally wended its way to the Supreme Court in 1993. The court decided someone doesn't have to prove economic or psychological injury to claim damages for sexual harassment. They need only to show it would be reasonably perceived as abusive—that, to put it clearly, someone's job is made harder than their fellow employees', solely because of their sex.

> The man who gets on best with women is the one who knows best how to get on without them.
>
> —Baudelaire, French poet

"The Harris case sorted it out for me," says Paskoff. "What is the practical message here? The message is that certain kinds of conduct create the possibility of legal risk. Since there's no real benefit to the conduct, just avoid it. What's so hard about that? If you thought of it like any other business issue—a safety rule, for instance—you'd just say, 'That's the rule, and I'll do it.' This is so simple, it's numbing to think that people don't get it."

Instead, says Paskoff, some people try to weasel around the rules by hairsplitting. They'll say, it's okay if I hug a person this way but not that way? This joke is okay but that joke isn't? Those people are still trying to indulge in risky conduct. The point is, don't hug people. Don't tell sex jokes.

If you're still nervous about this, worrying you'll make a wrong move, here are your options. You can buy every woman you work with an Harasser Flasher. Really. Some lady in Boston invented such a product. It's a lapel pin with green, yellow and red lights. The wearer, when confronted by a member of the opposite sex, can push the appropriate button. Push the red light and a siren wails.

Otherwise, just heed these guidelines and go about your business—treating fellow employees with the same respect you're supposed to lavish on customers nowadays, except nobody does that either.

No *quid pro quo*. That's Latin for, "You gimme that, I give you this." This is the ultimate in sexual harassment: sexual overtures accompanied by offers or threats, thinly veiled or not. Everyone agrees that a man who does this should go suck sewer scum. But sometimes a well-meaning fellow could appear to be sending this message to others by promoting the subordinate he's dating, or giving her the plum assignments.

Don't flirt. Especially with your subordinates, and most particularly with the PYTs (Pretty Young Things) you are most likely to fall all over yourself trying to impress. The older you are, the worse it looks. One study by a team of Arizona psychologists showed that attractive single men were less likely to be accused of sexual harassment than married men doing the very same thing. Besides, a reputation as the office wolf is not the stuff that normally launches a legendary career.

Don't touch. "I've handled several cases in which the meaning of allegedly harassing language attributed to a defendant was ambiguous and not necessarily harmful," recalls Des Moines, Iowa, attorney Frank Harty. "But then came testimony that the defendant had actually 'touched' the plaintiff. And juries take touching very seriously. In one case the defendant was accused of harassment because he patted the plaintiff on the back, and she claimed he had actually been feeling for her bra strap."

Don't refer to body parts. Your female colleague may have a terrific feature, but she may feel angry, humiliated and demeaned by your comment—even though you meant it as a compliment. The rule is that if you wouldn't say it to a guy, don't say it to a woman either. Another rule, and this applies to the second, third and fifth guidelines as well: One infraction won't sink you. Constant repetition inevitably will.

Don't tell sex jokes. Telling off-color jokes is bad enough. Trying to make your own jokes is usually worse. Someone always ends up as the butt of all those jokes, and your persistent teasing can be construed as creating a hostile environment. Somehow the lines that seem funny at the time sound awfully lame when repeated by a plaintiff's lawyer before a scowling jury.

Take complaints seriously. If you're a manager, it's your responsibility to nip harassment in the bud. The law firm of Baker and McKenzie failed to correct the behavior of a 49-year-old partner in its Palo Alto, California, office and got stuck with a $3.5 million verdict for damages.

Date with discretion. Especially if your company has a policy against dating. Such policies are upheld by courts if they're announced upon hiring and consistently enforced. They're often seen as unfair—the office these days is the most popular place to meet potential mates. Nonetheless, to the extent that you can keep your personal life out of the workplace (read: no getting caught in a smooch when the elevator doors open), you'll be applauded for your professionalism. If one of you directly supervises the other, that's much, much dicier. Your wisest move is to disclose your relationship to higher-ups. Now.

If you're being sexually harassed, you can file a complaint with the federal Equal Employment Opportunity Commission. You can file simultaneously with the agency in your state that handles civil rights violations. And you can file a civil suit against your place of business. But first you need an attorney who specializes in this area of the law. Yes, guys can sue for sexual harassment, too, although more women report being victimized. So keep this information handy in case your wife needs it. None of us wants our wives treated like Teresa Harris.

Especially when they make more money than we do.

WHAT DO MEN WANT?
We've Discovered Six Secret Desires

"Some men are not like all men," declares a 30-year-old optician. Well said. She's one of the women who answered our full-page survey that appeared in *Men's Health* magazine; it was good to hear this coming from a lady. Don't get suckered by stereotypes, she's saying. It reminds us to tread lightly before making sweeping generalizations about half the human race. Either half.

In our survey we asked, "Men are frequently accused of being clumsy or inconsiderate lovers. But in your experience, what is it about men's sexuality that women don't understand?" At times the responses all seemed to contradict each other. But the big-picture perspective is that they also express the contradictions that are within most men. Generalizations *are* hard to come by.

Nonetheless, a few strong themes did emerge from all the responses. We heard six broadly shared frustrations.

1. *Our eyes have it*. We stopped counting the number of times we read, "Men are more visually stimulated." At first your somewhat-thick authors wondered, why are all these guys telling us this not-so-fascinating little fact? But the more we thought about it, the more we realized it explains why a guy can be all hot and bothered when she's not yet. She needs to be stroked, but he's already been "stroked" by his vision of her. He's way ahead of her on the arousal curve.

   "A good deal of men's arousal is by visual stimulation, rather than by touch or tenderness," says a 36-year-old military man. "Women tend to be hurt when a man doesn't feel like a woman thinks he should feel."

   "They don't understand the power of images," says a 23-year-old teacher. "We like to see sex." A 25-year-old real estate investor feels the same way. "We want to have the lights on sometimes. We want to see them naked, not hidden under sheets."

2. *Sex is so physical.* We also stopped counting the number of times our respondents used the word "animal" to describe their sex drives. Men are every bit as horny as women think we are. Maybe hornier. "When I haven't had it in a few days, I just want to explode," says a 33-year-old paint sales representative. And a 35-year-old coal mining engineer talks about his "need to hump like a wild animal."

For most men the huge drag of it all is that the sexes' lusts are mismatched. "We crave sex more than our partners do," says a college student. "We like sex more often—like, all the time," complains a 39-year-old teacher. And a 27-year-old liquor sales manager had a most colorful way of putting it: "What women want in bed is a romance novel. Men want a pornographic movie. Isn't life set up great?"

Our hormonally driven need for sex lets us separate sex and love. "Sex can just be sex," says a 29-year-old chef. The differences in libido and the vastly separate paths that men and women follow to arousal very often lead to all sorts of misunderstandings. Sometimes you'd swear we *are* from different planets. "At times, sex is more of a need than a desire, a need to release tension," writes a 30-year-old police dispatcher. "When this is the case, my wife doesn't understand why I am in such a rush to have sex, rather than wait until she is totally ready." A 45-year-old rancher wonders how so many couples stay together: "For those people who only make love a couple of times a

> Men worldwide want physically attractive, young and sexually loyal wives who will remain faithful to them until death. These preferences cannot be attributed to Western culture, to capitalism, to white Anglo-Saxon bigotry, to the media or to incessant brainwashing by advertisers. They are universal across cultures and are absent in none.
>
> —David M. Buss, *The Evolution of Desire*

week or, God forbid, less often than that, how can a
female expect the male to control the biology of sexual
expression?"

This is why it's most helpful, for both men and
women, not to buy into the idea that we're all alike
except for a couple of minor plumbing differences.

3. *But we fool around and fall in love.* Elsewhere in this
book we quote a Cleveland psychiatrist's saying: The
penis is attached to the heart. Doesn't that contradict
what all those guys were saying above? Yes and no.
Regardless of the physical nature of our sex drive,
sooner or later the heart gets entangled. As a 46-year-
old therapist who responded to our magazine survey
says, "While the sexual part is sometimes needed, the
emotional connection enhances sex more than us guys
are given credit for."

Some men see themselves as having two distinctly
separate needs—and they suggest that two distinctly
separate acts are required. "Sometimes you must screw
and then make love," says a 43-year-old casino worker.
And a 34-year-old federal worker claims, "If a woman
helped him climax quickly, then more, longer, passionate love could follow."

An old saying is "Men use love to get sex, women
use sex to get love." But here's a 48-year-old chiropractor saying, "Men use lovemaking to gain intimacy." *Men* use sex to get love, too? Have we found
some common ground here? We heard from some
pretty tough guys, like a 38-year-old corrections officer who says, "Men are just as sentimental as women
are. We just need someone to help us out of our shell."
And a 22-year-old graduate student makes a good
point about how, for most men, their relationship with
a woman provides the only closeness they have. "Most
of us men go through the day very isolated," he
observes. "So when we get home or get alone with our
partner, we have an entire day's worth of emotional
and physical intimacy that we haven't gotten or shared
yet."

"Men need affection also," says a 63-year-old retired appliance store owner. "For many years I would start with my way of preparing for a good sexual act by attempting foreplay. In just a few minutes my wife would state very harshly, 'Do you want it? If so, let's go upstairs.' You'd better believe the turn-off this would cause."

"I know that many of us really try to balance our instincts with civilized skills to be caring and intimate lovers," says a 26-year-old program director. "We enjoy a loving touch or tender kiss just as much as any woman. We love to feel emotionally close to our partner and don't just want to get off."

Just because our drive is so physical, so seemingly detached from our brains, does not mean that our egos aren't on the line. We get nervous. We get embarrassed. And we spend a lot of energy trying to reconcile the contradictions inside ourselves.

4. *Is it good for her, too?* What's all this about men being inconsiderate lovers? These guys are dying to please! "Tell us," they say. "Encourage us. Men are not mind readers." Many men are not clumsy and inconsiderate—they're just confused. They need instructions. Especially because a woman's arousal tends to be much more individualized than a man's. "If you don't like our recipe for love, then give us some ingredients that will satisfy you," writes a 25-year-old warehouse loader. "Men are more eager to please than women think. We love directions! Women who are verbal in bed make me hornier. . . . Speak up ladies!"

Some of our respondents have noted women's hesitation to say something. "Even when I ask them directly what feels best, most of my partners were unable or unwilling to specify," says a 26-year-old insurance salesman.

Other respondents think they understand why. "Men need feedback during sex to enhance the experience, and my opinion is that women don't think a 'lady' should do that," says a 34-year-old computer systems analyst. Inevitably, this is a self-defeating inhibition. "Women sometimes allow men to do what the man wants," says a 45-year-old pharmaceutical sales representative. "Then later on they complain they are not getting what they need."

There is really no alternative to speaking up. As a 49-year-old helicopter pilot puts it, "No one is born knowing how to give pleasure."

5. *Let's take turns driving.* Would it be so impossible for more women to take charge of sex once in a while? If they did, they'd be fulfilling a major male fantasy. A common complaint is that most women are far too passive. "Men like to be openly seduced," says one. "Men want women to take more of a responsibility in love matters," agrees a 62-year-old social worker. And a 42-year-old dentist admits, "We wish they would be wilder in bed and take the initiative."

> Getting laid is just about the only thing men have left.
>
> —28-year-old builder and *Men's Health* magazine survey respondent

Oh, there are a few control freaks out there who might spazz out: "We are the aggressor and enjoy control," says one employee benefits manager. But most men are pleading, "Act slutty, honey!" A 31-year-old naval aviator says bluntly, "Some of us really want a woman to take us by the back of the neck."

6. *Women don't exactly get it either.* Men want women to understand us the same way women want us to understand them. "Women want to be wanted, chased and adored," says a 40-year-old Army sergeant. "But they forget that some of us men like to be treated in the same fashion." Other survey respondents make the same basic point: Women say they want to be touched and caressed more. Well, men like to be touched and caressed, too. Why don't women give what they want to get? They like surprises like flowers and cards? So do men! Wellll? The image of the

two genders standing far apart, demanding the exact same things of each other, amuses one 40-year-old antique shop owner to no end. "We're all such hypocrites when it comes to sex," he says.

And a 22-year-old student got it right when he wrote: "There are men in the world who are inconsiderate, but we do not have a corner on the market."

Some of our respondents complained that women can be clumsy lovers, too. They said women have no idea how to treat a penis. ("It ain't no stick shift!") They complain that women don't reciprocate in the oral sex department. And women don't realize how much our sexuality brings changes with the years. "This is especially true as I get older," says a 39-year-old insurance adjuster. "I used to have a perpetual erection, or could get one just looking at a woman. But now I find that a woman's reassurance, expressed appreciation and playful teasing all help. It is perhaps close to the same thing that women have been saying they need. The lovemaking starts at the beginning of the day with words, touches and attitudes and continues throughout the day. Not just at the moment when the clothes come off."

Seems like our advice comes right back at us. Speak up, gentlemen!

WHAT DO WOMEN WANT?
Answers to the Age-Old Question

In a legend from the days of knights and chivalry, King Arthur is asked a riddle by the evil Black Knight of Tarn Wathelyne. The riddle is: What is it in all the world that women most desire? King Arthur has a year to come up with the answer or he'll be killed. So he combs the kingdom, asking everyone. Idleness, some say. Riches. A fine husband. But in the end, he discovers the words that save his life (and, of course, free a good-looking princess from an evil enchantment): What women desire most in all the world is to get their own way.

Well, that's one answer (and a pretty good one, actually). A more recent one came from Priscilla Flood, an editor at *Vogue*, who set out to discover for an article what women really want in a man. Steering clear of old legends, sociological doublespeak and scholarly studies, she just got a bunch of her girlfriends together and yukked it up over dinner and a nice Chardonnay. Their conclusion: A woman looks for "rippling biceps, broad shoulders, strong legs, a flat stomach, clear eyes, a firm chin, straight teeth, long fingers, thick hair and a beautiful smile on a muscular, well-proportioned six-foot frame. Or a singularity that makes her forget all that."

Well, geez. Sounds like we might as well just pack it in right now.

Big Bucks, Big Brain

Another place to turn for an answer to the age-old question is the emerging field of evolutionary psychology, which has taken a bit of a longer view of things—looking, in fact, millions of years back into prehistory and at existing cultures all over the world. In his book *The Evolution of Desire*, David M. Buss, a psychology professor at the University of Michigan in Ann Arbor, reports on his landmark international study of 10,000 people in 37 cultures who were questioned about what they desired in a mate. There was amazing agreement among both women and men, from Australia to Zambia, New York to Nigeria. To Buss, this shows that human mating strategies are based on forces far older and more enduring than the mere 5,000 years we've been civilized. What do women want?

Bucks. Buss found that in virtually all these cultures, while men placed the highest value on physical attractiveness, women were after the bucks. Evidence from dozens of studies documents that modern American women value economic resources substantially more than men do, he reports. Almost 50 years of surveys that rated desirable characteristics in a potential mate all showed that women valued good financial prospects in a mate roughly twice as highly as men do.

Social status. Henry Kissinger once remarked that power is the most potent aphrodisiac. Well, says Buss, that's because social status, which generally means power, is a universal cue to control of resources. And a man who has resources is what a woman needs to take care of her and the kids. Virtually everywhere, whoever controls the resources gets all the good stuff: Better food, more territory, better health care, good seats at the Mets game. But again, in a variety of studies, women rate status more highly than men do.

> What this woman wants, with all due respect to Sigmund Freud, is for men to stop asking that question and to realize that women are human beings, not some alien species. They want the same things men want.
>
> —Diane White, newspaper columnist

Age. In all 37 cultures women preferred men who were older than they were (on average, 3½ years older). Why? Older guys almost always make more money than younger guys. They're also more stable and more mature.

Ambition. Again, women in the overwhelming majority of cultures rated ambition and industriousness much more highly than men did. Why? Same reason: The ambitious bird gets the worm.

Dependability and intelligence. Women rated emotional stability, a dependable character and intelligence very highly. (This was one thing men rated almost as highly as women.)

And, of course, love. What does it matter if the guy is smart, rich and ambitious, if he won't share the resources with her and her kids? That's why she's always looking for love and commitment. One of the most convincing signs of love, at least to her, is sexual fidelity. Another is, yup, really expensive gifts. In one study 89 percent of American women and 82 percent of Japanese women said that even if all the other traits were there in a man, without love they wouldn't marry.

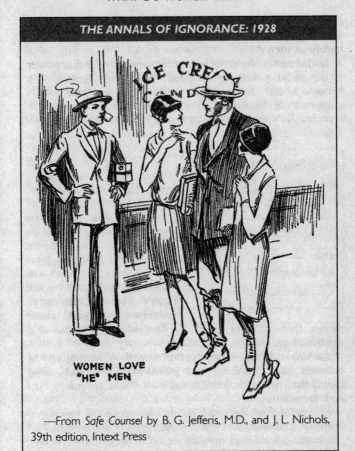

WOMEN LOVE
"HE" MEN

—From *Safe Counsel* by B. G. Jefferis, M.D., and J. L. Nichols, 39th edition, Intext Press

Lumped together, this whole array of terrific male traits is sometimes simply called dominance. In ape societies dominance is basically just size and aggressiveness; the biggest ape gets all the girls. But in human societies social dominance is mainly what counts—which is why intelligence, competence, daring and ambition are so important. Dominance, in fact, is the key factor in mate selection, Buss argues. That is what women want.

One controversial implication of all this is that since women worldwide tend to favor these hard-driving, success-obsessed guys, women also share responsibility, in an evolutionary sense, for selecting the macho traits that feminists denounce. Women say they want men to be soft and sensitive, but how many creampuffs are there on the Forbes 400 list?

The Return of Niceness

Well, nice little theory. But how does it play out in real life? To find out, researchers at Arizona State University in Tempe asked 327 male and female college students to rate the importance of 24 traits for selecting a potential partner (things like physical attractiveness, kindness and understanding, friendliness, sexiness, even good housekeeping). But the researchers added a little spin, also asking how they'd rate the partner for several different levels of involvement: a one-night stand, a single date, steady dating or marriage. The students were also asked to rate themselves on these traits.

> Why does a woman work ten years to change a man's habits and then complain that he's not the man she married?
>
> —Barbra Streisand

It turns out that, even for a one-night stand, women are a whole lot pickier than men are. In fact, on all but 1 of the 24 traits (physical attractiveness), guys were willing to set their standards lower than women in order to get laid. (Evolutionary psychologists would say this makes sense because men have a lower investment in brief sexual encounters—we've got a lot less to lose.) So the answer is that women want a lot, even if it's just for tonight. (In our own defense, the researchers also found that as the level of commitment increased, so did men's standards—so that when it comes to potential marriage partners, men and women are both about equally demanding.)

One other relevant finding is that women also tended to choose mates who matched their own self-ratings. That is, if a woman considered herself attractive and of high social status, she would choose someone equally good-looking and well-connected, no matter what level of involvement she was looking for. Men were inclined to be less concerned about all that, unless they were looking for a wife. So the answer is that if she thinks she's hot stuff, you'd better be, too.

Though they confirm the idea that women like dominant men, other studies have put a slightly softer spin on the whole thing. Turns out that another thing women really want is a nice guy.

In one study a team of psychologists at Texas A&M University in College Station set up an ingenious experiment to test 115 women on the attributes they found attractive in men. The researchers asked the women to evaluate the appeal of two men who acted out scripts on videotape in which they behaved in a forceful and dominating way, were weak and hesitant, displayed kindness and generosity and so on. The videotape was intentionally blurred to make sure the women weren't just picking the guy who was the cutest. The results showed that while dominance was an important part of what makes a man attractive to women, being nice and having a pleasant personality mattered even more.

Altruistic men were rated as more physically attractive, more sexually attractive, more socially desirable and more desirable as a date, relative to nonaltruistic men, the researchers concluded. Given past theory and research, we were surprised to find no evidence that dominant men were systematically more attractive to women than low-dominance men.

The Only Question That Matters

So there's a handful of answers for you. Yet, somehow, the question still seems unanswered, and perhaps it always will be. In the end every guy has probably had moments of profound sympathy for old Dr. Freud, when he muttered those famous words: "The great question, which I have not been able to answer despite my 30 years of research into the feminine soul, is, what does a woman want?"

Well, maybe that's the wrong question. (At least, that's the wrong question for the average guy simply trying to make a relationship work, not aspiring to become the Father of Modern Psychology.) Asking what do women want is really just a way of avoiding the only question that really matters: What does this particular woman want?

If you can figure that out, you're golden.

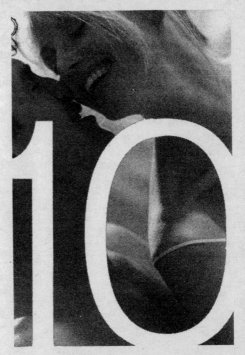

THE BEST SEX
I EVER HAD

AMAZING STORIES FROM
THE MEN OF AMERICA

"The worst I ever had was still on the money."

—Woody Allen

"The best sex I ever had was with my current girlfriend," one guy wrote us in response to the last question on our *Men's Health* magazine survey.

"One time she knew I'd had a bad day at work and invited me over to her place. I arrived to find her wrapped in a small quantity of opaque silk, a hot whirlpool bath bubbling, candles everywhere and my favorite red wine breathing. Dinner was fed to me by a smiling angel perched in my lap. She followed this by demonstrating previously undisclosed sexual talents that she later claimed were learned at a 'church social' during her girlhood in North Carolina. This led to an evening of passion that included four climaxes for me, six for her, both of us taking personal days from our jobs the next day and a trip to the chiropractor."

Now, the liars, braggarts and fishermen among you might be inclined to question whether such an event actually occurred. And we weren't too sure ourselves what we'd be getting into when we asked the question, "What's the best sex you've ever had?" What we received were plenty of responses: over 1,800 in all. By the time we finished reading the last of them, we were pretty sure that you, dear reader, would be interested in what your compadres had to say.

And, sure: A little bit of it was stupid, braggy, wink-and-a-nudge stuff. Some of it was pure raunch. A few guys even admitted they'd paid cash for the best sex they ever had. But what really surprised us was that for most of the men who answered, the best sex was loving sex. We were as likely to get long, gushing descriptions of a woman's personality as her uncanny technique or bodacious curves. And nobody—

nobody—parroted the old macho notion that men are meant to find 'em and forget 'em. If the responses we received could be turned into a song, it would sound like the ballads of Boyz II Men or Michael Bolton rather than Mick Jagger or misogynist gangsta rap.

What follows is the best of the best. Sure, we start with some tales of youthful conquest, strange locales, unbridled lust. But like the survey itself, sincere tales of devotion and love dominate. In all cases, we deleted material that was a little *too* descriptive. (An account of the effect of nibbling a strategically placed slice of peach had to go, unfortunately.) You can find salaciousness anywhere these days, and our point was not to compete with all that. Our point was simply to revisit some of the highest, richest, deepest, most unforgettable moments life has to offer in hopes that it might inspire you to new heights of your own. When these guys rejoice over the pure, sweet joy of sex, it's contagious, isn't it? By and large, they have a good attitude. As one respondent, a high school biology teacher, told us, "Sex is too much fun to be embarrassing."

Where was he when *we* took biology?

· I was 25; she was 36 and married. Her husband cheated on her and she wanted to get even.

She got even.

· It was 1988 at the theater-in-the-round I ran in college. She came to see me after a rehearsal of a play I was in. She had programmed the light-board earlier, did a striptease in the middle of the stage and the stagehands stumbled over us the next morning.

· I would have to say it was with my current partner. She is amazingly open and fun to be with. And she's constantly catching me off guard. We have had sex in closets at friends' parties. Ever get pulled into a closet by an arm coming out of the closet and made love while trying not to make a sound?

· I met a woman at a Halloween party, and we hit it off. We did it in a closet—masks on. To this day I don't know who she was.

• When I was a junior in high school my girlfriend and I drove to my grandfather's orchards and made love under a big old apple tree in the moonlight.

• In the open desert, under a full moon, on top of my Jeep.

• In the car—it was 92 in the shade and we still fogged the windshield.

• In a phone booth. We couldn't help it—they put us on hold.

• In a service elevator stopped between floors.

• On a rock in an icy cold stream in the Catskills.

• A cold, snowy night in Missoula, Montana. We now refer to sex as "doing the Missoula."

• I took my girlfriend to a cabin one year to go deer hunting. On the first night I got an oil rubdown in front of the fireplace. After making love, we went out to the hot tub. I never did make it hunting.

• She was an airline copilot, uninhibited, insatiable. Flew for Aeroflot. Aeroflot is history. So is Ludmila.

• In a cheap, no-tell motel when I was 17. She was the third person I had been with, and it was great. The best time was when the fans were all on, the room was cold and we had just gotten out of a hot shower. We clung together for warmth, and the closer we got, the more we moved, and the frostbite soon turned to sweat.

• It was when I was in Panama City. I was 21. I was in the Army. The woman took it upon herself to be my teacher. I was not a virgin, but I was a novice. We spent days together making love. She taught me timing, what a woman wants from a man in bed and, most of all, consideration.

• The best sex I ever had was on top of a movie theater that I used to work at before I joined the Navy. We went up a maintenance ladder to the roof and made love. (I had the keys to the building.) We could see everything up there, but you would need a helicopter to see us. We lived in a very small town, and the old theater was the tallest building. Stretched out on my red blanket, we held each other and slowly let nature take its course. There was no shaving cream, lingerie, honey or other sexual aids, but neither of us cared. The feeling of freedom and boldness was enough to

light us afire. Plus, that damn cold wind kept me active and
her close.

• My first love, my high school sweetheart, was in from
the Midwest visiting relatives, and she decided to ring me up.
I decided to take a mental health day, have a nice brunch and then do some shopping. I picked her up and we went for brunch. Afterward we drove to my summer house. I was only going to pass by, but she asked me to stop so she could use the bathroom. While showing her the house, she beckoned me to join her on the bed. Although initially I can't

> When you hear a woman sighing profoundly, and see her lips and ears become red ... this is the right moment for coition. If you penetrate her now your pleasure will be supreme.
>
> —The Perfumed Garden, a 2,000-year-old Indian love manual

really say I thought I was meeting her to make love, we spent
the next six hours in some of the most glorious lovemaking
I've ever experienced.

As teenagers we'd fumbled around, but on this sunny
afternoon we had such sweet, tender, passionate times that
I'll never forget it.

• She was a virgin when I met her, and we were together
for five years. She had waited until she was in her
midtwenties to have sex, mostly out of devotion to other
activities in her youth. When she did start having sex, she
was ravenous. We did it *everywhere*. On the beach, in the
car, in hot tubs . . . we would be on a trip and we'd have to
stop at a motel just to have sex before we could continue.
We expressed ourselves however we wanted—it was fantastic! We aren't together today because of differences in
our career goals, mostly. I regret being such a hardheaded
bastard back then.

• She was then and still is today a close friend. We had
previously been roommates, "platonically romantic," if you
will. By that I mean our cohabitation was initially for economic reasons. But it didn't take long for us to discover each

other's uncanny ability to arouse passion in the other. We were pals. We dated others but when those didn't work out, we always ended up together, very satisfied. But one particular night transcended all others.

We had taken a ferry from Seattle to an island in Puget Sound to party with friends at a local establishment. As I recall, we had argued over something on the way back (I'd drunk a fair amount, she does not, so it is likely I was evoking the finer points of one of my self-indulgent platforms). When we arrived at my apartment (we had parted living arrangements a few months earlier), I invited her in. She said, "If I come in, I won't be able to leave." And she didn't. Before we reached the top of the stairs, buttons were coming undone faster than Hillary Clinton's health care plan.

That night had an aura of hopeless addiction, as if raw, physical sex were a drug. We were so high on the passion that details escape me. She is a very verbal partner, and this night especially. That is like pouring gas on a fire for me.

Why am I not with her now? Perhaps because I was not able then to see beyond or to understand what was beyond the sex. We had "found common ground," but I was too stupid to recognize what we could build from such a foundation. I miss her now each time I have sex, and I now believe that the sex we had was founded on something stronger.

• My best sex was with a man. I'm not with him today because I opted for a "normal" sex life for social and religious reasons. Big mistake.

• My parents were away for the week and my ex-wife and I drove out to feed and ride the horses for them. The barn was old and a serious firetrap—we planned to tear it down when my father returned next week. I was in the house and my ex was outside. She called me on the intercom we had in the barn. All she said was that something weird was happening there and she was scared. It was a half-mile away. Since you needed a truck or horse to get there, I rode out bareback, only to see the barn start to smoke in the distance. When I arrived, she was in the barn laying naked on bales of hay. She'd fixed up a saddle blanket. The barn had just begun to catch fire good when she said, "Hurry and love me before the barn is gone." This barn was the first place we'd made love almost three years earlier.

We started our own fire and got out only moments before the roof collapsed. But sometimes I wonder whether the fuse box in the barn really did start sparking like she said.

• The best sex I ever had lasted 3½ weeks. She walked into my life, threw me around and left as quickly as she came in. That was three years ago. I don't miss her. If she had stayed any longer, I would be dead now.

• I dated a woman a couple of years ago that truly loved sex (a male dream). She was exciting, sexy and ready 90 percent of the time. I could ask her to do anything and she was game. Dating her was a sexual dream come true.

Emotionally, however, she was a nightmare. The rest of her life was a wreck. She moved from job to job, always blaming others. If she became upset, she would leave long hateful messages and then want to "make up." She was also as compulsive about spending money and drinking as she was about sex. Even though I will always miss the sex, I will never miss the craziness.

• When I was 22, I dated an older woman who reveled in experimenting with everything. Too bad she was a head case!

• I was a naive 17-year-old who had a one-timer with a 19-year-old girl on the beach in the surf. Only a half-dozen people saw us. Beaches are supposed to be desolate at 2:30 A.M.

• My girlfriend at the time and I went to the beach in Florida. We both found that being at the beach made us incredibly horny. The sun on our bodies, rubbing lotion on one another, the sound of the surf and all the people. Well, we got into the water and waded out about halfway up to my chest. She is quite a bit smaller so she got on my back. As I was walking out, she reached around and began to massage me. She took off her bottoms and began to grind into my hip. Well, it was more than I could stand so I dropped 'em and proceeded to pull her around front. At this point no one else could see below my chest so I "took the skin boat to tuna town." As we were making love, trying not to give ourselves away but not being very successful at it, we noticed another couple about 15 to 20 feet away in the same position that we were, with the girl hanging onto the front of the guy. We watched them for a few minutes and they watched us. The girl was talking to the guy and all of a sudden gave a huge shudder.

After my girlfriend and I both reached orgasm, we started walking toward the beach, and so did they. My girlfriend looked at the other girl and said, "Did you guys have fun out there?"

"Oh, yeah!"

We laughed and introduced ourselves and were bragging to one another about how cool it was that no one else noticed that we were having the time of our lives. Then we all had lunch.

• At the beach, at low tide, beyond the safety perimeter, with the lifeguard blowing his whistle at us the whole time.

• In college I met a woman. We fell in love quickly and inside of a month we were having sex regularly. The best sex we ever had, in my lowly opinion, was when we were in her dorm room the last day of school that spring. I was suspended from school because I spent most of my time thinking about sex. (She did just fine. Go figure.)

There was a kind of desperate quality to it that made it that much sweeter. We had no idea whether we would ever see each other again. Six years later we are still together.

• It's with my current girlfriend—because we talk. We tell each other what we want. We relax, we touch, we enjoy—and we tear the place apart.

We have made love in every room of my apartment and on almost every piece of furniture. The best sex I have with my lady love always seems to be the last time we were together.

The sex with my girlfriend is always good, but I remember a time that was particularly affectionate and loving. It was slow and it lasted a long time. We came together and woke up the next morning still holding on to each other.

• The best sex I ever had was one session where we made passionate love for eight hours without a break. We didn't plan this marathon or keep track of orgasms. Neither of us was thinking of anything other than our mutual pleasure—no work, no food, no pressures. Just riding wave after wave in this incredibly protracted moment.

• Last winter my girlfriend bought herself a mink coat. We had discussed the fantasy of making love with her wearing it—but she hadn't told me she'd bought it yet when I picked her up for a date. As I knocked on the door, she yelled to come in. I walked in and she's standing there wearing the coat with a pair of black high heels and stockings. She spun around several times asking me what I thought. Then she opened it up. The stockings were, well, stockings (not panty hose) and that was all she was wearing.

Another time, I showed up at her office with flowers. (Guys, don't ever underestimate the power of sending flowers!) She said I looked stressed to her. She closed the blinds in the window and proceeded to give me head in her office. Variety and spontaneity are key ingredients in good sex and lovemaking—for me, at least.

• It was my wife, who at the time was just my best friend. I was spending the night at her apartment and the next thing I knew, we were making love all weekend. I'm talking wearing-the-skin-off-the-genitals sex. It wasn't the sex as much as it was the acceptance. I'd wanted her since kindergarten.

• It was a sunny September Saturday afternoon. The baby was asleep upstairs and we were in our bedroom, both feeling horny. Trouble was, my father was ten feet away painting the garage. I begged her to stop, afraid he'd walk in on us. As we got into it, he began to ask me questions. Here I was in my bedroom, my wife was performing oral sex on me and my dad and I were carrying on a normal conversation. As we climbed into bed for some afternoon lovemaking, I don't know what made him stay out there painting away. But our lovemaking that afternoon was fast, furious, hot and sweaty.

• It was Valentine's Day when she accepted my engagement ring—we spent all day pleasing one another.

• The first time I made love with the woman I am going to marry.

• The best sex I've ever had has occurred during the past

two years, when my wife and I have put aside our hang-ups and devoted ourselves to being open and honest with each other. There is no one time to which I can point. We're in our midforties now, but our sex life is much better than when we were in our twenties. We make love three or four times a week but, just as importantly, we are erotic and loving with each other when we aren't having sex. Many mornings, for instance, I enjoy just sitting on the bed and watching my wife dress. Or she will wash the dishes while nude—or close to it.

• The best sex is right now. The kids are grown. We can make it anywhere and anytime we like. I'd like to have the physical stamina I had at age 17 but not the hang-ups and problems that go with that age. Now we're relaxed, we know each other and our turn-ons pretty well, and we stay inventive. We work hard at diet and keeping fit to be good sexual partners.

• A year ago at Christmas my wife and I took a quick trip to stay overnight out of town for a business dinner. We got to our hotel by noon. We walked into our room, dropped our bags and immediately locked the door and made love. We dozed off for about an hour in each other's arms and woke up to make love again. Then we went out to eat lunch and shop. Around 4 P.M. we stopped at Victoria's Secret and my wife bought a sexy little outfit. We immediately went back to the hotel for her to try it on. This time there was a bottle of champagne waiting for us in our room. We made love and showered together before dinner. After dinner that night we made love again before falling asleep. We woke again the next morning to one final session of lovemaking. That totals five times in two days—a record for us that will probably stand for some time. Not that I wouldn't mind another trip like that!

• My wife and I escape by kidnapping each other. The kidnapper coordinates with the other's boss.

• My wedding night and honeymoon—we were both virgins.

• My wedding night, slightly drunk and very happy. And this was after living together for seven years!

• My second honeymoon, a week when, alternating days, we would tell the other one exactly what we wanted to do—or what we wanted the other one to do—for hours and hours each day. We're together seven years.

• My wife and I on a weekend away, our tenth anniversary. In a 12-hour period we stayed in bed, ate shrimp, drank champagne and counted orgasms. We made love seven times.

• After 14 years it keeps getting better and better.

• I'm constantly having great sex with my wife of 15 years.

• I can honestly say that our sex life has improved over the 20 years we've been married, with the last 5 years being the best.

• Our 25th wedding anniversary. We had three glorious days and nights, and we used all 25 years of experience.

• My lovely wife of 44 years. It's so great to still have sex every day.

• My wife is a better lover than I could ever have hoped for. The best sex I ever had will change by next week.

ABOUT THE AUTHORS

Stefan Bechtel is the author of *The Practical Encyclopedia of Sex and Health*, which has sold more than 800,000 copies and been translated into Chinese and Korean. He is also the co-author of *Katherine, It's Time*, a nonfiction novel. He was a founding editor of *Men's Health* magazine and a former senior editor at *Prevention* magazine. His work has appeared in *Esquire, Reader's Digest, American Way* and other national magazines. He lives in Virginia.

Laurence Roy Stains has written for the *New York Times, Rolling Stone, GQ, Men's Health, Money, Worth, Boston Globe, Chicago Tribune, Christian Science Monitor, Philadelphia Inquirer Sunday Magazine* and elsewhere. He, too, was a founding editor of *Men's Health* magazine and also helped launch *New Shelter* magazine. He lives outside Philadelphia.

ACKNOWLEDGMENTS

This book, more than most books, has been a collaborative effort. We owe thanks, first of all, to the dozens of doctors, research scientists and therapists who took time out of their busy days and nights to explain the developments in their fields, especially Jerome H. Check, M.D., Donald S. Coffey, Ph.D., Irwin Goldstein, M.D., Joseph Khoury, M.D., and John D. Perry, Ph.D., and therapists Donald Strassberg, Ph.D., Shirley Zussman, Ed.D., and Judith Seifer, Ph.D. Thanks, too, to our reviewers, E. Douglas Whitehead, M.D., and Bernie Zilbergeld, Ph.D., for their helpful comments and suggestions.

At Rodale Press we'd like to thank Charles Beasley, designer; copy editors John D. Reeser and Amy K. Fisher; Ann Gossy Yermish, Sheryl Loeffler, Liz Wolbach and

Rebecca Theodore for their research assistance. Thanks to Debora T. Yost, vice president and editorial director of health and fitness books; Mike Lafavore, editor of *Men's Health* magazine and C. E. Brietzke for their support.

Finally, we'd like to thank Mark Bricklin, whose creative leadership has blessed us all, and our unflappable editor, Neil Wertheimer, for his encouragement, guidance, wisdom, decency and diligence.

INDEX

Note: **Boldfaced** page references indicate primary discussion.
Underscored page references indicate illustrations.